Mosby's Pocket Guide to
Nursing Skills
& Procedures

EIGHTH EDITION

Anne Griffin Perry, EdD, RN, FAAN
Interim Dean and Professor
School of Nursing
Southern Illinois University—Edwardsville
Edwardsville, Illinois

Patricia A. Potter, PhD, RN, FAAN
Director of Research
Patient Care Services
Barnes-Jewish Hospital
St. Louis, Missouri

Subject Matter Expert
Paul L. Desmarais, PhD, RN, CCRN
Lecturer
College of Nursing
University of Central Florida
Orlando, Florida

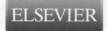

ELSEVIER
MOSBY

3251 Riverport Lane
St. Louis, Missouri 63043

MOSBY'S POCKET GUIDE TO NURSING SKILLS 978-0-323-18741-1
AND PROCEDURES

Previous editions copyrighted 2011, 2007, 2003, 1998, 1994, 1990, 1986

International Standard Book Number 978-0-323-18741-1

Content Development Manager, Education: Jean Sims Fornango
Associate Content Development Specialist: Savannah Davis
Publishing Services Manager: Deborah L. Vogel
Senior Project Manager: Jodi M. Willard
Design Direction: Brian Salisbury

Printed in China
Last digit is the print number:
9 8 7 6 5 4 3 2 1

Working together
to grow libraries in
developing countries

www.elsevier.com • www.bookaid.org

Mosby's Pocket Guide to Nursing Skills and Procedures, eighth edition, is a practical, portable reference for students and practitioners in the clinical setting. Grouped alphabetically, 85 commonly performed skills are presented in a clear, step-by-step format that includes:

- Purpose for performing each skill
- Guidelines to help students in delegating tasks to assistive personnel
- List of equipment required
- Rationales to explain why specific techniques are used
- Full-color photographs and drawings to provide visual reinforcement

In addition, Safety Alerts are included in the skills to highlight important information about patient safety and effective performance. Current Standard Precautions guidelines from the Centers for Disease Control and Prevention are incorporated throughout. Preprocedure and postprocedure protocols are conveniently located on the inside back cover.

Features of This Edition

- Glove logo identifies when gloves should be worn.
- Information is completely updated for every skill and procedure.
- Unexpected Outcomes and Related Interventions present commonly occurring complications and the appropriate responses for patient care.
- Completely updated, full-color illustrations throughout.

This pocket guide is also available in formats compatible with handheld electronic devices. For a more complete discussion of information presented in this book, refer to Perry and Potter: *Clinical Nursing Skills and Techniques,* eighth edition.

CONTENTS

H

I

M

N

O

P

W

Appendix: Overview of CDC Hand Hygiene Guidelines, 637

Bibliography, 640

Acapella Device

The Acapella is a handheld airway clearance device that provides positive expiratory pressure (PEP) with oral airway oscillations to aid sputum clearance. PEP stabilizes airways and improves aeration of the distal lung areas. During exhalation, pressure from the airways is transmitted to the Acapella device, which helps mucus dislodge from the airway walls, thereby preventing airway collapse, accelerating expiratory flow, and moving mucus toward the trachea. This device combines resistive features of PEP and vibration to mobilize airway secretions. The Acapella device is easy to use as patients are able to perform airway clearance independently. Patients with chronic conditions such as cystic fibrosis appear to receive the greatest benefit from this type of treatment.

Delegation Considerations

The skill of using an Acapella device can be delegated to nursing assistive personnel (NAP). The nurse is responsible for performing respiratory assessment, determining that the procedure is appropriate and that a patient can tolerate it, and evaluating a patient's response to the procedure. The nurse directs the NAP to:

- Be alert for the patient's tolerance of procedure, such as comfort level and changes in breathing pattern, and to immediately report changes to the nurse.
- Use specific patient precautions, such as positioning restrictions related to disease or treatment.

Equipment

- Stethoscope
- Pulse oximeter
- Water and glass
- Chair
- Tissues and paper bag
- Clear, graduated, screw-top container
- Suction equipment (if patient cannot cough and clear own secretions)
- Acapella device
- Clean gloves
- Patient education materials

Implementation

STEP	RATIONALE
1 Complete preprocedure protocol.	
2 🦅 Prepare Acapella device (Fig. 1-1):	
a Turn Acapella frequency adjustment dial counterclockwise to lowest resistance setting. As patient improves or is more proficient, adjust proper resistance level upward by turning dial clockwise.	This initial setting helps patient adjust to device and benefit from treatment.
b If aerosol drug therapy is ordered, attach a nebulizer to the end of the Acapella valve.	
3 Instruct patient to:	
a Sit comfortably.	
b Take in breath that is larger than normal but not to fill lungs completely.	
c Place mouthpiece into the mouth, maintaining tight seal.	
d Hold breath for 2 to 3 seconds.	
e Try not to cough and to exhale slowly for 3 to 4 seconds through the device while it vibrates.	
f Repeat cycle for 5 to 10 breaths as tolerated.	
g Remove mouthpiece and perform one or two "huff" coughs.	
h Repeat Steps a through g as ordered.	

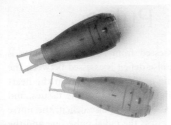

Fig. 1-1 Acapella device.
(Used with permission,
Smithmedical.com.)

STEP	RATIONALE
4 Auscultate lung fields; obtain vital signs and pulse oximetry. Inspect color, character, and amount of sputum. Help patient with oral hygiene.	
5 Complete postprocedure protocol.	

Recording and Reporting

- Record level of resistance and patient's tolerance.

UNEXPECTED OUTCOMES	RELATED INTERVENTIONS
1 Patient cannot maintain exhalation for 3 to 4 seconds.	• Adjust dial clockwise to allow patient to exhale at a lower flow rate.

Apical-Radial Pulse

The difference between pulses assessed from two different sites is known as a *pulse deficit*. When a pulse deficit is assessed between the apical and radial pulses, the volume of blood ejected from the heart may be inadequate to meet the circulatory needs of the tissues, and intervention may be required. To assess for a pulse deficit, the nurse and a second health care provider assess the radial pulse rate and the apical pulse rate simultaneously and compare the measurements.

Delegation Considerations

The skill of assessing an apical-radial pulse deficit cannot be delegated to nursing assistive personnel (NAP). Collaboration between the nurse and a second health care provider is required to determine an apical-radial pulse deficit.

Equipment

- Stethoscope
- Watch with second hand or digital display
- Pen and vital sign flow sheet or electronic health record (EHR)
- Alcohol swab

Implementation

STEP	RATIONALE
1 Complete preprocedure protocol.	
2 Assist patient to supine or sitting position. Move aside bedclothes and gown to expose sternum and left side of chest.	
3 Locate apical and radial pulse sites. Nurse auscultates apical pulse while second provider palpates radial pulse.	Simultaneous measurement allows for comparison of the two pulse rates.
4 Nurse begins pulse count by calling out loud when to begin counting pulses.	Ensures that pulse rates are measured simultaneously.

STEP	RATIONALE
5 Each nurse completes a 60-second pulse count simultaneously. The count ends when the nurse taking the apical pulse states "stop."	Sixty seconds is required when discrepancy between pulse sites is expected or rhythm is irregular.
6 Subtract radial rate from apical rate to obtain pulse deficit.	If the pulse count differs by more than 2, a pulse deficit exists. The pulse deficit reflects number of ineffective cardiac contractions in 1 minute.
7 If pulse deficit is noted, assess for other signs and symptoms of decreased cardiac output.	
8 Discuss findings with patient as needed.	
9 Complete postprocedure protocol.	

Recording and Reporting

- Record apical pulse, radial pulse and site, and pulse deficit in nurses' notes and EHR.
- Inform nurse in charge, physician, or health care provider of pulse deficit.

UNEXPECTED OUTCOMES	RELATED INTERVENTIONS
1 Pulse deficit exists.	• Report findings to health care provider/physician. • Anticipate physician's order for an electrocardiogram. • Reassess for deficit at next scheduled assessment.

Aquathermia and Heating Pads

A water-flow pad such as an aquathermia pad, electric heating pads, and commercial heat packs are common forms of dry heat therapy. Dry heat devices are applied directly to the surface of the skin; for this reason you need to take extra precautions to prevent burns, dry skin, and loss of body fluids. The aquathermia pad (water-flow pad) used in health care settings consists of a waterproof rubber or plastic pad connected by two hoses to an electrical control unit that has a heating element and motor. Distilled water circulates through hollowed channels in the pad to the control unit where water is heated (or cooled). In most health care facilities, the central supply department sets the temperature regulators to the recommended temperature. A temperature of 40°C (104°F) is safe for skin exposure for a long duration.

A conventional heating pad used in the home care setting consists of an electric coil enclosed in a waterproof cover. A cotton or flannel cloth covers the outer pad. The pad connects to an electrical cord that has a temperature-regulating unit for high, medium, or low settings. Because it is so easy to readjust temperature settings on heating pads, instruct patients not to turn the setting higher once they have adapted to the temperature. Instruct patient and family not to use the highest setting.

Delegation Considerations

The skill of applying dry heat can be delegated to nursing assistive personnel (NAP). The nurse must assess and evaluate the condition of the skin and tissues in the area that is treated and explain the purpose of the treatment. If there are risks or expected complications, this skill cannot be delegated. The nurse directs the NAP about:

- Specific positioning and time requirements to keep the application in place based on health care provider order or agency policy.
- What to observe and report immediately, such as excessive redness and pain during application.
- Reporting when treatment is complete so the patient's response can be evaluated.

Equipment

- Aquathermia or commercial heat pack
- Distilled water (for aquathermia pad)

- Bath towel or pillowcase
- Tape ties or gauze roll

Implementation

STEP	RATIONALE
1 Complete preprocedure protocol.	
2 Check electrical plugs and cords for obvious fraying or cracking.	Prevents injury from accidental electrical shock.
3 Determine patient's or family members' knowledge of procedure, including steps for application and safety precautions.	Determines extent of health teaching required.
4 Apply dry heat device:	
a For aquathermia, cover or wrap area to be treated with bath towel or enclose the pad with pillowcase.	Prevents heated surface from touching patient's skin directly and increasing risk for injury to patient's skin.
b For commercially prepared heat pack, break pouch inside larger pack (follow manufacturer's guidelines).	Activates chemicals within pack to warm outer surface.

SAFETY ALERT Do not pin the wrap to the pad, because this may cause a leak in the device.

5 Place pad over affected area (Fig. 3-1), and secure with tape, tie, or gauze as needed.	Pad delivers dry, warm heat to injured tissues. Pad should not slip onto different body part.

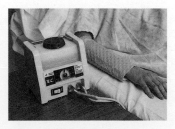

Fig. 3-1 Aquathermia pad applied.

STEP	RATIONALE

SAFETY ALERT Never position the patient so that he or she is lying directly on the pad. This position prevents dissipation of heat and increases risk for burns.

STEP	RATIONALE
6 Turn on aquathermia unit and check temperature setting.	Prevents exposure of patient to temperature extremes.
7 Monitor condition of skin every 5 minutes during application, and question patient regarding sensation of burning.	Determines if heat exposure is causing any burn, blistering, or injury to underlying skin.
8 After 20 to 30 minutes (or time ordered by physician), remove pad and store.	Continued exposure results in burns.
9 Complete postprocedure protocol.	

SAFETY ALERT Do not have patient actively exercise muscle to evaluate results of therapy. Active exercise can aggravate muscle strain.

STEP	RATIONALE
10 Observe patient or family caregiver apply pad to be used in home.	Measures level of learning.

Recording and Reporting

- Record type of application, temperature and duration of therapy, and patient's response.
- Describe any instruction given and patient's/family caregiver's success in demonstrating procedure.
- Report pain level, range of motion (ROM) of body part, skin integrity, color, temperature, sensitivity to touch, blistering, or dryness.

UNEXPECTED OUTCOMES	RELATED INTERVENTIONS
1 Skin is reddened and sensitive to touch. Extreme warmth caused burning of skin layer.	• Discontinue application immediately. • Verify proper temperature, or check device for proper functioning. • Notify health care provider and, if there is a burn, complete an incident report.
2 Patient complains of burning and discomfort.	• Reduce temperature. • Assess for skin breakdown. • Notify health care provider.
3 Body part is painful to move. Movement stretches burn-sensitive nerve fibers in skin.	• Discontinue aquathermia or heat pack use. Wait for swelling to resolve before attempting to reapply. • Notify nurse in charge, or contact health care provider.
4 Patient applies pad incorrectly or cannot explain precautions.	• Reinstruct patient or family caregiver as necessary. Consider possible home health referral.

Aspiration Precautions

The ability to swallow effectively and safely is a basic human need. Any alteration or delay in the swallowing process causes dysphagia (difficulty swallowing). Aspiration pneumonia can be a fatal complication of dysphagia. The goal of dysphagia evaluation and management is to ensure that a patient will be able to swallow oral fluids and food safely. The single most important measure to prevent aspiration is to place the patient on NPO status until a swallowing evaluation determines that dysphagia poses no substantial risk. Bedside screening for dysphagia includes giving the patient water or foods with different textures and observing for coughing, gagging, choking, and voice alteration.

Dysphagia management includes dietary modification by altering the consistency of foods and liquids and is most effective when implemented using a multidisciplinary approach. The speech-language pathologist (SLP) and registered dietitian (RD) are central to dysphagia management.

Four levels comprise the National Dysphagia Diet: dysphagia puree, dysphagia mechanically altered, dysphagia advanced, and regular (Table 4-1). Thin liquids create safety risks in swallowing because of their speed and decreased texture for patients with impaired oral motor control. Thickened liquids are commonly prescribed to prevent aspiration pneumonia. Nectarlike liquids (medium viscosity) are liquids that are thickened but drip off a spoon at a slower rate than thin liquids. Honeylike liquids (high viscosity) are thickened so the liquid drips off a spoon at a much slower rate. Spoon-thick viscosity liquids include foods that do not easily drip off a spoon. It is important to remember that the desired thickness of a liquid depends on the patient's swallowing deficit.

Delegation Considerations

The assessment of a patient's risk for aspiration and determination of positioning cannot be delegated to nursing assistive personnel (NAP). However, NAP may feed patients after receiving instruction on aspiration precautions. The nurse directs the NAP to:

- Position patient upright or according to medical restrictions during and after feeding.
- Use aspiration precautions while feeding patients who need assistance.
- Immediately report any onset of coughing, gagging, or a wet voice or pocketing of food.

TABLE 4-1 Stages of National Dysphagia Diet

Stage	Description	Examples
NDD 1: Dysphagia pureed	Uniform, pureed, cohesive, pudding-like texture	Smooth, hot cereals cooked to a "pudding" consistency; mashed potatoes; pureed meat and vegetables; pureed pasta or rice; yogurt
NDD 2: Dysphagia mechanically altered	Moist, soft-textured; easily forms a bolus	Cooked cereals; dry cereals moistened with milk; canned fruit (except pineapple), moist ground meat; well-cooked noodles in sauce/gravy; well-cooked, diced vegetables
NDD 3: Dysphagia advanced	Regular foods (except very hard, sticky, or crunchy foods)	Moist breads (e.g., butter, jelly); well-moistened cereals, peeled soft fruits (peach, plum, kiwi); tender, thin-sliced meats; baked potato (without skin); tender, cooked vegetables
Regular	All foods	No restrictions

Data from National Dysphagia Diet Task Force: *National dysphagia diet: standardization for optimal care,* Chicago, 2002, American Dietetic Association.
NDD, National Dysphagia Diet.

Equipment
- Upright chair or bed in high-Fowler's position
- Thickening agents as designated by SLP (rice, cereal, yogurt, gelatin, commercial thickener)
- Tongue blade
- Penlight
- Oral hygiene supplies
- Pulse oximeter
- Suction equipment
- Clean gloves

Implementation

STEP	RATIONALE
1 Complete preprocedure protocol.	

STEP	RATIONALE
2 Perform a nutritional assessment.	Patients with dysphagia alter their eating patterns or choose foods that do not provide adequate nutrition (see Table 4-1).
3 Assess mental status, including alertness, orientation, and ability to follow simple commands.	If orientation and command-following are impaired, risk for aspiration is higher.
4 Determine if patient has an increased risk for aspiration, and assess for signs and symptoms of dysphagia (Box 4-1). Use a dysphagia screening tool if available.	Performing an assessment before feeding determines when referral to SLP is necessary. Interventions to minimize aspiration and possible pneumonia can be implemented.
5 ✋ Apply clean gloves, if needed, and assess patient's oral health.	Poor oral hygiene can result in decayed teeth, plaque, and periodontal disease and cause growth of bacteria in the mouth, which can be aspirated.
6 Observe patient during mealtime for signs of dysphagia such as coughing, dyspnea, or drooling. Note during and at end of meal if patient tires.	Indicates swallowing impairment and possible aspiration. Chewing and sitting up for feeding accelerate onset of fatigue. Fatigue increases risk for aspiration.
7 Indicate on patient's chart and Kardex that dysphagia/aspiration risk is present.	Identifying patient as dysphagic reduces risk for his or her receiving oral nutrients without supervision.
8 Position patient in an upright (90 degrees) position or highest position allowed by medical condition during mealtimes.	Uses gravity to facilitate safe swallowing and enhances esophageal motility. Side-lying position is an option if patient cannot have head elevated.
9 Using penlight and tongue blade, gently inspect mouth for pockets of food.	Pockets of food in the mouth indicate difficulty swallowing.

BOX 4-1 Criteria for Dysphagia Referral

Before Referral:

If the answer is "yes" to either of the following two questions, referral at this time is not appropriate:

- Is patient unconscious or drowsy?
- Is patient unable to sit in an upright position for a reasonable length of time?

Consider the Next Two Questions Before Making the Referral:

- Is patient near the end of life?
- Does patient have an esophageal problem that will require surgical intervention?

When Observing the Patient or Giving Mouth Care, Look for the Following:

- Open mouth (weak lip closure)
- Drooling liquids or solids
- Poor oral hygiene/thrush
- Facial weakness
- Tongue weakness
- Difficulty with secretions
- Slurred, indistinct speech
- Change in voice quality

- Poor posture or head control
- Weak involuntary cough
- Delayed cough (up to 2 minutes after swallow)
- General frailty
- Confusion/dementia
- No spontaneous swallowing movements

If any of the above is present, the patient may have swallowing problems and need referral to a speech-language pathologist.

STEP	RATIONALE
10 Have patient assume a chin-tuck position. Have patient swallow twice or repeatedly, and monitor for swallowing and respiratory difficulty.	Chin-tuck or chin-down position helps reduce aspiration (Brady, 2008). Double or repeat-swallowing requires patient to use additional swallows to help clear any remaining food from an unprotected airway (Garcia and Chambers, 2010).

STEP	RATIONALE
11 Add thickener to thin liquids to create desired consistency per SLP evaluation.	Increasing viscosity or thickness of liquid slows movement through mouth and pharynx and protects airway (Brady, 2008).
12 Encourage patient to feed self. Tell patient not to tilt head backward when eating or while drinking out of a glass or cup.	Promotes independence and may help patient initiate more natural swallow (Brady, 2008). Backward head tilt extends neck; thus food and liquid are more likely to be misdirected into airway (Ney et al., 2009).
13 If patient cannot feed self, place $\frac{1}{2}$ to 1 teaspoon of food on unaffected side of mouth, allowing utensils to touch the mouth or tongue.	Small bites help patient's ability to swallow (Grodner et al., 2012). Provides a tactile cue to begin eating (Brady, 2008).
14 Provide verbal cueing while feeding. Remind patient to chew and think about swallowing. Avoid mixing food of different textures in same mouthful. Minimize distractions, and do not rush patient. Use sauces, condiments, and gravies to facilitate cohesive food bolus formation.	Helps elicit normal swallow and prevent aspiration (Brady, 2008). Single textures are easier to swallow than multiple textures. Environmental distractions and conversations during mealtime increase risk for aspiration (Chang and Roberts, 2011).
15 Report signs and symptoms of dysphagia or aspiration to health care provider.	
16 Ask patient to remain sitting upright for at least 30 to 60 minutes after the meal.	Reduces the chance of aspiration by allowing food particles remaining in pharynx to clear (Frey and Ramsberger, 2011).
17 Complete postprocedure protocol.	

Recording and Reporting

- Document in patient's medical record assessment findings, patient's tolerance of liquids and food textures, amount of assistance required, position during meal, absence or presence of any symptoms of dysphagia during feeding, fluid intake, and amount eaten.
- Report any coughing, gagging, choking, or swallowing difficulties to health care provider.

UNEXPECTED OUTCOMES	RELATED INTERVENTIONS
1 Patient coughs, gags, complains of food "stuck in throat," or has pockets of food in mouth.	• Stop feeding immediately and place patient on NPO. Notify health care provider, and suction as needed. • Anticipate consultation with SLP for swallowing exercises and techniques to improve swallowing.
2 Patient experiences weight loss.	• Consult with health care provider and RD about increasing frequency of meals or providing oral nutritional supplements or alternative feeding methods such as tube feedings.

Assistive Device Ambulation (Use of Crutches, Cane, and Walker)

Patients who are immobile for even a short time may require assistance with ambulation. Whenever assisting a patient up and out of bed or a chair, there is a risk for fainting. Use safety precautions to control for orthostatic hypotension and subsequent falling. Use of an assistive device increases stability. These devices range from standard canes to crutches and walkers (Pierson and Fairchild, 2008).

Delegation Considerations

The skill of assisting patients with ambulation can be delegated to nursing assistive personnel (NAP). The nurse directs the NAP by:

- Instructing them to have a patient dangle at the side of the bed before ambulation.
- Instructing them to immediately return a patient to the bed or chair if the patient is nauseated, dizzy, pale, or diaphoretic and to report these signs and symptoms to the nurse immediately.
- Discussing the importance of applying safe, nonskid shoes and ensuring that the environment is free of clutter and there is no moisture on the floor before ambulating the patient.

Equipment

- Ambulation device (crutch, walker, cane)
- Safety device (gait belt)
- Well-fitting, flat, nonskid shoes for patient
- Robe
- Goniometer *(optional)*

Implementation

STEP	RATIONALE
1 Complete preprocedure protocol.	

STEP	RATIONALE
2 Assess degree of assistance patient needs.	For safety, another person may be needed initially to assist with patient ambulation.
3 Prepare patient for procedure:	Teaching and demonstration enhance learning, reduce anxiety, and encourage cooperation.
a Explain reasons for exercise, and demonstrate specific gait technique.	
b Decide with patient how far to ambulate.	Determines mutual goal.
c Schedule ambulation around patient's other activities.	Scheduled rest periods between activities reduce patient fatigue.
d Place bed in low position, and slowly assist patient to upright Fowler's position. If in chair, have patient sit upright with feet flat on floor.	Allows a few minutes for circulation to equilibrate. Prevents orthostatic hypotension and potential injuries.
e Assist patient in bed to dangling position on side of bed (Fig. 5-1). Apply gait belt. Assist sitting patient to standing	Movement of legs in dangling position promotes venous return (Eanarroch, 2007).

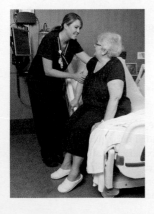

Fig. 5-1 Assisting patient to side of bed.

STEP	RATIONALE
position, and allow to stand until balance is gained. Support by holding gait belt.	
f Ask if patient feels dizzy or light-headed. If patient appears light-headed, set patient back down and recheck blood pressure.	Allows nurse to detect orthostatic hypotension before ambulation begins.
g Care must be taken if patient has intravenous (IV) tubing or a Foley catheter. Obtain IV pole with wheels that can be pushed as patient walks. Urinary catheter drainage bags must stay at or below level of bladder. A second person may be needed to assist.	Allows patient to ambulate unencumbered. Urine in tubing must not reenter bladder, which increases infection risk.

SAFETY ALERT Remove obstacles, including throw rugs, from pathways, and wipe up any spills immediately. Avoid crowds. Crowds increase the risk for the crutch, cane, or walker being kicked or jarred and patient losing balance.

4 Determine the appropriate height of ambulation device, if used:	
a **Crutch measurement:** Includes three areas— patient's height, distance between crutch pad and axilla, and angle of elbow flexion. Use one of two methods:	Promotes optimal support and stability.
(1) *Standing:* Position crutches with crutch tips at 15 cm (6 inches) to side and 15 cm in front of	Radial nerve passes under axillary area superficially. If crutch is too long, it can cause pressure on axilla and radial nerve, leading to paralysis of

STEP	RATIONALE
patient's feet and crutch pads 5 cm (2 inches) below axilla (Pierson and Fairchild, 2008).	elbow and wrist extensors (crutch palsy). Also, if crutch is too long, shoulders are forced upward and patient cannot push body off ground. If ambulation device is too short, patient will be bent over and uncomfortable.
(2) *Supine:* Crutch pad should be approximately 5 cm (2 inches) or two to three finger widths under axilla with crutch tips positioned 15 cm (6 inches) lateral to patient's heel (Pierson and Fairchild, 2008) (Figs. 5-2 and 5-3).	
(3) Instruct patient to report any tingling or numbness in upper torso.	May mean that crutches are being used incorrectly or that they are wrong size.
(4) With either measurement method, elbows should be flexed 15 to 30 degrees. Elbow flexion is verified with goniometer (Fig. 5-4).	Angle ensures that arms can push body off ground.

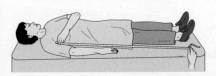

Fig. 5-2 Supine method.

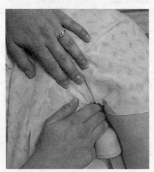

Fig. 5-3 Top of crutch.

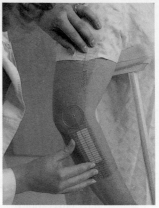

Fig. 5-4 Elbows flexed. Verification of elbow flexion using goniometer.

STEP	RATIONALE
(5) In addition to overall *length* of axillary crutch, *height* of handgrip is important. Adjust handgrip so that patient's elbow is slightly flexed.	If handgrip is too low, radial nerve can be damaged even if overall crutch length is correct. Extra length between handgrip and axillary bar can force bar up into axilla as patient stretches down to reach handgrip. If handgrip is too high, patient's elbow is sharply flexed and strength and stability of arms are decreased.
b **Cane measurement:** Patient holds cane on uninvolved side 10 to 15 cm (4 to 6 inches) to side of foot. Cane extends from greater trochanter to floor while cane is held 15 cm (6 inches) from foot. Allow approximately 15 to 30 degrees of elbow flexion.	Offers most support when cane is placed on stronger side of body. Cane and weaker leg work together with each step. If cane is too short, patient will have difficulty supporting weight and be bent over and uncomfortable. As weight is taken on by hand and affected leg is lifted off floor, complete extension of elbow is necessary.

STEP	RATIONALE
c **Walker measurement:** Top of walker should match crease in wrist when patient stands up straight (American Academy of Orthopaedist Surgeons, 2011). Elbows are flexed at approximately 15 to 30 degrees when patient is standing inside walker with hands on handgrips.	Walker should be at proper height so patient does not bend forward.
5 Make sure ambulation device has rubber tips.	Prevents device from slipping.
6 Make sure surface that patient walks on is clean and dry. Remove any obstacles or objects that might obstruct pathway.	Prevents injuries.
7 Ambulation with crutches: a Assist patient in crutch-walking by choosing appropriate crutch gait:	To use crutches, patient supports self with hands and arms; therefore strength in arm and shoulder muscles, ability to balance body in upright position, and stamina are necessary. Type of gait patient uses depends on amount of weight patient can support with one or both legs.
(1) Four-point gait:	This is most stable of crutch gaits. Requires bearing weight on both legs. Each leg moves alternately with each opposing crutch so that three points of support are on floor all the time.

STEP	RATIONALE
(a) Begin in tripod position. Place crutches 15 cm (6 inches) in front and 15 cm to side of each foot. Have patient place weight on handgrips, not under arms (Fig. 5-5).	Improves patient's balance by providing wide base of support. Patient should have posture of erect head and neck, straight vertebrae, and extended hips and knees.
(b) Move right crutch forward 10 to 15 cm (4 to 6 inches) (Fig. 5-6, *A*).	Crutch and foot position is similar to arm and foot position during normal walking.
(c) Move left foot forward to level of left crutch (Fig. 5-6, *B*).	
(d) Move left crutch forward 10 to 15 cm (4 to 6 inches) (Fig. 5-6, *C*).	
(e) Move right foot forward to level of right crutch (Fig. 5-6, *D*).	
(f) Repeat above sequence.	
(2) Three-point gait:	Requires patient to bear all weight on uninvolved leg and then on both crutches. Affected leg does not touch ground during early phase of three-point gait. May be useful for patient with broken leg or sprained ankle.

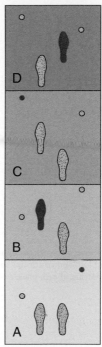

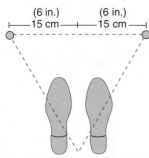

Fig. 5-5 Tripod position.

Fig. 5-6 Four-point gait. Solid feet and crutch tips show foot and crutch tip movement in each of the four phases. **A,** Right tip moves forward. **B,** Left foot moves toward left crutch. **C,** Left crutch tip moves forward. **D,** Right foot moves toward right crutch.

STEP	RATIONALE
(a) Begin in tripod position (Fig. 5-7, *A*). (b) Advance both crutches and affected leg (Fig. 5-7, *B*).	Improves patient's balance by providing wide base of support.

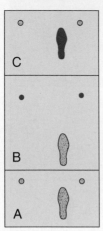

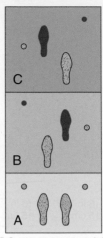

Fig. 5-7 Three-point gait with weight borne on unaffected right leg. Solid foot and crutch tips show weight bearing in each phase.

Fig. 5-8 Two-point gait. Solid areas indicate weight-bearing leg and crutch tips.

STEP	RATIONALE
(c) Move stronger leg forward, stepping on floor (Fig. 5-7, *C*).	
(d) Repeat sequence.	
(3) Two-point gait:	Requires at least partial weight bearing on each foot. Requires more balance because only two points support body at one time (Hoeman, 2007).
(a) Begin in tripod position (Fig. 5-8, *A*).	Improves patient's balance by providing wide base of support.
(b) Move left crutch and right foot forward (Fig. 5-8, *B*).	Crutch movements are similar to arm movement during normal walking as patient moves crutch at same time as opposing leg.

STEP	RATIONALE
(c) Move right crutch and left foot forward (Fig. 5-8, *C*).	
(d) Repeat sequence.	
(4) Swing-to gait:	Frequently used by patients whose lower extremities are paralyzed or who wear weight-supporting braces on their legs. This is the easier of the two swinging gaits. It requires ability to partially bear body weight on both legs.
(a) Begin in tripod position.	
(b) Move both crutches forward.	
(c) Lift and swing legs to crutches, letting crutches support body weight.	
(d) Repeat two previous steps.	
(5) Swing-through gait:	Requires that patient have ability to bear partial weight on both feet. Improves patient's balance by providing wide base of support. Initial placement of crutches is to increase patient's base of support so that when body swings forward, patient is moving center of gravity toward additional support provided by crutches.
(a) Begin in tripod position.	
(b) Move both crutches forward.	
(c) Lift and swing legs through and beyond crutches.	
b Assist patient in climbing stairs with crutches:	
(1) Begin in tripod position.	Improves patient's balance by providing wide base of support.
(2) Patient transfers body weight to crutches (Fig. 5-9).	Prepares patient to transfer weight to unaffected leg when ascending first stair.
(3) Patient advances unaffected leg to stair (Fig. 5-10).	Crutch adds support to affected leg. Patient then shifts weight from crutches to unaffected leg.

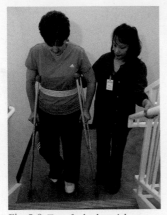

Fig. 5-9 Transfer body weight to crutches.

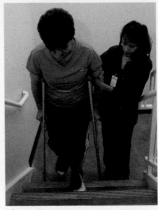

Fig. 5-10 Advance unaffected leg to stair.

STEP	RATIONALE
(4) Both crutches are aligned with unaffected leg on stairs (Fig. 5-11).	Maintains balance and provides wide base of support.
(5) Repeat sequence until patient reaches top of stairs.	
c Assist patient in descending stairs with crutches:	
(1) Begin in tripod position.	Improves patient's balance by providing wide base of support.
(2) Patient transfers body weight to unaffected leg (Fig. 5-12).	Prepares patient to release support of body weight maintained by crutches.
(3) Move crutches to stair, and instruct patient to begin to transfer body weight to crutches (Fig. 5-13) and move affected leg forward.	Maintains patient's balance and base of support.

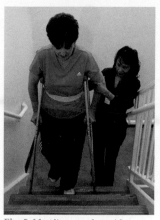

Fig. 5-11 Align crutches with unaffected leg.

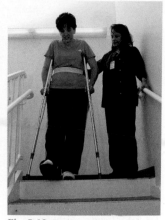

Fig. 5-12 Body weight is transferred to unaffected leg.

STEP	RATIONALE
(4) Patient moves unaffected leg to stair and aligns with crutches (Fig. 5-14). (5) Repeat sequence until stairs are descended.	Maintains balance and provides base of support.
8 Ambulation with walker: Walker is used by patients who are able to bear partial weight.	Patient needs sufficient strength to be able to pick up walker. Four-wheeled model does not need to be picked up; however, it is not as stable.
a Have patient stand in center of walker and grasp handgrips on upper bars.	Patient balances self before attempting to walk.
b Have patient lift walker, move it 15 to 20 cm (6 to 8 inches) forward, and then set it down, making sure all four feet of walker stay on floor. Take step forward with either foot. Then follow through with other leg.	Provides broad base of support between walker and patient. Patient then moves center of gravity toward walker. Keeping all four feet of walker on floor is necessary to prevent tipping of walker.

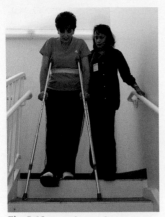

Fig. 5-13 Transfer weight to crutches.

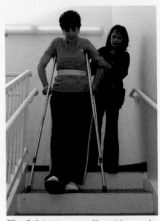

Fig. 5-14 Move unaffected leg, and align with crutches.

STEP	RATIONALE
c If there is unilateral weakness, after walker is advanced, instruct patient to step forward with weaker leg, support self with arms, and follow through with uninvolved leg. If patient cannot bear weight on one leg, after advancing walker have patient swing into it, supporting weight on hands.	
9 Ambulation with cane (same steps are taught for standard or quad cane) (Fig. 5-15):	
a Begin by placing cane on side of strong leg.	Provides added support for weak or impaired side.
b Place cane forward 15 to 25 cm (6 to 10 inches), keeping body weight on both legs.	Distributes body weight equally.

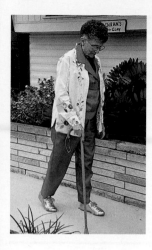

Fig. 5-15 Patient walking properly with cane.

STEP	RATIONALE
c Move strong leg forward, even with cane.	Body weight is supported by cane and uninvolved leg.
d Advance strong leg past cane.	Body weight is supported by cane and involved leg.
e Move involved leg forward, even with uninvolved leg.	Aligns patient's center of gravity. Returns patient's body weight to equal distribution.
f Repeat these steps.	
10 Complete postprocedure protocol.	

Recording and Reporting

- Record in the nurses' notes and electronic health record (EHR) the type of gait patient used, assistive device, amount of assistance required, distance walked, and activity tolerance.
- Immediately report to nurse in charge or health care provider any injury sustained during attempts to ambulate, alteration in vital signs, or inability to ambulate.

UNEXPECTED OUTCOMES	RELATED INTERVENTIONS
1 Patient is unable to ambulate.	• Possible reasons include fear of falling, physical discomfort, upper body muscles that are too weak to use ambulation device, and lower extremities that are too weak to support body.
	• Initiate isometric exercise program to strengthen upper body muscles.
	• Provide analgesic if needed.
2 Patient sustains injury.	• Notify health care provider. Return patient to bed if injury is stable.

Automated External Defibrillator

Defibrillation is the electrical attempt to stop a lethal dysrhythmia such as ventricular fibrillation. An automated external defibrillator (AED) allows for individuals trained only in basic life support to defibrillate. The AED is a defibrillator that incorporates a rhythm analysis system. The device attaches to a patient by two adhesive pads and connecting cables. Most AEDs are stand-alone boxes with a very simple three-step function and verbal prompts to guide the responder. After rhythm identification, some AEDs automatically provide a verbal warning, followed by an electrical shock. Other AEDs recommend a shock, if needed, and then prompt the responder to press the shock button.

Delegation Considerations

Basic life support certification provides hands-on training with an AED for laypersons, nursing assistive personnel (NAP), and licensed health care professionals. Most hospitals using AEDs have given the authority to use an AED to all cardiopulmonary resuscitation (CPR)–certified personnel, including NAP. Refer to specific hospital policies for use of the AED.

Equipment

- AED
- Pair of AED adhesive pads

Implementation

STEP	RATIONALE
1 Establish unresponsiveness, and call for help.	This information assists in determining if patient is unresponsive rather than asleep, intoxicated, hearing impaired, or postictal. Rapid response by qualified professionals ensures ongoing resuscitation support.

STEP	RATIONALE
2 Establish absence of respirations and lack of circulation: no pulse, no respirations, no movement.	Indicates need for emergency measures, including AED.

SAFETY ALERT An AED should be applied only to a patient who is unconscious, not breathing, and pulseless. For children younger than 8 years, AED pads designed for children should be used. If child pads are not available, use adult AED pads (Berg et al., 2010).

STEP	RATIONALE
3 Activate code team in accordance with hospital policy and procedure.	First available person to bring resuscitation cart and AED.
4 Start chest compressions, and continue until AED is attached to patient and verbal prompt of device advises you, "Do not touch the patient."	To minimize interruption time of chest compressions, continue CPR while AED is being applied and turned on.
5 Place AED next to patient near chest or head.	Ensures easy access to device.

SAFETY ALERT If the AED is immediately available, attach it to patient as soon as possible. The faster defibrillation is delivered, the better the survival rate (Ewy and Kern, 2009).

STEP	RATIONALE
6 Turn on power (Fig. 6-1).	Turning on power begins verbal prompts to guide you through next steps.
7 Attach device. Place the first AED pad on the upper right sternal border directly below the clavicle. Place the second AED pad lateral to the left nipple with the top of the pad a few inches below the axilla. Ensure that cables are connected to the AED.	Alternative pad placement of AED pads is not recommended. AEDs analyze most heart rhythms using lead II. If the AED pads are placed as directed, patient's heart rhythm will be analyzed in lead II. Patients with large amount of chest hair may require shaving to obtain adequate pad contact.

SAFETY ALERT Do not attach pads to a wet surface, over a medication patch, or over a pacemaker or implanted defibrillator. Wet surfaces, implanted defibrillators, and medication patches reduce the effectiveness of the defibrillation attempt and result in complications.

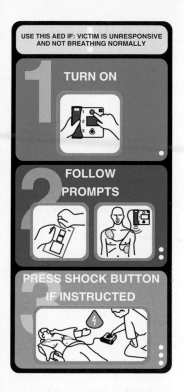

Fig. 6-1 AED power panel with prompts. (Courtesy Philips Medical Systems.)

STEP	RATIONALE
8 When AED prompts you, stop touching patient. Do *NOT* touch patient after this prompt. Direct rescuers and bystanders to avoid touching patient by announcing "Clear!" Allow the AED to analyze the rhythm. Some devices require that an analysis button be pressed. The AED takes approximately 5 to 15 seconds to analyze the rhythm.	Each brand of AED is different, so familiarity with model is important. Not touching the victim prevents artifact errors, avoids all movement during analysis (Link et al., 2010), and prevents shock from being delivered to bystanders.

STEP	RATIONALE
9 Before pressing the shock button, announce loudly to clear the victim and perform a visual check to ensure that no one is in contact with victim.	Clearing the patient ensures safety for those involved in rescue efforts.
10 Immediately begin chest compression after the shock, and continue for 2 minutes.	Continues cardiac perfusion.
11 Deliver two breaths using mouth-to-mouth with barrier device or mouth-to-mask device or bag-mask device. Watch for chest rise and fall. Deliver 10 to 12 breaths/min.	In a hospital setting where protected methods of artificial ventilation are available, mouth-to-mouth without a barrier device is not recommended because of risk for microbial contamination.
12 After 2 minutes of CPR, the AED will prompt you not to touch patient and will resume analysis of patient's rhythm. This cycle will continue until patient regains a pulse or physician determines death.	
13 Inspect pad adhesion to chest wall. If pads are not in good contact with chest wall, remove them and apply a new set. Attach new set of pads to the AED.	Poor pad-skin contact reduces the effectiveness of the shock, causes skin burns, or increases chance of shocking those involved in the rescue efforts. Always apply a new set of pads. Do *NOT* reuse.
14 Continue resuscitative efforts until patient regains pulse or until physician determines death.	

Recording and Reporting

- Immediately report arrest via the hospital-wide communication system, indicating exact location of victim.
- Cardiopulmonary arrest requires precise documentation. Most hospitals use a form designed specifically for in-hospital arrests.
- Record in nurses' notes and electronic health record (EHR) or on designated CPR worksheet: onset of arrest, time and number of AED shocks (you will not know the exact energy level used by the AED), time and energy level of manual defibrillations, medications given, procedures performed, cardiac rhythm, use of CPR, and patient's response.

UNEXPECTED OUTCOMES	RELATED INTERVENTIONS
1 Patient's heart rhythm does not convert into stable rhythm with pulse after defibrillation.	• Assess pad contact on patient's chest wall. • Do not touch patient during AED's rhythm analysis. • Avoid placing AED pads over medication patches, pacemaker, or implantable defibrillator generators.
2 Patient's skin has burns under AED pads.	• Assess AED pad contact on chest. • Ensure that chest is dry before applying pads to chest.

Bladder Volume Measurement

A bladder scanner is a noninvasive device that creates an ultrasound image of the bladder for measuring the volume of urine in the bladder. The device makes calculations to report accurate urine volumes, especially lower volumes (Al-Shaikh et al., 2009). Use a bladder scanner to assess bladder volume whenever inadequate bladder emptying is suspected. The most common use for the bladder scan is to measure postvoid residual (PVR)—the volume of urine in the bladder after a normal voiding. To obtain the most reliable reading, measure PVR within 10 minutes of voiding (Newman and Wein, 2009). A volume less than 50 mL is considered normal. Two or more PVR measurements greater than 100 mL require further investigation (Newman and Wein, 2009).

Delegation Considerations

The skill of measuring bladder volume by bladder scan can be delegated to nursing assistive personnel (NAP). The nurse must first determine the timing and frequency of the bladder scan measurement and interpret the measurements obtained. The nurse also assesses the patient's ability to toilet before measuring PVR and, if urinary retention is suspected, assesses the patient's abdomen for distention. The nurse directs the NAP to:

- Follow manufacturer's recommendations for the use of the device.
- Measure PVR volumes 10 minutes after helping the patient to void.
- Report and record bladder scan volumes.

Equipment

- BladderScan or bladder ultrasound device (Fig. 7-1)
- Ultrasound transmission gel
- Cleaning agent for scanner head, such as an alcohol pad

Implementation

STEP	RATIONALE
1 Complete preprocedure protocol.	

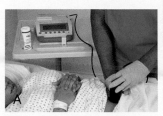
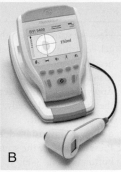

Fig. 7-1 **A,** Correct placement of BladderScan head. **B,** BladderScan reading.
(Courtesy Verathon, Inc., Bothell, Wash.)

STEP	RATIONALE
2 Use bladder scanner to assess PVR:	
a Assist patient to a supine position with head slightly elevated.	
b Expose the patient's lower abdomen.	
c Turn on the scanner per manufacturer's guidelines.	
d Set gender designation per manufacturer's guidelines. Women who have had a hysterectomy should be designated as male.	
e Wipe the scan head with an alcohol pad or other cleaner and allow to air dry.	
f Palpate the patient's symphysis pubis (pubic bone), and apply a generous amount of ultrasound gel (or a bladder scan gel pad) to midline abdomen about 2.5 to 4 cm (1 to 1½ inches) above symphysis pubis.	Allows for correct positioning of scanner.

STEP	RATIONALE
g Place the scan head on the gel, ensuring that scanner head is oriented per manufacturer's guidelines.	Use of gel improves the clarity of the scanned image.
h Apply light pressure, keep the scanner head steady, and point it slightly downward toward bladder. Press and release the scan button (see Fig. 7-1).	
i Verify accurate aim (refer to manufacturer's guidelines). Complete scan, and print image (if needed).	
3 Remove ultrasound gel from patient's abdomen with paper towel.	
4 Remove ultrasound gel from scanner head and wipe with alcohol pad or other cleaner; allow to air dry.	
5 Complete postprocedure protocol.	

Recording and Reporting

- Record and report amount voided before scan as well as scan volume.

Blood Administration

Transfusion therapy or blood replacement is the intravenous (IV) administration of whole blood, its components, or plasma-derived product for therapeutic purposes. Transfusions are used to restore intravascular volume with whole blood or albumin, to restore oxygen-carrying capacity of blood with red blood cells (RBCs), and to provide clotting factors and/or platelets. Despite precautions, transfusion therapy carries risks. Compatibility of the patient and donor is essential.

A health care provider's order is required for the administration of a blood product. A nurse is responsible for understanding which components are appropriate in various situations.

Delegation Considerations

You cannot delegate the skill of initiating blood therapy to nursing assistive personnel (NAP). After the transfusion has been started and the patient is stable, monitoring of a patient by NAP does not relieve the nurse of the responsibility and accountability to continue to assess the patient during the transfusion. Instruct NAP about:

- Frequency of vital sign monitoring.
- What to observe, such as complaints of shortness of breath, hives, and/or chills, and the importance of reporting this information to the nurse.
- Obtaining blood components from the blood bank (if agency allows).

Equipment

- Y-type blood administration set (in-line filter) (**NOTE:** Depending on blood product, special tubing and filter are necessary.)
- Prescribed blood product
- 250-mL bag 0.9% NaCl (normal saline) IV solution
- Antiseptic wipes (chlorhexidine based)
- Clean gloves
- Tape
- Vital sign equipment: thermometer, blood pressure cuff, and stethoscope
- Signed transfusion consent form

Optional Equipment

- Rapid infusion pump
- Electronic infusion device (EID) (Verify that pump can be used to deliver blood and blood products.)

- Leukocyte-depleting filter
- Blood warmer
- Pressure bag
- Pulse oximeter

Implementation

STEP	RATIONALE
1 Complete preprocedure protocol.	
2 Verify that IV cannula is patent and that complications such as infiltration or phlebitis are not present:	Patent IV ensures that transfusion will be initiated and infused within established time guidelines. Gauge of IV cannula should be appropriate for accommodating infusion of blood and/or blood components (Infusion Nurses Society [INS], 2011a). Large cannulas, such as 18 gauge, promote optimal flow of blood components. Use of smaller cannulas, such as 24 gauge, may require blood bank to divide unit so that each half can be infused within allotted time or may require pressure-assisted devices.
a Administer blood or blood components to an adult, using a 14- to 24-gauge short peripheral catheter.	
b Transfuse a neonate or pediatric patient using a 22- to 24-gauge device (INS, 2011a).	
c A 1.9 Fr is the smallest central venous access device (CVAD) that can be used (INS, 2011a).	
3 Check that patient has properly completed and signed transfusion consent before retrieving blood, and assess laboratory values such as hematocrit, coagulation values, platelet count.	Most agencies require patients to sign consent forms before receiving blood component therapy because of the inherent risks (INS, 2011a). Pretransfusion laboratory values provide a baseline for later evaluation of patient response to the transfusion.
4 Obtain and record pretransfusion vital signs (temperature, pulse, respirations, and blood pressure).	Change from baseline vital signs during infusion will alert nurse to a potential transfusion reaction or adverse effect of therapy (INS, 2011a).

STEP	RATIONALE
5 Preadministration:	
a Obtain blood component from blood bank following agency protocol. Blood transfusion must be initiated within 30 minutes after release from laboratory or blood bank (INS, 2011a).	Timely acquisition ensures product is safe to administer. Agency protocol usually encompasses safeguards to ensure quality control throughout transfusion process.
b Verbally compare and correctly verify patient, blood product, and type with another person considered qualified by your agency (e.g., RN or LPN):	Strict adherence to verification procedures before administration of blood or blood components reduces risk for administering the wrong blood to patient (INS, 2011a).
(1) Identify patient using two identifiers (e.g., name and birthday or name and account number) according to agency policy. Compare identifiers with information on patient's MAR or medical record.	Ensures correct patient. Complies with The Joint Commission requirements for patient safety (TJC, 2014).
(2) Check that transfusion record number and patient's identification number match.	Prevents accidental administration of wrong component.
(3) Check that the patient's name is correct on all documents.	
(4) Check unit number on blood bag with blood bank form to ensure that they are the same.	

STEP	RATIONALE
(5) Verify that blood type matches on transfusion record and blood bag. Verify that component received from blood bank is the same component physician or health care provider ordered (e.g., packed red cells, platelets).	Ensures that patient receives correct therapy. One of the most common causes of a patient receiving the incorrect transfusion is obtaining the wrong blood component from the blood bank (Alexander et al., 2009; Gabriel, 2008; INS, 2011a).
(6) Check that patient's blood type and Rh type are compatible with donor blood type and Rh type.	Verifies accurate donor blood type and compatibility.
(7) Check expiration date and time on unit of blood.	Never use expired blood, because the cell components deteriorate and may contain excess citrate ions (Alexander et al., 2009; American Association of Blood Banks [AABB], 2011; INS, 2011a).
c Empty urine drainage collection container, or have patient void.	If a transfusion reaction occurs, a urine specimen containing urine produced after initiation of the transfusion will be sent to the laboratory.

SAFETY ALERT Initiate the blood transfusion within 30 minutes from time of release from blood bank. If you cannot do this, immediately return the blood to the blood bank, and retrieve it when you can administer it.

6 Administration:

a ✋ Perform hand hygiene, and apply clean gloves.	Using Standard Precautions reduces risk for transmission of microorganisms.

STEP	RATIONALE
b Open Y-tubing blood administration set.	Y-tubing facilitates maintenance of IV access in case a patient will need more than 1 unit of blood.
c Set all clamps to "off" position.	Setting clamps to "off" position prevents accidental spilling and wasting of product.
d Spike 0.9% normal saline IV bag with one of Y-tubing spikes (Fig. 8-1). Hang the bag on an IV pole, and prime tubing. Open the upper clamp on normal saline side of tubing, and squeeze the drip chamber until fluid covers the filter and one third to one half of the drip chamber.	Prime tubing with fluid to eliminate air in Y-tubing. Closing the clamp prevents spillage and waste of fluid.
e Maintain clamp on blood product side of Y-tubing in "off" position. Open common tubing clamp to finish priming the tubing to the distal end of tubing connector. Close tubing clamp when tubing is filled with saline. All three tubing clamps should be closed. Maintain protective sterile cap on tubing connector.	Prime the tubing with saline so that the IV line is ready to be connected to the patient's vascular access device (VAD).
f Prepare blood component for administration. Gently agitate blood unit bag. Remove protective covering from access port. Spike blood component unit with other Y connection (Fig. 8-2).	Gentle agitation suspends the red blood cells in the anticoagulant. A protective barrier drape may be used to catch any potential blood spillage. The tubing is primed with the blood unit and ready for transfusion into the patient.

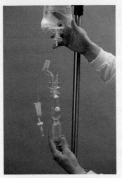

Fig. 8-1 Blood administration set is primed with normal saline.

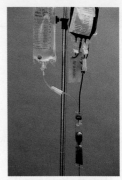

Fig. 8-2 Unit of blood connected to Y-tubing.

STEP	RATIONALE
Close normal saline clamp above filter, and open clamp above filter to blood unit and prime tubing with blood. Blood will flow into the drip chamber. Tap the filter chamber to ensure residual air is removed. Allow saline in tubing to flow into receptacle, being careful to ensure any blood spillage is contained in Blood Precaution container.	

SAFETY ALERT Normal saline is compatible with blood products, unlike solutions that contain dextrose, which causes coagulation of donor blood.

g	Maintaining asepsis, attach primed tubing to patient's VAD. Open common tubing clamp, and regulate blood infusion to allow only 2 mL/min to infuse in the initial 15 minutes.	Initiates infusion of blood product into patient's vein.

STEP	RATIONALE
h Remain with patient during the first 15 minutes of a transfusion. Initial flow rate during this time should be 2 mL/min, or 20 gtt/min.	Most transfusion reactions occur within the first 15 minutes of a transfusion (Snyder et al., 2008). Infusing a small amount of blood component initially minimizes the volume of blood to which the patient is exposed, thereby minimizing the severity of a reaction.

SAFETY ALERT If signs of a transfusion reaction occur, stop the transfusion, start normal saline with new primed tubing directly to the VAD at keep-vein-open (KVO) rate, and notify the physician immediately.

i Monitor patient's vital signs at 5 minutes, 15 minutes, and every 30 minutes until 1 hour after transfusion (AABB, 2011) or per agency policy.	Frequent monitoring of vital signs will help to quickly alert nurse to a transfusion reaction (Alexander et al., 2009; Gabriel, 2008; INS, 2011a).
j If there is no transfusion reaction, regulate rate of transfusion according to physician's orders. Check the drop factor for the blood tubing.	Maintaining the prescribed rate of flow decreases risk for fluid volume excess while restoring vascular volume. In most cases, drop factor for blood tubing is 10 gtt/mL.

SAFETY ALERT Do not let a unit of blood hang for more than 4 hours, because bacterial growth can occur (INS, 2011a). Never store blood in a facility's refrigerator.

SAFETY ALERT Never inject medication into the same IV line with a blood component because of the risk for contaminating the blood product with pathogens and the possibility of incompatibility. A separate IV access must be maintained if the patient requires IV solutions or medications (INS, 2011a).

k After blood has infused, clear IV line with 0.9% normal saline and discard blood bag according to agency policy.	Infusing IV saline solution infuses remainder of blood in IV tubing and keeps IV line patent for supportive measures in case of a transfusion reaction (INS, 2011a).

STEP	RATIONALE
l Appropriately dispose of all supplies. Remove gloves, and perform hand hygiene.	Standard Precautions during a transfusion reduce transmission of microorganisms.
m Monitor IV site and status of infusion each time vital signs are taken.	Detects presence of infiltration or phlebitis and verifies continuous and safe infusion of blood product.
n Observe for any changes in vital signs and for chills, flushing, itching, dyspnea, rash, or other signs of transfusion reaction.	Compare presenting signs and symptoms with baseline assessment of patient before transfusion. These are early signs of a transfusion reaction.
o Complete postprocedure protocol.	

Recording and Reporting

- Record pretransfusion medications, vital signs, location and condition of IV site, and patient education.
- Record the type and volume of blood component, blood unit/donor/recipient identification, compatibility, and expiration date according to agency policy, along with patient's response to therapy. Document on the transfusion record, nurses' notes, electronic health record (EHR), medication administration record, flow sheet, and/or intake and output sheet, depending on agency policy.
- Record volume of normal saline and blood component infused.
- Report signs and symptoms of a transfusion reaction immediately to the health care provider.
- Record amount of blood received by autotransfusion and patient's response to therapy.
- Report to health care provider any intratransfusion/posttransfusion deterioration in cardiac, pulmonary, and/or renal status.
- Record vital signs before, during, and after transfusion.

UNEXPECTED OUTCOMES	RELATED INTERVENTIONS
1 Patient displays signs and symptoms of transfusion reaction.	• Stop transfusion immediately. • Disconnect blood tubing at VAD hub, and cap distal end with sterile connector to maintain sterile system.

UNEXPECTED OUTCOMES	RELATED INTERVENTIONS
	• Connect normal saline–primed tubing at VAD hub to prevent any subsequent blood from infusing from tubing.
	• Keep vein open with slow infusion of normal saline at 10 to 12 gtt/min to ensure venous patency and maintain venous access for medication or to resume transfusion.
	• Notify health care provider.
2 Patient develops infiltration or phlebitis at venipuncture site.	• Remove IV and insert new VAD at different site. Restart the product if remainder can be infused within 4 hours of initiation of transfusion.
	• Institute nursing measures to reduce discomfort at infiltrated or infected site.
3 Rate of infusion slows in the absence of infiltration.	• Verify IV catheter is patent and all clamps are open. Gently flush IV line with normal saline, or use a pressure bag or EID to increase flow rate.
4 Fluid overload occurs, and/or patient exhibits difficulty breathing or has crackles upon auscultation.	• Slow or stop transfusion, elevate head of bed, and inform health care provider of physical findings.
	• Administer diuretics, morphine, and/or oxygen as ordered by health care provider.
	• Continue frequent assessments, and closely monitor vital signs, intake and output.

Blood Glucose Testing

Blood glucose monitoring allows patients with diabetes mellitus to self-manage their disease. Obtaining capillary blood by skin puncture is less painful than venipuncture, and the ease of the skin puncture method makes it possible for patients to perform this procedure. Glucose levels can be evaluated by performing a skin puncture and using either a visually read test (e.g., Chemstrip bG, Glucostix) or a reflectance meter. Measurement by a visually read test may not be accurate but can be useful for screening. Blood glucose reflectance meters are lightweight and run on batteries (e.g., Accu-Chek III, One-Touch) (Fig. 9-1). After a drop of blood from the skin puncture is dropped or wicked onto a reagent strip, the meter provides an accurate measurement of blood glucose level in 5 to 50 seconds. The various methods allow measurement of blood glucose between 20 and 800 mg/dL, thus providing a sensitive measurement of blood glucose level.

Delegation Considerations

Assessment of a patient's condition cannot be delegated to nursing assistive personnel (NAP). When the patient's condition is stable, the skill of obtaining and testing a sample of blood for blood glucose level can be delegated to NAP. The nurse informs the NAP by:

- Explaining appropriate sites to use for puncture and when to obtain glucose levels.
- Reviewing expected blood glucose levels and when to report unexpected glucose levels to the nurse.

Equipment

- Antiseptic swab
- Cotton ball
- Lancet device, either self-activating or button activated
- Blood glucose meter (e.g., Accu-Chek III, OneTouch)
- Blood glucose test strips appropriate for meter brand used
- Clean gloves
- Paper towel

Implementation

STEP	RATIONALE
1 Complete preprocedure protocol.	

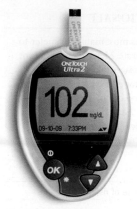

Fig. 9-1 Blood glucose monitor. (Courtesy LifeScan, Milpitas, CA.)

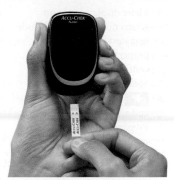

Fig. 9-2 Load test strip into meter. (Courtesy Accu-Chek Glucometer.)

STEP	RATIONALE
2 Perform hand hygiene. Instruct adult to perform hand hygiene, including forearm (if applicable) with soap and water. Rinse and dry. Position patient.	Promotes skin cleansing and vasodilation at selected puncture site. Reduces transmission of microorganisms.
3 Remove reagent strip from vial and tightly seal cap. Check code on test strip vial. Use only test strips recommended for glucose meter. Some newer meters do not require code and/or have disk or drum with 10 or more test strips.	Protects strips from accidental discoloration caused by exposure to air or light. Code on test strip vial must match code entered into glucose meter.
4 Insert strip into meter (refer to manufacturer's directions) (Fig. 9-2).	Some machines must be calibrated; others require zeroing of timer. Each meter is adjusted differently.

STEP	RATIONALE
5 Meter displays code on screen that must match code from test strip vial. Press proper button on meter to confirm matching codes. Meter is ready for use.	Codes must match for meter to operate. Meters have different messages that confirm that meter is ready for testing and blood can be applied.
6 🖐 Perform hand hygiene and apply clean gloves. Prepare single-use lancet or multiple-use lancet device.	Reduces transmission of microorganisms.

SAFETY ALERT Never reuse a lancet because of risk for infection.

STEP	RATIONALE
7 Obtain blood sample:	
a Wipe patient's finger or forearm lightly with antiseptic swab. Choose vascular area for puncture site. In stable adults, select lateral side of finger. Avoid central tip of finger, which has denser nerve supply (Pagana and Pagana, 2011).	Removes microorganisms from skin surface. Side of finger is less sensitive to pain.
b Hold area to be punctured in dependent position. Do not milk or massage finger site.	Increases blood flow to area before puncture. Milking may hemolyze specimen and introduce excess tissue fluid (Pagana and Pagana, 2011).
c Hold tip of lancet device against area of skin chosen for test site (Fig. 9-3). Press release button on device. Some devices allow you to see blood sample forming. Remove device.	Placement ensures that lancet enters skin properly.

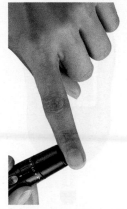

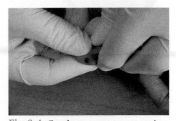

Fig. 9-3 Prick side of finger with lancet. (Courtesy Accu-Chek Glucometer.)

Fig. 9-4 Gently squeeze puncture site until drop of blood forms.

STEP	RATIONALE
d With some devices a blood sample begins to appear. Otherwise, gently squeeze or massage fingertip until round drop of blood forms (Fig. 9-4).	Adequate-size blood sample is needed to test glucose.
8 Obtain test results:	
a Be sure that meter is still on. Bring test strip in meter to drop of blood. Blood will be wicked onto test strip (Fig. 9-5). Follow specific meter instructions to be sure that you obtain adequate sample.	Blood enters strip, and glucose device shows message on screen to signal that enough blood is obtained.
b Blood glucose test result will appear on screen (Fig. 9-6). Some devices "beep" when completed.	

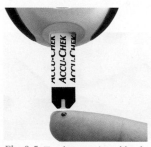

Fig. 9-5 Touch test strip to blood drop. Blood wicks into test strip. (Courtesy Accu-Chek Glucometer.)

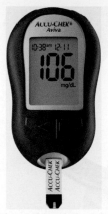

Fig. 9-6 Results appear on meter screen. (Courtesy Accu-Chek Glucometer.)

STEP	RATIONALE
9 Turn meter off. Some meters turn off automatically. Dispose of test strip, lancet, and gloves in proper receptacles.	Meter is battery powered. Proper disposal reduces risk for needlestick injury and spread of infection.
10 Complete postprocedure protocol.	

Recording and Reporting

- Record procedure and glucose level in nurses' notes or special flow sheet. Record action taken for abnormal range.
- Describe patient response, including appearance of puncture site, in nurses' notes.
- Describe explanations or teaching provided in nurses' notes.
- Record and report abnormal blood glucose levels.

UNEXPECTED OUTCOMES	RELATED INTERVENTIONS
1 Puncture site is bruised or continues to bleed.	• Apply pressure. • Notify health care provider if bleeding continues.

UNEXPECTED OUTCOMES	RELATED INTERVENTIONS
2 Blood glucose level is above or below target range.	• Continue to monitor patient. • Check if there are medication orders for deviations in glucose level. • Notify health care provider. • Administer insulin or carbohydrate source as ordered, depending on glucose level.
3 Glucose meter malfunctions.	• Review instructions for troubleshooting glucose meter. • Repeat test.
4 Patient expresses misunderstanding of procedure and results.	• Repeat instructions to patient. • Have patient demonstrate procedure.

Blood Pressure by Auscultation: Upper Extremities, Lower Extremities, Palpation

The most common technique of measuring blood pressure is auscultation with a sphygmomanometer and stethoscope. As the sphygmomanometer cuff is deflated, the five different sounds heard over an artery are called *Korotkoff phases*. The sound in each phase has unique characteristics (Fig. 10-1). Blood pressure is recorded with the systolic reading (first Korotkoff sound) before the diastolic (beginning of the fifth Korotkoff sound). The difference between systolic and diastolic pressure is the pulse pressure. For a blood pressure of 120/80, the pulse pressure is 40.

Delegation Considerations

The skill of blood pressure measurement can be delegated to nursing assistive personnel (NAP) unless the patient is considered unstable (e.g., hypotensive). The nurse instructs the NAP by:

- Explaining the appropriate limb for measurement, blood pressure cuff size, and equipment (manual or electronic) to be used.
- Communicating the frequency of measurement and factors related to the patient's history, such as risk for orthostatic hypotension.
- Reviewing the patient's usual blood pressure values and significant changes or abnormalities to report to the nurse.

Equipment

- Aneroid sphygmomanometer
- Cloth or disposable vinyl pressure cuff of appropriate size for patient's extremity
- Stethoscope
- Alcohol swab
- Pen and vital sign flow sheet or electronic health record (EHR)

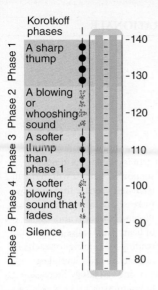

Fig. 10-1 The sounds auscultated during blood pressure (BP) measurement can be differentiated into five Korotkoff phases. In this example, the BP is 140/90 mm Hg.

Implementation

STEP	RATIONALE
1 Complete preprocedure protocol.	
2 Assess for factors that influence blood pressure: Age, gender, daily (diurnal) variation, position, exercise, weight, medications, smoking, ethnicity	Acceptable values for blood pressure vary throughout life. Blood pressure varies throughout the day.
3 Determine best site for blood pressure assessment. Avoid applying cuff to extremity where intravenous (IV) fluids are infusing, an arteriovenous shunt or fistula is present, or breast or axillary surgery has been performed on that side. In addition, avoid applying cuff to extremity that has been traumatized or diseased or requires a cast or bulky	Inappropriate site selection may result in poor amplification of sounds, causing inaccurate readings. Application of pressure from inflated bladder temporarily impairs blood flow and can further compromise circulation in extremity that already has impaired blood flow. Use of improper-size cuff causes false-low or false-high reading.

STEP	RATIONALE
bandage. Use lower extremities when brachial arteries are inaccessible. Select appropriate cuff size (Fig. 10-2), and ensure that other equipment is in the patient's room.	
4 Assess blood pressure by auscultation:	
a Upper extremity: With patient sitting or lying, position his or her forearm at heart level with palm turned up. If sitting, instruct patient to keep feet flat on floor without legs crossed. If supine, patient should not have legs crossed. Lower extremity: With patient prone, position patient so knee is slightly flexed.	If arm is extended and not supported, patient will perform isometric exercise that can increase diastolic pressure. Placement of arm above level of heart causes false-low reading—2 mm Hg for each inch above heart level. Leg crossing can falsely increase blood pressure.
b Expose extremity (arm or leg) fully by removing constricting clothing.	Ensures proper cuff application. Do not place blood pressure cuff over clothing.

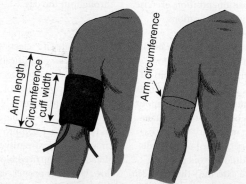

Fig. 10-2 Guidelines for proper blood pressure cuff size. Cuff width = 20% more than upper arm diameter, or 40% of circumference and two thirds of upper arm length.

STEP	RATIONALE
c Palpate brachial artery (Fig. 10-3, *A*) or popliteal artery (Fig. 10-3, *B*). With cuff fully deflated, apply bladder of cuff above artery by centering arrows marked on cuff over artery (Fig. 10-3, *C*). If cuff does not have any center arrows, estimate center of bladder and place this center over artery. Position cuff 2.5 cm (1 inch) above site of pulsation (antecubital or popliteal space). With cuff fully deflated, wrap it evenly and snugly around upper arm (Fig. 10-3, *D*).	Placing bladder directly over artery ensures that you apply proper pressure during inflation. Loose-fitting cuff causes false-high readings. Popliteal artery is just below patient's thigh, behind knee. Placing bladder directly over artery ensures that you apply proper pressure during inflation.
d Position manometer gauge vertically at eye level. You should be no farther than 1 meter (approximately 1 yard) away.	Looking up or down at scale can result in distorted readings.

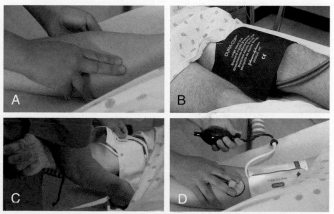

Fig. 10-3 **A,** Palpating brachial artery. **B,** Blood pressure cuff applied around thigh. **C,** Aligning blood pressure cuff arrow with brachial artery. **D,** Blood pressure cuff wrapped around upper arm.

STEP	RATIONALE
e Measure blood pressure.	
(1) **Two-step method:**	
(a) Relocate brachial pulse. Palpate artery distal to cuff with fingertips of nondominant hand while inflating cuff rapidly to a pressure 30 mm Hg above point at which pulse disappears. Slowly deflate cuff and note point at which pulse reappears. Deflate cuff fully and wait 30 seconds.	Estimating prevents false-low readings. Determine maximal inflation point for accurate reading by palpation. If unable to palpate artery because of weakened pulse, use an ultrasonic stethoscope. Completely deflating cuff prevents venous congestion and false-high readings.
(b) Place stethoscope earpieces in ears and be sure that sounds are clear, not muffled.	Ensure that each earpiece follows angle of ear canal to facilitate hearing.
(c) Relocate brachial artery, and place bell or diaphragm chest piece of stethoscope over it. Do not allow chest piece to touch cuff or clothing.	Proper stethoscope placement ensures best sound reception. The bell provides better sound reproduction, whereas the diaphragm is easier to secure with fingers and covers a larger area.
(d) Close valve of pressure bulb clockwise until tight. Quickly	Tightening valve prevents air leak during inflation. Rapid inflation ensures accurate measurement of systolic pressure.

STEP	RATIONALE
inflate cuff to 30 mm Hg above patient's estimated systolic pressure.	
(e) Slowly release pressure bulb valve and allow manometer needle to fall at rate of 2 to 3 mm Hg/ second.	Too-rapid or too-slow a decline causes inaccurate readings.
(f) Note point on manometer at which you hear first clear sound. The sound will slowly increase in intensity.	First Korotkoff sound reflects systolic blood pressure.
(g) Continue to deflate cuff gradually, noting point at which sound disappears in adults. Note pressure to nearest 2 mm Hg. Listen for 20 to 30 mm Hg after last sound and allow remaining air to escape quickly.	Beginning of fifth Korotkoff sound is indication of diastolic pressure in adults (National High Blood Pressure Education Program [NHBPEP], 2003). Fourth Korotkoff sound involves distinct muffling of sounds and is indication of diastolic pressure in children.
(2) One-step method:	
(a) Place stethoscope earpieces in ears and be sure that sounds are clear, not muffled.	Earpieces should follow angle of ear canal to facilitate hearing.

STEP	RATIONALE
(b) Relocate brachial artery and place bell or diaphragm chest piece of stethoscope over it. Do not allow chest piece to touch cuff or clothing.	Proper stethoscope placement ensures optimal sound reception.
(c) Close valve of pressure bulb clockwise until tight. Quickly inflate cuff to 30 mm Hg above patient's usual systolic pressure.	Tightening valve prevents air leak during inflation. Inflation above systolic level ensures accurate measurement of systolic pressure.
(d) Slowly release pressure bulb valve and allow manometer needle to fall at rate of 2 to 3 mm Hg/second. Note point on manometer at which you hear first clear sound. Sound will slowly increase in intensity.	Too-rapid or too-slow a decline in mercury level causes inaccurate readings. First Korotkoff sound reflects systolic pressure.
(e) Continue to deflate cuff gradually, noting point at which sound disappears in adults. Note pressure to nearest 2 mm Hg. Listen for 10 to 20 mm Hg after	Beginning of fifth Korotkoff sound is indication of diastolic pressure in adults (NHBPEP, 2003). Fourth Korotkoff sound involves distinct muffling of sounds and is indication of diastolic pressure in children (NHBPEP, 2003).

STEP	RATIONALE
last sound and allow remaining air to escape quickly.	
(f) The Joint National Committee (NHBPEP, 2003) recommends the average of two sets of blood pressure measurements 2 minutes apart. Use second set of blood pressure measurements as patient's baseline.	Two sets of blood pressure measurements help prevent false-positive readings based on patient's sympathetic response (alert reaction). Averaging minimizes effect of anxiety, which often causes first reading to be higher than subsequent measures (NHBPEP, 2003).
5 Assess systolic blood pressure by palpation:	
a Follow Steps 1a through 1d of auscultation method.	
b Locate and then continually palpate brachial, radial, or popliteal artery with fingertips of one hand. Inflate cuff to a pressure 30 mm Hg above point at which you can no longer palpate pulse.	Ensures accurate detection of true systolic pressure once pressure valve is released.

SAFETY ALERT If unable to palpate artery because of weakened pulse, use a Doppler ultrasonic stethoscope.

c Slowly release valve and deflate cuff, allowing manometer needle to fall at rate of 2 mm Hg/second. Note point on manometer at which pulse is again palpable.	Too-rapid or too-slow a decline results in inaccurate readings. Palpation helps identify systolic pressure only.

STEP	RATIONALE
d Deflate cuff rapidly and completely. Remove cuff from patient's extremity unless you need to repeat measurement.	Continuous cuff inflation causes arterial occlusion, resulting in numbness and tingling of extremity.
e Help patient return to comfortable position and cover extremity if previously clothed.	Restores comfort and promotes sense of well-being.
f If assessing blood pressure for the first time, establish baseline blood pressure if it is within acceptable range.	Used to compare future blood pressure measurements.
g Compare blood pressure reading with patient's previous baseline and usual blood pressure for patient's age.	Allows nurse to assess for change in condition. Provides comparison with future blood pressure measurements.
6 Complete postprocedure protocol.	

Recording and Reporting

- Record blood pressure and site assessed on vital sign flow sheet, nurses' notes, and electronic health record [EHR].
- Document measurement of blood pressure after administration of specific therapies in nurses' notes and EHR.
- Record any signs or symptoms of blood pressure alterations in nurses' notes and EHR.
- Report abnormal findings to nurse in charge or health care provider.

UNEXPECTED OUTCOMES	RELATED INTERVENTIONS
1 Patient's blood pressure is above acceptable range.	• Repeat measurement in other extremity and compare findings. • Verify correct selection and placement of blood pressure cuff. • Have another nurse repeat measurement in 1 to 2 minutes.

UNEXPECTED OUTCOMES	RELATED INTERVENTIONS
	• Observe for related symptoms that are not apparent unless blood pressure is extremely high, including headache, facial flushing, nosebleed, and fatigue in older patient.
	• Report blood pressure to nurse in charge or health care provider to initiate appropriate evaluation and treatment.
	• Administer antihypertensive medications as ordered.
2 Patient's blood pressure is not sufficient for adequate perfusion and oxygenation of tissues.	• Compare blood pressure value with baseline.
	• Position patient in supine position to enhance circulation, and restrict activity that decreases blood pressure further.
	• Repeat measurement with sphygmomanometer. Electronic blood pressure devices are less accurate in low-flow conditions.
	• Assess for signs and symptoms associated with hypotension, including tachycardia; weak, thready pulse; weakness; dizziness; confusion; and cool, pale, dusky, or cyanotic skin.
	• Assess for factors that contribute to a low blood pressure, including hemorrhage, dilation of blood vessels, or medication side effects.

Continued

UNEXPECTED OUTCOMES	RELATED INTERVENTIONS
	• Report blood pressure to nurse in charge or health care provider to initiate appropriate evaluation and treatment.
	• Increase rate of IV infusion or administer vasoconstriction drugs if ordered.
3 Unable to obtain blood pressure reading.	• Determine that no immediate crisis is present by obtaining pulse and respiratory rate.
	• Assess for signs and symptoms of decreased cardiac output; if present, notify nurse in charge or health care provider immediately.
	• Use alternative sites or procedures to obtain blood pressure; use Doppler ultrasonic instrument; palpate systolic blood pressure.
4 Patient experiences orthostatic hypotension.	• Maintain patient safety.
	• Return patient to safe position in bed or chair.

Blood Pressure:
Automatic

Many different styles of electronic blood pressure (BP) machines are available to determine BP automatically. Electronic BP machines rely on an electronic sensor to detect the vibrations caused by the rush of blood through an artery. Although electronic BP machines are fast, the nurse must consider the advantages and limitations of electronic BP machines. The devices are used when frequent assessment is required, such as in critically ill or potentially unstable patients, during or after invasive procedures, or when therapies require frequent monitoring.

Delegation Considerations

The use of an electronic BP machine can be delegated to nursing assistive personnel (NAP) unless the patient is considered unstable (e.g., hypotensive). The nurse instructs the NAP by:

- Communicating the frequency and extremity for measurement.
- Reviewing how to select appropriate-size blood pressure cuff for designated extremity and appropriate cuff for the machine.
- Reviewing patient's usual blood pressure and instructing NAP to report significant changes or abnormalities to the nurse.

Equipment

- Electronic blood pressure machine
- Source of electricity
- BP cuff of appropriate size, as recommended by manufacturer
- Pen and vital sign flow sheet or electronic health record

Implementation

1 Complete preprocedure protocol.
2 Determine the appropriateness of using electronic BP measurement. Patients with irregular heart rate, peripheral vascular disease, seizures, tremors, or shivering are not candidates for this device.
3 Determine best site for cuff placement.
4 Perform hand hygiene. Assist patient to comfortable position, either lying or sitting. Plug in and place device near patient, ensuring that connector hose between cuff and machine will reach.
5 Locate on/off switch, and turn on machine to enable device to self-test computer systems (Fig. 11-1).

Fig. 11-1 Digital electronic
blood pressure display.
(Courtesy Welch Allyn.)

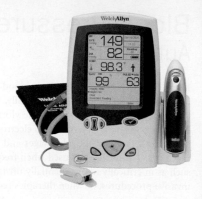

6 Select appropriate cuff size for patient extremity (see Skill 10)
   and appropriate cuff for machine. Electronic BP cuff and
   machine must be matched by manufacturer and are not
   interchangeable.
7 Expose extremity by removing constricting clothing to ensure
   proper cuff application. Do not place BP cuff over clothing.
8 Prepare BP cuff by manually squeezing all the air out of the cuff
   and connecting cuff to connector hose.
9 Wrap flattened cuff snugly around extremity, verifying that only
   one finger can fit between cuff and patient's skin. Make sure the
   "artery" arrow marked on the outside of the cuff is placed
   correctly.
10 Verify that connector hose between cuff and machine is not
   kinked. Kinking prevents proper inflation and deflation of cuff.
11 Following manufacturer's directions, set the frequency control for
   automatic or manual and then press the start button. The first
   BP measurement will pump the cuff to a peak pressure of about
   180 mm Hg. After this pressure is reached, the machine begins a
   deflation sequence that determines the BP. The first reading
   determines the peak pressure inflation for additional
   measurements.
12 When deflation is complete, digital display will provide most
   recent values and flash time in minutes that has elapsed since the
   measurement occurred.

SAFETY ALERT If unable to obtain BP with electronic device, verify
machine connections (e.g., plugged into working electrical outlet, hose-
cuff connections tight, machine on, correct cuff). Repeat electronic blood
pressure; if unable to obtain, use auscultatory technique (see Skill 10).

13 Set frequency of BP measurements and upper and lower alarm limits for systolic, diastolic, and mean BP readings. Intervals between BP measurements can be set from 1 to 90 minutes. The nurse determines frequency and alarm limits based on patient's acceptable range of BP, nursing judgment, and health care provider order.

14 Obtain additional readings at any time by pressing the start button. Pressing the cancel button immediately deflates the cuff.

15 If frequent measurements are required, the cuff may be left in place. Remove cuff at least every 2 hours to assess underlying skin integrity and, if possible, alternate BP sites. Patients with abnormal bleeding tendencies are at risk for microvascular rupture from repeated inflations. When the patient no longer requires frequent BP monitoring, remove and clean BP cuff according to facility policy to reduce transmission of microorganisms.

16 Discuss findings with patient. Perform hand hygiene.

17 Compare electronic BP readings with auscultatory BP measurements to verify the accuracy of electronic BP device.

18 Record BP and site assessed on vital sign flow sheet, electronic health record (EHR), or nurses' notes; record any signs or symptoms of BP alterations in narrative form in EHR and nurses' notes; report abnormal findings to nurse in charge or health care provider.

Central Venous Access Device Care: Central Venous Catheter, Ports

A central vascular access device (CVAD) differs from short peripheral or midline catheters in relation to the final catheter tip location. A CVAD has a final tip location in the junction of the right atrium (Fig. 12-1). The final tip placement of CVADs inserted in the femoral region should be in the inferior vena cava above the level of the diaphragm.

Valve-tipped devices are those in which the tip is configured with a three-way pressure-activated valve (e.g., Groshong) or the hub of the device has a pressure-activated valve, which reduces the risk for hemorrhage, air embolism, and occlusion. CVADs can have single or multiple lumens (Fig. 12-2). With the exception of the implanted venous port, each of these devices is accessed using the hub, which is located on the end of each of the external lumen(s).

Implanted venous ports are located within the reservoir pocket. To use the implanted venous port, the septum is palpated and a special noncoring needle is inserted through the skin into a self-sealing injection port (Fig. 12-3).

Primary complications associated with CVADs are usually related to *central line–associated bloodstream infections (CLABSIs)* (Alexander et al., 2009). The Institute for Healthcare Improvement (IHI) Central Line Bundle is a group of evidence-based interventions for patients with intravascular central catheters (IHI, 2011). The key components of the IHI Central Line Bundle are: hand hygiene, maximal barrier precautions upon insertion, chlorhexidine skin antisepsis, optimal catheter site selection with avoidance of the femoral vein for central venous access in adult patients, and daily review of line necessity with prompt removal of unnecessary lines

Delegation Considerations

The skill of caring for a CVAD cannot be delegated to nursing assistive personnel (NAP). Delegation to licensed practical nurses (LPNs) varies by state Nurse Practice Act. The nurse instructs the NAP to:

- Report the following to the nurse immediately: patient's dressing becomes damp or soiled, catheter line appears to be pulled out farther than original insertion position, IV line becomes

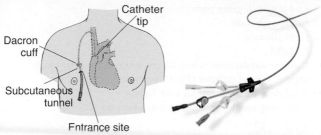

Fig. 12-1 Catheter tip of central venous access device (CVAD) lies in superior vena cava.

Fig. 12-2 Peripherally inserted central catheter (PICC) showing three access ports to individual lumens. (Courtesy and copyright © Bard Access Systems.)

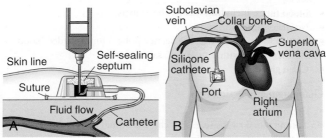

Fig. 12-3 **A,** Cross section of implantable port showing access of the port with noncoring needle. **B,** Implanted port and catheter.

disconnected, patient has a fever, patient complains of pain at the site.

- Help with positioning patient during insertion and care.

Equipment

Site Care and Dressing Change

- CVAD dressing change kit, which includes:
  - Sterile gloves
  - Mask
  - Antimicrobial swabs (e.g., 2% chlorhexidine [IHI, 2011] [see agency policy])
  - Transparent semipermeable membrane (TSM)

- 4 × 4–inch gauze pads
- Tape measure
- Sterile tape
- Label
- Catheter stabilization device (if not sutured) for peripherally inserted central catheter (PICC) or nontunneled catheters
- Needleless injection cap for each lumen
- Noncoring needle for implanted venous port

Blood Sampling

- Clean gloves
- Antimicrobial swabs (e.g., 2% chlorhexidine, alcohol)
- 5-mL Luer-Lok syringes
- 10-mL Luer-Lok syringes
- Vacutainer system or blood transfer device (see agency policy)
- Preservative-free saline flush (0.9% normal saline solution [NSS])
- Blood tubes, including waste tubes, labels
- Needleless injection cap
- Syringe (5 mL or 10 mL; see agency policy) for discarded blood
- 10-mL syringe with 5 to 10 mL saline flush
- Clean gloves

Changing the Injection Cap

- Clean gloves
- Antimicrobial swabs (e.g., 2% chlorhexidine)
- Needleless injection cap(s)
- 10-mL syringe with 10 mL normal saline (NS) flush (0.9% NSS)

Flushing a Positive-Pressure Device

- Clean gloves
- Alcohol swabs
- Positive-pressure injection cap
- 10-mL prefilled saline syringe

Discontinuation of a Nontunneled Catheter or PICC

- CVAD dressing change kit
- Tape
- Antimicrobial solution: 2% chlorhexidine (IHI, 2011)
- Suture removal kit (if sutures are in place)
- Goggles, gown, mask, and clean gloves

Implementation

STEP	RATIONALE
1 Complete preprocedure protocol.	
2 When CVAD is in place, assess the type of device. Review manufacturer's directions concerning the catheter and maintenance.	Care and management depend on type and size of catheter or port, number of lumens, purpose of therapy.
3 Assess if any lumens require flushing or site needs dressing change by referring to medical record, nurses' notes, agency policies, and manufacturer's recommended guidelines for use.	Provides guidelines for maintaining catheter patency and preventing infection.
4 Insertion site care:	
a Position patient in comfortable position with head slightly elevated. In the case of a PICC or midline device, have arm extended.	Provides access to patient. Infusion port requires palpation.
b *Gauze dressing:* Provide insertion site care every 48 hours and as needed. *Transparent dressings:* Provide insertion site care every 5-7 days and as needed.	Transparent semipermeable membrane dressings have the advantage of allowing visualization of the IV site. Gauze is preferable to TSM if the patient is diaphoretic or if the site is oozing or bleeding (INS, 2011a).
c Perform hand hygiene, and apply mask.	Reduces transfer of microorganisms; prevents spread of airborne microorganisms over CVAD insertion site.
d Apply clean gloves. Remove old dressing by lifting and removing either TSM or tape and gauze in the direction of the catheter insertion. Discard in appropriate biohazard container.	Stabilizes catheter as you remove dressing.

STEP	RATIONALE
e Remove catheter stabilization device if used. Must be removed with alcohol.	Allows clear visualization of insertion site and surrounding skin (INS, 2011a).

SAFETY ALERT If sutures are used for initial catheter stabilization and become loosened or are no longer intact, alternative stabilization measures should be used (INS, 2011a). Recent recommendation includes use of stabilization device because of the increased risk for infection when the catheter is sutured (Alexander et al., 2009).

STEP	RATIONALE
f Inspect catheter, insertion site, and surrounding skin. Measure mid-arm circumference above insertion site.	Insertion site requires regular inspection for complications. Measure of mid-arm circumference assesses for thrombosis.
g Remove and discard clean gloves; perform hand hygiene. Open CVAD dressing kit using sterile technique and **apply sterile gloves.**	Sterile technique is required to apply new dressing.
h Cleanse site:	
(1) 2% chlorhexidine (preferred). Apply using back-and-forth motion vertically and horizontally for at least 30 seconds; allow to dry for 30 seconds.	Allowing antiseptic solutions to air-dry completely effectively reduces microbial counts (INS, 2011a). Drying allows time for maximum microbicidal activity of agents (INS, 2011b).
(2) Povidone-iodine may be used in some settings (see agency policy).	
i Apply skin protectant to entire area. Allow to dry completely so that skin is not tacky.	Protects irritated or fragile skin from the dressing. It must be used if a catheter stabilization device is used.

STEP	RATIONALE
j Apply new catheter stabilization device per manufacturer's instructions if the catheter is not sutured in place.	Provides catheter stability to minimize dislodgment.
k Apply sterile, transparent semipermeable dressing or gauze dressing over insertion site.	Transparent dressing allows for clear visualization of catheter site between dressing changes.
l Apply label with date, time, and your initials.	Provides information about next dressing change.
m Dispose of soiled supplies and used equipment. Remove gloves, and perform hand hygiene.	Reduces transmission of microorganisms.
5 **Blood sampling:**	
a Perform hand hygiene.	Reduces transmission of microorganisms.
b ✎ Apply clean gloves.	Prevents transfer of body fluids.
c Turn off any infusion for at least 1 minute before drawing blood. **NOTE:** If you cannot stop infusion, draw blood from a peripheral vein.	Prevents interruption of critical fluid therapy.
d When drawing through multilumen catheters, the distal lumen (or one recommended by manufacturer) is preferred.	Distal lumen typically is largest-gauge lumen (Alexander et al., 2009).
e Clean injection cap with antiseptic solution and allow to dry completely. Attach syringe and flush port with 3-5 mL of preservative-free 0.9% sodium chloride, per agency policy. Do not flush before drawing blood for blood cultures.	Determines catheter patency and clears IV.

STEP	RATIONALE
f Syrine Method: **NOTE:** Check agency policy for use of Vacutainer with CVADs. (1) Remove end of IV tubing or injection cap from catheter hub. Keep end of tubing sterile.	
(2) Disinfect catheter hub with antiseptic solution.	Reduces risk for microorganisms.
(3) Attach an empty 10-mL syringe, unclamp catheter (if necessary), and withdraw blood 1.5 to 2 times fill volume (4 to 5 mL) of catheter for the discard sample.	Discard sample reduces risk for drug concentrations or diluted specimen (Alexander et al., 2009).
(4) Reclamp catheter (if necessary); remove syringe with blood and discard in appropriate biohazard container.	Open and valved CVADs differ in recommendations for clamping before removal of injection cap and syringe(s) (e.g., Hickman versus Groshong) (INS, 2011a).
(5) Clean hub with another antiseptic solution.	
(6) Attach second syringe(s) to obtain required volume of blood needed for specimen ordered.	Multiple syringes may be required, depending on specimens required and number of blood tubes needed.
(7) Unclamp catheter (if necessary) to withdraw blood.	

STEP	RATIONALE
(8) Once specimens are obtained, reclamp catheter (if necessary) and remove syringe.	
(9) Clean catheter hub with antiseptic solution.	
(10) Attach prefilled injection cap (attached to 10-mL syringe filled with 0.9% sodium chloride) to catheter, unclamp (if necessary), and flush. Reclamp catheter (if necessary).	Flushing with 10 mL of 0.9% sodium chloride after blood draw is minimum volume of solution recommended (INS, 2011a). Reduces risk for catheter clotting after procedure.
(11) Remove syringe and discard into appropriate biohazard container.	Reduces transmission of microorganisms.

SAFETY ALERT If blood cultures have been ordered, do not discard any blood. Use initial specimen for blood cultures.

---

g	Transfer blood using transfer vacuum device.	Reduces risk for blood exposure.
h	Flush catheter port with syringe containing heparin solution (check agency policy).	Heparin flush volume and concentration vary by agency and type of catheter. Flush Groshong catheters with 0.9% sodium chloride only.

SAFETY ALERT Always use a 10-mL syringe on central lines to minimize pressure during injection.

---

i	Remove syringe. Attach new sterile cap or IV tubing, and resume infusion.	Maintains sterile seal to catheter.

STEP	RATIONALE
j Dispose of soiled equipment and used supplies. Remove gloves, and perform hand hygiene.	Reduces transmission of microorganisms.
6 Changing injection cap:	
a Determine if injection caps should be changed.	Injection caps are usually changed with each administration set change, at least every 7 days for catheter maintenance, if residual blood is present, and when integrity is compromised (INS, 2011a).
b Prepare new injection cap(s):	
(1) Remove cap from package, and cleanse septum with alcohol using friction.	
(2) Keep the protective cap on the tip of the injection cap.	Maintains sterility.
(3) Prime the injection cap by flushing with 0.9% normal saline through cap until fluid is seen in the protective cap. Keep syringe attached.	Removes air from the system.
c If required based on device type, clamp catheter lumens one at a time by using slide or squeeze clamp.	Prevents air from entering system when opened. Patient can also perform Valsalva maneuver during cap changes.
d 🖐 Apply clean gloves.	Prevents transmission of microorganisms by nurse's hands.
e Remove old injection caps using aseptic technique.	Routine injection cap changes decrease catheter infections.

STEP	RATIONALE
f Cleanse catheter hub with antiseptic swab. Connect new injection cap(s) on catheter hub.	Allowing antiseptic solutions to air-dry completely effectively reduces microbial counts (INS, 2011a). Drying allows time for maximum microbicidal activity of agents.
g Flush catheter with 10-mL syringe of 0.9% sodium chloride followed by heparin solution as required by manufacturer.	Prevents clot formation.
h Dispose of all soiled supplies and used equipment. Remove gloves, and perform hand hygiene.	Reduces spread of microorganisms.
7 **Discontinuing nontunneled catheters or PICCs:**	
a Verify health care provider's order to discontinue line. See agency policy because most require physician to discontinue CVAD. In some settings, critical care nurses are certified for removal of line.	Verifies appropriateness of procedure. Only a competent health care professional can remove a CVAD.
b If IV fluids are to continue, prepare to convert them to a short peripheral or midline before CVAD discontinuation. Be aware of pH and osmolarity of solution for appropriateness of conversion.	
c Position patient in 10-degree Trendelenburg's position.	Position promotes venous filling and prevents air embolus during catheter removal.

STEP	RATIONALE
d Perform hand hygiene, and turn off IV fluids infusing through central line.	
e ⬛ Apply gown, mask, goggles, and clean gloves.	Prevents transmission of microorganisms and nurse's exposure to bloodborne pathogens.
f Gently remove CVAD dressing. Discard in biohazard container. Inspect catheter and insertion site.	Prevents skin tears. Disposal prevents transmission of microorganisms. Provides information about catheter and site before removal.
g Remove gloves and perform hand hygiene; open CVAD dressing change kit and suture removal kit (if sutures in place), and apply sterile gloves.	Prevents transfer of organisms on soiled dressing to catheter insertion site.
h Cleanse CVAD site using combination antiseptic or chlorhexidine swabs (see agency policy). Begin at insertion site and move outward in a circular motion, or, with chlorhexidine only, use a back-and-forth scrub method, vertical, horizontal, and circular, for 3 seconds. Allow to dry completely.	Removes microorganisms from skin surrounding insertion site. Allowing antiseptic solutions to air-dry completely effectively reduces microbial counts (INS, 2011a).
i If catheter securement device is present, carefully disconnect catheter from device and remove device with alcohol. If sutures are present, remove clean gloves and open suture removal kit.	Alcohol aids in removal of securement device.

STEP	RATIONALE
j To remove sutures with nondominant hand, grasp suture with forceps. Using dominant hand, carefully cut suture with sterile scissors; avoid damaging skin or catheter. Lift suture out and discard. Continue until all sutures are removed.	Technique prevents pulling contaminated end of suture through patient's skin.
k Using nondominant hand, apply sterile 4 × 4–inch gauze to site. Instruct patient to take a deep breath and hold it as you withdraw catheter.	Valsalva maneuver reduces the risk for air embolus by decreasing negative pressure in respiratory system.
l With dominant hand, remove catheter in a smooth, continuous motion an inch at a time. Note any resistance while removing the catheter. Inspect catheter for intactness, especially along tip. Keeping fingers near insertion site, immediately apply pressure to site until bleeding stops.	Gentle removal of catheter prevents stretching and breaking of the catheter. Damaged catheter may break off and leave a piece of catheter in patient's arm. Direct pressure reduces risk for bleeding and hematoma formation.

SAFETY ALERT It is often necessary to apply pressure longer if patient is receiving anticoagulants.

m Apply antiseptic ointment to exit site (*option*: see agency policy). Apply sterile occlusive dressing such as transparent dressing or sterile gauze to site.	Reduces chance of bacterial growth at old insertion site. Decreases chance of bleeding and infection.
n Label dressing with date, time, and your initials.	Identifies date of catheter removal and need for dressing change.

STEP	RATIONALE
o Inspect catheter integrity, and discard in biohazard container. **NOTE:** Catheter cultures should be performed when catheter is removed for suspected catheter-related bloodstream infections (CRBSIs). Catheter cultures should not be obtained routinely (INS, 2011a; Mermel et al., 2009).	Prevents transmission of microorganisms. If catheter tip is broken or compromised, place in container and label for possible follow-up.
p Return patient to comfortable position. Be sure peripheral IV is infusing at correct rate.	Maintains IV fluid therapy.
q Complete postprocedure protocol.	

Recording and Reporting

- Immediately notify health care provider of signs and symptoms of any complications.
- Document catheter site care in nurses' notes: size of catheter, change of injection caps, appearance of site, condition and type of securement device, date and time of dressing change.
- Document in nurses' notes and electronic health record (EHR) the condition of exit site or port insertion site, including skin integrity, signs of infection, and placement, integrity, and functionality of catheter.
- Document in nurses' notes and EHR catheter removal: patient position, appearance of site, length of catheter removed, integrity of catheter after removal, dressing applied, patient's tolerance of procedure, presence/absence of bleeding from site every 15 minutes for 1 hour, and any problems with removal.
- Document in nurses' notes and EHR blood draw: date, time, sample drawn.
- Document in nurses' notes unexpected outcomes, health care provider notification, interventions, and patient response to treatment.

UNEXPECTED OUTCOMES	RELATED INTERVENTIONS
1 Catheter damage, breakage	• Clamp the catheter near insertion site, and place sterile gauze over break or hole until repaired. • Use permanent repair kit, if available. • Remove catheter.
2 Occlusion: thrombus, precipitation, malposition	• Reposition patient • Have patient cough and deep breathe. • Raise patient's arm overhead. • Obtain venogram if ordered. • Administer thrombolytics if ordered. • Remove catheter (CVAD requires order). • Obtain x-ray examination as ordered. • If precipitate, try hydrochloric acid or ethanol solution per orders. • Do not use a 1-mL syringe to instill saline because pressure exceeds 200 psi.
3 Infection and sepsis: exit site, tunnel, thrombus, port pocket	• Obtain blood cultures first, from peripheral and CVAD if ordered. • Administer antibiotic therapy as ordered. • Remove catheter (CVAD requires order). • Administer thrombolytic agent if ordered. • Replace catheter.

Continued

UNEXPECTED OUTCOMES	RELATED INTERVENTIONS
4 Infiltration, extravasation	• Apply cold/warm compresses according to specific vesicant protocol. • Provide emotional support. • Obtain x-ray examination if ordered. • Use antidotes per protocol. • Discontinue IV fluids.
5 Pneumothorax, hemothorax, air emboli, hydrothorax	• Administer oxygen as ordered. • Elevate feet. Aspirate air, fluid. • If air emboli suspected, place patient on left side with head elevated slightly. Remove catheter as ordered. • Assist with insertion of chest tubes as ordered.
6 Incorrect placement	• Stop all fluid administration until placement is confirmed. Discontinue catheter (central venous catheter [CVC] requires order). • Obtain x-ray examination and electrocardiogram (for PICC and CVAD). Administer support medications as ordered.

Chest Tube Care

A chest tube is a large catheter inserted through the thorax to remove fluid (effusions), blood (hemothorax), and/or air (pneumothorax). The location of the chest tube indicates the type of drainage expected. Apical (second or third intercostal space) and anterior chest tube placement promotes removal of air. Chest tubes placed low (usually in the fifth or sixth intercostal space) and posterior or lateral drain fluid (Fig. 13-1). A mediastinal chest tube is placed in the mediastinum, just below the sternum (Fig. 13-2), and is connected to a drainage system. This tube drains blood or fluid, preventing its accumulation around the heart. This skill reviews the nursing responsibilities and interventions related to the safe management of chest tubes. Review the roles and responsibilities of the health care provider for chest tube placement (Table 13-1). There are two types of commercial drainage systems: the water-seal and the waterless systems.

Delegation Considerations

The skill of chest tube management cannot be delegated to nursing assistive personnel (NAP). The nurse directs the NAP about:

- Proper positioning of the patient with chest tubes to facilitate chest tube drainage and optimal functioning of the system.
- How to ambulate and transfer patient with chest drainage.
- Measuring vital signs and reporting to the nurse immediately any abnormal changes in vital signs, any complaints of chest pain or sudden shortness of breath, or excessive bubbling in water-seal chamber.
- The danger of any disconnection of system, change in type and amount of drainage, sudden bleeding, or sudden cessation of bubbling, and the importance of notifying the nurse immediately.

Equipment

- Prescribed chest drainage system
- Suction source and setup (wall canister or portable)
  - *Water-seal system*: Add sterile water or normal saline (NS) solution to cover the lower 2.5 cm (1 inch) of the water-seal U tube. Or pour sterile water or NS into the suction control chamber if suction is to be used (see manufacturer's directions)
  - *Waterless system*: Add vial of 30 to 45 mL of sterile sodium chloride or water (for diagnostic air-leak indicator), 20-mL syringe, 21-gauge needle, and antiseptic swab
  - Dry suction system

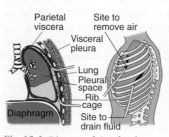

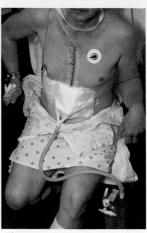

Fig. 13-1 Diagram of sites for chest tube placement.

Fig. 13-2 Mediastinal chest tube.

TABLE 13-1 Physician's or Advanced Practice Nurse's Role in Chest Tube Placement

Role	Purpose
Explain purpose, procedure, and possible complications to the patient, and have patient sign consent form.	Provides informed consent.
Have pain medication available to administer before or immediately after chest tube insertion as appropriate according to patient's condition.	Analgesia improves patient comfort throughout the procedure and assists patient in taking appropriate deep breaths to promote lung reexpansion and drainage of fluid in the pleural space.
Perform hand hygiene. Cleanse chest wall with antiseptic.	Reduces transmission of microorganisms.
Apply mask and gloves.	Maintains surgical asepsis.
Drape area of chest tube insertion with sterile towels.	Maintains surgical asepsis.
Inject local anesthetic, and allow time to take effect.	Decreases pain during procedure.

TABLE 13-1 Physician's or Advanced Practice Nurse's Role in Chest Tube Placement—cont'd

Role	Purpose
Make a small incision over the rib space where tube is to be inserted. Thread a clamped chest tube through the incision. Health care provider clamps chest tube until system is connected to water seal.	Inserts chest tube into the intrapleural space. Clamping prevents entry of atmospheric air into the chest and worsening of the pneumothorax.
Suture chest tube in place if suturing is policy or health care provider preference.	Secures chest tube in place.
Cover the chest insertion site with sterile 4 × 4–inch gauze and large dressing to form an occlusive dressing supported with an elastic bandage (Elastoplast). Sterile petrolatum gauze is used around the tube.	Holds chest tube in place and occludes site around chest tube. Helps stabilize chest tube and holds dressing tightly in place. Sterile petrolatum gauze helps prevent bacteria entry and air leak.
Water-Seal System	
Remove connector cover from patient's end of chest drainage tubing with sterile technique. Secure drainage tubing to the chest tube and drainage system.	Health care provider is responsible for making certain that the system is set up properly, the proper amount of water is in the water seal, the dressing is secure, and the chest tube is securely connected to the drainage system.
Water-Seal Suction	
Connect system to suction or supervise a nurse connecting it to suction if suction is to be used.	The health care provider is responsible for determining and checking the amount of fluid that is to be added to the suction control chamber and prescribing the suction setting.
Waterless System	
Remove connector cover from patient's end of chest drainage tubing with sterile technique. Secure drainage tubing to the chest tube and drainage system.	Health care provider is responsible for making certain that the system is set up properly and the chest tube is securely connected to the drainage system.

Continued

TABLE 13-1 Physician's or Advanced Practice Nurse's Role in Chest Tube Placement—cont'd

Role	Purpose
Waterless Suction	
Turn on suction source. Set float ball level to prescribed setting.	Health care provider is responsible for prescribing level of float ball and prescribing the suction setting.
The health care provider or nurse adds sterile water or normal saline (NS) to diagnostic indicator.	Allows quick assurance that the system is functioning properly.
Unclamp the chest tube.	Connects chest tube to drainage.
In both systems, the health care provider orders and reviews chest x-ray studies.	Verifies correct chest tube placement.

- Clean gloves
- Sterile gauze sponges
- Local anesthetic, if not an emergent procedure
- Chest tube tray (all items are sterile): Knife handle (1), chest tube clamp, small sponge forceps, needle holder, knife blade No. 10, 3-0 silk sutures, tray liner (sterile field), curved 8-inch Kelly clamps (2), 4 × 4–inch sponges (10), suture scissors, hand towels (3), sterile gloves
- Dressings: Petrolatum gauze, split chest-tube dressings, several 4 × 4–inch gauze dressings, large gauze dressings (2), and 4-inch tape or elastic bandage (Elastoplast)
- Head cover
- Face mask/face shield
- Sterile gloves
- Two rubber-tipped hemostats (shodded) for each chest tube
- 1-inch adhesive tape for taping connections or plastic zip ties
- Stethoscope, sphygmomanometer, and pulse oximeter

Implementation

STEP	RATIONALE
1 Complete preprocedure protocol.	

STEP	RATIONALE
2 Measure vital signs and pulse oximetry.	Provides baseline to determine patient's response to chest tube.
3 Perform a complete respiratory assessment.	Patients in need of chest tubes have impaired oxygenation and ventilation.
4 Assess patient for known allergies. Ask patient if he or she has had a problem with medications, latex, or anything applied to the skin.	Povidone-iodine and chlorhexidine are antiseptic solutions used to cleanse the skin (Durai et al., 2010). Lidocaine is a local anesthetic administered to reduce pain. The chest tube will be held in place with tape.
5 Review patient's medication record for anticoagulant therapy, including aspirin, warfarin (Coumadin), heparin, or platelet aggregation inhibitors such as ticlopidine (Ticlid) or dipyridamole (Persantine).	Anticoagulation therapy can increase procedure-related blood loss.
6 For patients who have chest tubes, observe:	
a Chest tube dressing and site surrounding tube insertion.	Ensures that dressing is intact and occlusive seal remains without air or fluid leaks and that area surrounding insertion site is free of drainage or skin irritation.
b Tubing for kinks, dependent loops, or clots.	Maintains a patent, freely draining system, preventing fluid accumulation in chest cavity. Subcutaneous emphysema can occur if the tubing is blocked or kinked. When the tubing is coiled, looped, or clotted, the drainage is impeded and risk for a tension pneumothorax or surgical emphysema is increased (Briggs, 2010).

STEP	RATIONALE
c Chest drainage system should remain upright and below level of tube insertion.	An upright drainage system facilitates drainage and maintains the water seal.
7 Set up water-seal system (or dry system with suction); see manufacturer guidelines:	
a Obtain chest drainage system. Remove wrappers, and prepare to set up the system.	
b While maintaining sterility of the drainage tubing, stand the system upright and add sterile water or NS to the appropriate compartments:	Reduces possibility of contamination.
(1) *For a two-chamber system (without suction):* Add sterile solution to the water-seal chamber (second chamber), bringing fluid to required level as indicated.	Water-seal chamber acts as one-way valve so air cannot enter pleural space (Briggs, 2010).
(2) *Three-chamber system (with suction):* Add sterile solution to water-seal chamber (middle chamber). Add amount of sterile solution prescribed by health care provider to the suction control (third chamber), usually 20 cm (8 inches). Connect tubing from suction control chamber to suction source.	Depth of rod below fluid level dictates highest amount of negative pressure that can be present within system. Any additional negative pressure applied to the system is vented into the atmosphere through suction control vent. This safety device prevents damage to pleural tissues from an unexpected surge of negative pressure from suction source.

STEP	RATIONALE
(3) *Dry suction system:* Fill the water-seal chamber with 2 cm of sterile solution. Adjust the suction control dial to the prescribed level of suction; suction ranges from −10 to −40 cm of water pressure. The suction control chamber vent is never occluded when suction is used.	The automatic control valve on the dry suction control device adjusts to changes in patient air leaks and fluctuation in suction source and vacuum to deliver the prescribed amount of suction.
8 Prepare a waterless drainage system (see manufacturer's guidelines):	
a Remove sterile wrappers, and prepare to set up.	Maintains sterility of the system for use in sterile operating room conditions.
b For a two-chamber system (without suction), nothing is added or needs to be done to the system.	Waterless two-chamber system is ready for connecting to the patient's chest tube after opening the wrappers.
c For a three-chamber waterless system with suction, connect tubing from suction control chamber to the suction source.	The suction source provides additional negative pressure to the system.
d Instill 15 to 45 mL of sterile water or NS into the diagnostic indicator injection port located on top of the system.	Allows observation of the rise and fall in the diagnostic air-leak window. Constant left-to-right bubbling or rocking is abnormal and may indicate an air leak.
9 Secure all tubing connections with tape in double-spiral fashion using 2.5-cm (1-inch)	Prevents atmospheric air from leaking into system and patient's intrapleural space. Provides chance to

STEP	RATIONALE
adhesive tape or use zip ties (nylon cable) with a clamp (Bauman and Handley, 2011). Check system for patency by: a Clamping drainage tubing that will connect to patient's chest tube. b Connecting tubing from float ball chamber to suction source. c Turning on suction to prescribed level.	ensure airtight system before connection to patient.
10 Turn off suction source and unclamp drainage tubing before connecting patient to system. Make a second check to be sure that drainage tubing is not excessively long. Suction source is turned on again after patient is connected.	Having patient connected to suction when it is initiated could damage pleural tissues from sudden increase in negative pressure. Tubing that is coiled or looped may become clotted and cause a tension pneumothorax.
11 Administer premedication such as sedatives or analgesics as ordered.	Reduces patient anxiety and pain during procedure.

SAFETY ALERT During procedure, carefully monitor patient for changes in level of sedation.

12 Provide psychological support to patient (Durai et al., 2010): a Reinforce preprocedure explanation. b Coach and support patient throughout procedure.	Reduces patient anxiety and helps complete procedure efficiently.
13 ![hand] Perform hand hygiene, and apply clean gloves. Position patient for tube	Reduces transmission of microorganisms.

STEP	RATIONALE
insertion so that side in which tube is to be inserted is accessible to health care provider.	
14 Help health care provider with chest tube insertion by providing needed equipment and systemic analgesic. Health care provider will anesthetize skin over insertion site, make a small skin incision, insert a clamped tube, suture it in place, and apply occlusive dressing.	Ensures smooth insertion.
15 Help health care provider attach drainage tube to chest tube; remove clamp. Turn on suction to prescribed level.	Connects drainage system and suction (if ordered) to chest tube.
16 Tape or zip-tie all connections between chest tube and drainage tube. (**Note:** Chest tube is usually taped by health care provider at time of tube placement; check agency policy.)	Secures chest tube to drainage system and reduces risk for air leak that causes breaks in airtight system.
17 Check systems for proper functioning. Health care provider will order a chest x-ray film.	Verifies intrapleural placement of tube.
18 After tube placement, position patient: a Use semi-Fowler's or high-Fowler's position to evacuate air (pneumothorax). b Use high-Fowler's position to drain fluid (hemothorax).	Permits optimum drainage of fluid and/or air.

STEP	RATIONALE
19 Check patency of air vents in system.	
a Water-seal vent must have no occlusion.	Permits displaced air to pass into atmosphere.
b Suction control chamber vent is not occluded when suction is used.	Provides safety factor of releasing excess negative pressure into atmosphere.
c Waterless systems have relief valves without caps.	Provides safety factor of releasing excess negative pressure.
20 Position excess tubing horizontally on mattress next to patient. Secure with clamp provided so it does not obstruct tubing.	Prevents excess tubing from hanging over edge of mattress in dependent loop. Drainage collected in loop can occlude drainage system, which predisposes patient to a tension pneumothorax (Briggs, 2010).
21 Adjust tubing to hang in straight line from chest tube to drainage chamber.	Promotes drainage and prevents fluid or blood from accumulating in pleural cavity.

SAFETY ALERT Frequent gentle lifting of the drain allows gravity to assist blood and other viscous material to move to the drainage bottle. Patients with recent chest surgery or trauma need to have the chest drain lifted based on assessment of the amount of drainage; some patients might need chest tube drains lifted every 5 to 10 minutes until drainage volume decreases. However, when coiled or dependent looping of tubing is unavoidable, the tubing is lifted every 15 minutes at a minimum to promote drainage (Briggs, 2010).

22 Place two rubber-tipped hemostats (for each chest tube) in an easily accessible position (e.g., taped to top of patient's headboard). These should remain with patient when ambulating.	Chest tubes are double clamped under specific circumstances: (1) to assess for an air leak (Table 13-2), (2) to empty or quickly change disposable systems, or (3) to assess if patient is ready to have tube removed.

SAFETY ALERT In the event of a chest tube disconnection and risk for contamination, submerge the tube 2 to 4 cm (1 to 2 inches) below the surface of a 250-mL bottle of sterile water or NS until a new chest tube unit can be set up (Bauman and Handley, 2011).

TABLE 13-2 Troubleshooting with Chest Tubes

Assessment	Intervention
Air leak can occur at insertion site, connection between tube and drainage, or within drainage device itself. Determine when the air leak occurs during respiratory cycle (e.g., inspiration or expiration). Continuous bubbling that is noted in water-seal chamber and water seal indicates a leak during the inspiratory and expiratory phases (Cerfolio, 2005).	Check all connections between the chest tube and drainage system. Locate leak by clamping tube at different intervals along the tube. Leaks are corrected when constant bubbling stops. If present on chest drainage system, such as the Sahara S 1100a Pleur-evac, observe the air leak meter to determine the size of the leak.
Assess for location of leak by clamping chest tube with two rubber-shod or toothless clamps close to the chest wall. If bubbling stops, air leak is inside patient's thorax or at chest insertion site.	Unclamp tube, reinforce chest dressing, and notify health care provider immediately. Leaving chest tube clamped can cause collapse of lung, mediastinal shift, and eventual collapse of other lung from buildup of air pressure within the pleural cavity.
If bubbling continues with the clamps near the chest wall, gradually move one clamp at a time down drainage tubing away from patient and toward suction control chamber. When bubbling stops, leak is in section of tubing or connection between the clamps.	Replace tubing, or secure connection and release clamps.
If bubbling still continues, this indicates the leak is in the drainage system.	Change the drainage system. Make sure chest tubes are patent: remove clamps, eliminate kinks, or eliminate occlusion.

Continued

TABLE 13-2 Troubleshooting with Chest Tubes—cont'd

Assessment	Intervention
Assess for tension pneumothorax, indicated by: • Severe respiratory distress • Low oxygen saturation • Chest pain • Absence of breath sounds on affected side • Tracheal shift to unaffected side • Hypotension and signs of shock • Tachycardia	Obstructed chest tubes trap air in intrapleural space when air leak originates within the thorax. Notify health care provider immediately, and prepare for another chest tube insertion. A flutter (Heimlich) valve or large-gauge needle may be used for short-term emergency release of pressure in the intrapleural space. Have emergency equipment, oxygen, and code cart available because condition is life threatening.
Water-seal tube is no longer submerged in sterile fluid because of evaporation.	Add sterile water to water-seal chamber until distal tip is 2 cm under surface level.

STEP	RATIONALE
23 Dispose of sharps in proper container, dispose of used supplies, and then perform hand hygiene.	Reduces transmission of microorganisms.
24 Care of patient after chest tube insertion: a ⚡ Perform hand hygiene, and apply clean gloves. Assess vital signs; oxygen saturation; skin color; breath sounds; rate, depth, and ease of respirations; and insertion site every 15 minutes for first 2 hours and then at least every shift.	Provides immediate information about procedure-related complications such as respiratory distress and leakage.

STEP	RATIONALE
b Monitor color, consistency, and amount of chest tube drainage every 15 minutes for first 2 hours. Indicate level of drainage fluid, date, and time on write-on surface of chamber:	Provides baseline for continuous assessment of type and quantity of drainage. Ensures early detection of complications.
(1) Expect less than 100 mL/hr from a mediastinal tube immediately after surgery and no more than 500 mL in first 24 hours.	Sudden gush of drainage may result from coughing or changing patient's position that releases pooled/collected blood rather than indicating active bleeding.
(2) Expect between 100 and 300 mL in the first 3 hours after insertion of posterior chest tube, with total of 500 to 1000 mL expected in first 24 hours. Drainage is grossly bloody during first several hours after surgery and changes to serous.	Acute bleeding indicates hemorrhage. Health care provider should be notified if there is more than 250 mL of bloody drainage in an hour (Durai et al., 2010).
(3) Expect little or no output from anterior chest tube that is inserted for a pneumothorax.	
c Observe chest dressing for drainage.	Drainage around tube may indicate blockage.
d Palpate around tube for swelling and crepitus (subcutaneous emphysema) as noted by crackling.	Indicates presence of air trapping in subcutaneous tissues. Small amounts are commonly absorbed. Large amounts are potentially dangerous. ›

STEP	RATIONALE
e Check tubing to ensure that it is free of kinks and dependent loops.	Promotes drainage.
f Observe for fluctuation of drainage in tubing and water-seal chamber during inspiration and expiration. Observe for clots or debris in tubing.	If fluctuation or tidaling stops, it means that either the lung is fully expanded or system is obstructed (Bauman and Handley, 2011). In nonmechanically ventilated patient, fluid rises in water-seal or diagnostic indicator (waterless system) with inspiration and falls with expiration. The opposite occurs in patient who is mechanically ventilated. This indicates that system is functioning properly (Lewis et al., 2011).
g Keep drainage system upright and below level of patient's chest.	Promotes gravity drainage and prevents backflow of fluid and air into pleural space.
h Check for air leaks by monitoring bubbling in water-seal chamber: Intermittent bubbling is normal during expiration when air is being evacuated from pleural cavity, but continuous bubbling during both inspiration and expiration indicates leak in system.	Absence of bubbling may indicate that lung is fully expanded in patient with a pneumothorax. Check all connections and locate sources of air leak (see Table 13-2).
i Remove gloves and dispose of used soiled equipment in appropriate biohazard container. Perform hand hygiene.	Prevents accidents involving contaminated equipment.

Recording and Reporting

- Record respiratory assessment, type of drainage device, amount of suction if used, amount of drainage in chamber, and presence or absence of an air leak. Record patient teaching and validation of understanding in nurses' notes and electronic health record (EHR).
- Record level of patient comfort and baseline vital signs, including oxygen saturation. If postoperative patient, record vital signs and oxygen saturation every 15 minutes for at least 2 hours after surgery.
- Record integrity of dressing and presence of drainage on dressing.
- Report any unexpected outcomes immediately to nurse in charge or health care provider.

UNEXPECTED OUTCOMES	RELATED INTERVENTIONS
1 Patient develops respiratory distress. Chest pain, a decrease in breath sounds over affected and nonaffected lungs, marked cyanosis, asymmetric chest movements, presence of subcutaneous emphysema around tube insertion site or neck, hypotension, tachycardia, and/or mediastinal shift are critical and indicate a severe change in patient status, such as excessive blood loss or tension pneumothorax.	• Notify health care provider immediately. • Collect set of vital signs and pulse oximetry. • Prepare for chest x-ray. • Provide oxygen as ordered.
2 Air leak unrelated to patient's respirations occurs.	• Locate source (see Table 13-2). • Notify health care provider.

Continued

UNEXPECTED OUTCOMES	RELATED INTERVENTIONS
3 There is no chest tube drainage.	• Observe for kink in chest drainage system.
	• Observe for possible clot in chest drainage system.
	• Observe for mediastinal shift or respiratory distress (medical emergency).
	• Notify health care provider.
4 Chest tube is dislodged.	• Immediately apply pressure over chest tube insertion site.
	• Have assistant apply occlusive gauze dressing and tape three sides.
	• Notify health care provider.
5 Substantial increase in bright red drainage occurs.	• Obtain vital signs.
	• Monitor drainage.
	• Assess patient's cardiopulmonary status.
	• Notify health care provider.

Cold Applications

There are a variety of cold (cryotherapy) modalities, such as moist cold compresses, chemical or cold packs, electromechanical or compression devices, or cold soak immersion of a body part. Cold therapy treats localized inflammatory responses that lead to edema, hemorrhage, muscle spasm, or pain (Table 14-1). Cold exerts a profound physiological effect on the body, reducing inflammation caused by injuries to the musculoskeletal system (Markert, 2011). Because reduction of inflammation is the primary goal, cryotherapy is the treatment of choice for the first 24 to 48 hours after an injury (Gottschalk, 2011). When used appropriately, cold applications significantly lessen pain and immobility by reducing swelling of injured tissues (Physiotherapy Canada, 2010). This is an important point for nurses to know when choosing heat or cold for the treatment of acute injuries. Cold is also indicated as an adjunct analgesic for chronic pain and spasticity control.

Delegation Considerations

The skill of applying cold applications can be delegated to nursing assistive personnel (NAP) in special situations (see agency policy). The nurse must assess and evaluate the patient and explain the purpose of the treatment. If there are risks or complications, the skill is not delegated. Direct NAP to:

- Keep the application in place for only the length of time specified in the health care provider's order.
- Immediately report to the nurse any excessive redness on the skin, increase in pain, or decrease in sensation.
- Report when treatment is complete so that a nurse can evaluate the patient's response.

Equipment

All Compresses, Bags, and Packs

- Clean gloves (if blood or body fluids are present)
- Cloth tape or ties or elastic wrap bandage
- Soft cloth cover: towel, pillowcase, or stockinette
- Bath towel or blanket and waterproof pad

Cold Compress

- Absorbent gauze (clean or sterile) folded to desired size
- Basin
- Prescribed solution at desired temperature

TABLE 14-1 Pathophysiological Effects of Hot and Cold Applications

	COLD	HOT
Pain	↓	↓
Spasm	↓	↓
Metabolism	↓	↑
Blood flow	↓	↑
Inflammation	↓	↑
Edema	↓	↑
Extensibility	↓	↑

Modified from Garner A, Fendius A: Temperature physiology, assessment and control, *Br J Neurosci Nurs* 6(8):397, 2010; Superficial heat, *Physiother Can* 62(5):47, 2010, DOI:10.3138/ptc 2009-09-s6.

Ice Bag or Gel Pack

- Ice bag
- Ice chips and water
- Reusable commercial gel pack (cold pack)
- Disposable commercial chemical cold pack

Electrically Controlled Cooling Device

- Cool water flow pad or cooling pad (e.g., aquathermia pad) and electrical pump
- Gauze roll or elastic wrap

Implementation

STEP	RATIONALE
1 Complete preprocedure protocol.	
2 Position patient carefully, keeping body part in proper alignment and exposing only area to be treated, and drape patient with bath blankets.	Prevents further injury to body part. Avoids unnecessary exposure of body parts, maintaining patient's comfort and privacy.
3 Place towel or absorbent pad under area you will treat.	Prevents soiling of bedclothes.
4 Apply clean gloves.	Reduces spread of infection.

STEP	RATIONALE
5 Apply cold compress:	
a Check temperature of solution, and submerge gauze into basin filled with cold solution; wring out excess moisture.	Extreme temperature can cause tissue damage.
b Apply compress to affected area, molding it gently over site.	Ensures that cold is directed over site of injury.
c Remove, remoisten, and reapply to maintain temperature as needed.	
6 Apply ice pack or bag:	
a Fill bag with water, secure cap, and invert.	Ensures that there are no leaks.
b Empty water, and fill bag two-thirds full with small ice chips and water.	Bag is easier to mold over body part when it is not full.
c Express excess air from bag, secure bag closure, and wipe bag dry.	Excess air interferes with cold conduction. Allows bag to conform to area and promotes maximum contact.
d Squeeze or knead commercial ice pack.	Releases alcohol-based solution to create cold temperature.
e Wrap pack or bag with towel, pillowcase, or stockinette. Apply over injury. Secure with tape as needed.	Protects patient's tissue and absorbs condensation. Prevents direct exposure of cold against patient's skin.
7 Apply commercial gel pack:	
a Remove from freezer.	
b Wrap pack with towel, pillowcase, or stockinette. Apply pack directly over injury (Fig. 14-1).	Protects patient's tissue and absorbs condensation. Prevents direct exposure of cold against patient's skin.

STEP	RATIONALE
c Secure with gauze, cloth tape, or ties as needed.	

SAFETY ALERT Do not reapply ice pack to red or bluish areas; continual use of ice pack causes ischemia sores.

STEP	RATIONALE
8 Apply electrically controlled cooling device:	
a Wrap flow pad in towel or pillowcase.	Prevents adverse reactions from cold such as burn or frostbite.
b Wrap cool water flow pad around body part (Fig. 14-2).	Ensures even application of cold temperature.
c Turn pad on, and be sure correct temperature is set.	Ensures effective therapy.
d Secure with elastic wrap bandage, gauze roll, or ties.	

Fig. 14-1 Commercial ice pack.

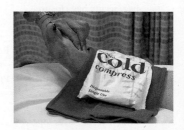

Fig. 14-2 Aquathermia pad.

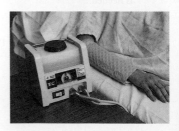

STEP	RATIONALE
9 Remove gloves and dispose of in proper container.	Reduces transfer of microorganisms.
10 Check condition of skin every 5 minutes for duration of application.	Determines if there are adverse reactions to cold (e.g., mottling, redness, burning, blistering, and numbness) (Physiotherapy Canada, 2010).
a If area is edematous, sensation may be reduced; use extra caution during cold therapy and assess more often.	
b Numbness and tingling are common sensations with cold applications and indicate adverse reactions only when severe and coupled with other symptoms. Stop when patient complains of burning sensation or skin begins to feel numb.	When applying cold, skin will initially feel cold, followed by relief of pain. As cryotherapy continues, patient will feel a burning sensation, then pain in the skin, and finally numbness (Physiotherapy Canada, 2010).
11 ![icon] After 15 to 20 minutes (or as ordered by the physician), apply clean gloves, remove compress or pad, and gently dry off any moisture.	Drying prevents maceration of skin.

SAFETY ALERT Areas with little body fat (e.g., knee, ankle, or elbow) do not tolerate cold as well as fatty areas (e.g., thigh or buttocks). For bony areas, decrease time of cold application to lower ranges.

STEP	RATIONALE
12 Assist patient to comfortable position.	Maintains relaxing environment.
13 Complete postprocedure protocol.	Reduces transfer of microorganisms.

Recording and Reporting

- Record procedure, including type, location, and duration of application and patient's response.
- Describe any instruction given and patient's success in demonstrating procedure.
- Report any sensations of burning, numbness, or unrelieved skin color changes to health care provider.

UNEXPECTED OUTCOMES	RELATED INTERVENTIONS
1 Skin appears mottled, reddened, or bluish purple as a result of prolonged exposure.	• Stop the treatment. • Notify nurse in charge or health care provider. • Injury from prolonged exposure requires different therapy.
2 Patient complains of burning type of pain and numbness.	• Stop the treatment because these are signs of ischemia. • Notify nurse in charge or health care provider.
3 Patient is unable to describe application or use compress correctly.	• Reinstruction and clarification are necessary.

Condom Catheter

The external urinary catheter, also called a *condom catheter* or *penile sheath,* is a soft, pliable condomlike sheath that fits over the penis, providing a safe and noninvasive way to contain urine. Most external catheters are made of soft silicone, which reduces friction. Latex catheters are still available and used by some patients. The catheters come in a variety of styles and sizes. For the best fit and correct application it is important to refer to manufacturer's guidelines.

Delegation Considerations

Assessment of the skin of a patient's penile shaft and determination of a latex allergy are done by a nurse before catheter application. The skill of applying a condom catheter can be delegated to nursing assistive personnel (NAP). The nurse directs the NAP to:

- Follow the manufacturer's directions for applying the condom catheter and securing the device.
- Monitor urine output, and record intake and output (I&O) if applicable.
- Immediately report any redness, swelling, skin irritation, or breakdown of glans or penile shaft.

Equipment

- Condom catheter kit (condom sheath of appropriate size, securing device, skin preparation solution [per manufacturer's directions])
- Urinary collection bag with drainage tubing or leg bag and straps
- Basin with warm water and soap
- Towels and washcloth(s)
- Bath blanket
- Clean gloves
- Scissors, hair guard or paper towel

Implementation

STEP	RATIONALE
1 Complete preprocedure protocol.	

STEP	RATIONALE
2 Assess condition of penis. Use the manufacturer's measuring guide to measure the diameter of penis in a flaccid state.	Provides baseline to compare changes in condition of skin after condom catheter application. Condom catheters can be applied only to intact skin (Newman and Wein, 2009). Measurement of the penile shaft aids in determining appropriate catheter size.
3 Prepare urinary drainage collection bag and tubing. Clamp off drainage bag port. Place nearby ready to attach to condom after applied.	Provides easy access to drainage equipment after applying condom catheter.
4 ✋ Apply clean gloves. Provide perineal care. Dry thoroughly before applying device. In uncircumcised patient, ensure that foreskin has been replaced to normal position. Do not apply barrier cream.	Prevents skin breakdown from exposure to secretions. Removes any residual adhesives. Perineal care minimizes skin irritation and promotes adhesion of new external catheter. Barrier creams prevent sheath from adhering to penile shaft (Pomfret, 2008).
5 Clip hair at base of penis as necessary before application of condom sheath. Some manufacturers provide a hair guard that is placed over penis before applying device. Remove hair guard after applying catheter. An alternative to hair guard is to tear a hole in a paper towel, place it over penis, and remove after application of device.	Hair adheres to condom and is pulled during condom removal or may get caught in adhesive as external catheter is applied.

SAFETY ALERT The pubic area should not be shaved because it may increase risk for skin irritation (Pomfret, 2008).

STEP	RATIONALE
6 Apply condom catheter. With nondominant hand, grasp penis along shaft. With dominant hand, hold rolled condom sheath at tip of penis and smoothly roll sheath onto penis. Allow 2.5 to 5 cm (1 to 2 inches) of space between tip of glans penis and end of condom catheter (Fig. 15-1).	Excessive wrinkles or creases in external catheter sheath after application may mean that patient needs smaller size (Newman and Wein, 2009).
7 Apply appropriate securing device as indicated in manufacturer's directions:	Condom must be secured firmly so it is snug and stays on but not tight enough to cause constriction of blood flow. Application of gentle pressure ensures adherence of adhesive with penile skin.
a Self-adhesive condom catheters: After application, apply gentle pressure on penile shaft for 10 to 15 seconds to secure catheter.	
b Outer securing strip-type condom catheters: Spiral-	Using spiral-wrap technique allows supplied elastic adhesive

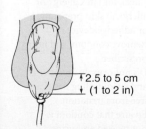

Fig. 15-1 Distance between end of penis and tip of condom.

2.5 to 5 cm
(1 to 2 in)

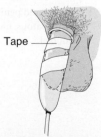

Tape

Fig. 15-2 Tape applied in spiral fashion.

STEP	RATIONALE
wrap penile shaft with strip of supplied elastic adhesive. Strip should not overlap itself. Elastic strip should be snug, not tight (Fig. 15-2).	to expand so blood flow to penis is not compromised.
8 Remove hair guard or paper towel if used. Connect drainage tubing to end of condom catheter. Be sure condom is not twisted. If using large drainage bag, place excess tubing on bed and secure to bottom sheet.	Allows urine to be collected and measured. Keeps patient dry. Twisted condom obstructs urine flow, causing urine pooling; skin irritation; and weakening and deterioration of adhesive, causing catheter to come off (Pomfret, 2008).
9 Place patient in safe, comfortable position. Lower bed, and place side rails up as required.	Promotes safety and comfort.
10 Complete postprocedure protocol.	Reduces spread of microorganisms.

Recording and Reporting

- Record condom application; condition of penis, skin, and scrotum; urinary output; and voiding pattern in nurses' notes and electronic health record (EHR).
- Report penile erythema, rashes, and/or skin breakdown.

UNEXPECTED OUTCOMES	RELATED INTERVENTIONS
1 Skin around penis is erythematous, ulcerated, or denuded.	• Check for latex allergy or allergy to skin preparation or adhesive device. • Remove condom, and notify prescriber. • Do not reapply until penis and surrounding tissue are free from irritation. • Ensure that condom is not twisted and urine flow is unobstructed after reapplication.

UNEXPECTED OUTCOMES	RELATED INTERVENTIONS
2 Penile swelling or discoloration occurs.	• Remove external catheter. • Notify health care provider. • Reassess current condom size. See manufacturer's size chart.
3 Condom does not stay on.	• Ensure that catheter tubing is anchored and that patient understands to not pull or tug on catheter. • Reassess condom catheter size. Refer to manufacturer's guidelines for sizing. • Observe whether outlet is kinked and urine is pooling at tip of condom. Reapply as necessary, and avoid catheter obstruction. • Assess need for another brand of external catheter (i.e., one that is self-adhesive).
4 Frequency and amount of urination are reduced.	• Check for bladder distention. • Observe whether urine is pooling at tip of condom and bathing penis in urine. Reapply as necessary. • Check for kinks in tubing or in condom catheter.

Continuous Passive Motion Machine

The continuous passive motion (CPM) machine is designed to exercise various joints such as the hip, ankle, knee, shoulder, and wrist. The CPM machine is most commonly used after knee surgery. It is usually prescribed on the day of surgery or the first postoperative day, depending on the surgeon's preference and patient's condition. The purpose of the CPM machine is to mobilize the joint to prevent contractures, muscle atrophy, venous stasis, and thromboembolism. It helps alleviate pain, edema, stiffness, and dislocation and potentially can shorten a patient's hospital stay.

Delegation Considerations

The skill of using the CPM machine cannot be delegated to nursing assistive personnel (NAP). The nurse directs the NAP by:
- Instructing them to immediately report increase in patient's pain, skin breakdown, or joint inflammation.

Equipment
- CPM machine
- Clean gloves

Implementation

STEP	RATIONALE
1 Complete preprocedure protocol.	
2 Provide analgesic 20 to 30 minutes before CPM machine is needed.	Pain control assists patient in tolerating exercise.
3 ✄ Wear clean gloves if wound drainage is present.	Reduces nurse's risk for exposure to bloodborne viruses or bacteria.
4 Place elastic hose on patient if ordered (see Skill 67).	Elastic stockings promote venous return from lower extremities.
5 Place CPM machine on bed.	

STEP	RATIONALE
6 Set limits of flexion and extension as prescribed by health care provider, and set speed control to slow or moderate range.	Prevents injury by setting machine at safe limits.
7 Put machine through one full cycle.	Ensures CPM machine is working properly.
8 Stop CPM machine when in extension. Place sheepskin on CPM machine.	Ensures all exposed hard surfaces are padded to prevent rubbing and chafing of patient's skin.
9 Support patient's joints while placing extremity in CPM machine (Fig. 16-1).	
10 Adjust CPM machine to patient's extremity. Lengthen and shorten appropriate sections of frame.	
11 Center patient's extremity on frame.	Avoids pressure areas on extremity.
12 Align patient's joint with CPM's mechanical joint.	
13 Secure patient's extremity on CPM machine with Velcro straps. Apply loosely.	Protects skin from irritation.
14 Start machine. When it reaches flexed position, stop machine and check degree of flexion.	Prevents possible complications and ensures correct settings.

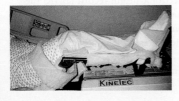

Fig. 16-1 Patient's extremity properly placed and secured on CPM machine.

Fig. 16-2 Nurse observes several cycles of CPM machine.

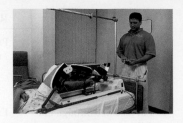

STEP	RATIONALE
15 Start CPM machine, and observe for two full cycles (Fig 16-2).	Ensures CPM machine is fully operational at the preset extension and flexion modes.
16 Make sure patient is comfortable.	
17 Instruct patient to turn CPM machine off if malfunctioning or if he or she is experiencing pain. Instruct him or her to notify nurse immediately.	Prevents excessive stress on joint.
18 Provide patient with on/off switch.	Allows patient to turn CPM machine on and off if it malfunctions or discomfort develops.
19 Complete postprocedure protocol.	

Recording and Reporting

- Record in nurses' notes and electronic health record (EHR) the patient's tolerance for CPM machine, rate of cycles per minute, degree of flexion and extension used, condition of extremity and skin, condition of operative site if present, length of time CPM machine in use.
- Report immediately to nurse in charge or health care provider any resistance to range of motion; increased pain; swelling, heat, or redness in joint.

UNEXPECTED OUTCOMES	RELATED INTERVENTIONS
1 Patient does not tolerate increase in flexion or extension.	• Consult with health care provider and physical therapist to plan additional therapies to increase flexion and extension of joint. • Provide rest periods throughout day to rest the joint. • Consider need for analgesia before CPM machine is used.
2 Patient experiences increased pain when using CPM machine.	• Determine efficacy of current analgesic, and obtain new orders to change dosage or medication. • Determine cause of increased pain.
3 Patient develops reddened areas on bony prominences or extremity.	• Determine if hard surfaces on CPM machine are well padded. • Monitor patient's alignment and positioning at least every 2 hours. • Provide skin care at least every 2 hours.

Continuous Subcutaneous Infusion

The continuous subcutaneous infusion (CSQI or CSCI) route of medication administration is used for selected medications (e.g., opioids, insulin). The route is also effective with medications to stop preterm labor (e.g., terbutaline [Brethine]) and to treat pulmonary hypertension (e.g., treprostinil sodium [Remodulin]) (Box 17-1). One factor that determines the infusion rate of CSQI is the rate of medication absorption. Most patients can absorb 3 to 5 mL/hr of medication (Infusion Nurses Society [INS], 2011ab; Justad, 2009).

Use a small-gauge (25 to 27) winged butterfly intravenous (IV) needle or special commercially prepared Teflon cannula to deliver medications. Use the needle with the shortest length and the smallest gauge necessary to establish and maintain the infusion.

Use the same anatomical sites as for subcutaneous injections (see Skill 71), as well as the upper chest. Site selection depends on a patient's activity level and the type of medication delivered. Always avoid sites where the pump's tubing could be disturbed. Rotate sites used for medication administration at least every 2 to 7 days or whenever complications such as leaking occur (INS, 2011ab).

Delegation Considerations

The skill of administering CSQI medications cannot be delegated to nursing assistive personnel (NAP). The nurse instructs the NAP about:

- Potential medication side effects or reactions and to report their occurrence to the nurse.
- Reporting complications (e.g., leaking, redness, discomfort) at the CSQI needle insertion site to the nurse.
- Obtaining any required vital signs and reporting them to the nurse.

Equipment

Initiation of CSQI Therapy

- Clean gloves
- Alcohol swab
- Antibacterial skin preparation such as chlorhexidine
- Small-gauge (25 to 27) winged IV catheter with attached tubing or CSQI–designed catheter (e.g., Sof-Set)
- Infusion pump

BOX 17-1 Benefits Associated with Pain Management Delivered by Continuous Subcutaneous Infusion

- Benefits patients with poor venous access.
- Provides pain relief to patients who cannot tolerate oral pain medications.
- Allows patients greater mobility.
- Onset of action takes about 20 minutes.
- Better pain control than IM injections.
- Costs are almost half of costs associated with IV infusions.

IM, Intramuscular; *IV,* intravenous.
Modified from Ellershaw J, Wilkinson S: *Care of the dying,* ed 2, Oxford, 2010, Oxford University Press.

- Occlusive, transparent dressing
- Tape
- Medication in appropriate syringe or container
- Medication administration record (MAR) or computer printout

Discontinuing CSQI

- Clean, nonsterile gloves
- Small, sterile gauze dressing
- Tape or adhesive bandage
- Alcohol swab and chlorhexidine *(optional)*
- Puncture-proof container

Implementation

STEP	RATIONALE
1 Complete preprocedure protocol.	
2 Check accuracy and completeness of each MAR or computer printout.	The prescriber's order is the most reliable source and legal record of patient's medications. Ensures that patient receives correct medications.
3 Perform hand hygiene. Prepare medication using aseptic technique, or check dose on prefilled syringe. Connect syringe and prime	*This is the first check for accuracy* and ensures that correct medication is administered.

STEP	RATIONALE
tubing with medication, being careful not to lose any medication. Compare label of the medication with the MAR or computer printout two times.	
4 Obtain and program medication administration pump. Place syringe in pump.	Ensures that medication dose is administered accurately.
5 Read label on prefilled syringe, and compare with MAR or computer printout.	*This is the second check for accuracy.*
6 Identify patient using two identifiers (e.g., name and birthday or name and account number) according to agency poilcy. Compare identifiers with information on patient's MAR or medical record.	Ensures correct patient. Complies with The Joint Commission requirements for patient safety (TJC, 2014). Some agencies are now using a bar-code system to help with patient identification.
7 At patient's bedside, again compare MAR or computer printout with names of medications on medication labels and patient name. Ask patient if he or she has allergies.	*This is the final check for accuracy* and ensures that patient receives correct medication. Confirms patient's allergy history.
8 Discuss purpose of each medication, action, and possible adverse effects. Allow patient to ask any questions. Tell patient that needle insertion will cause slight burning or stinging.	Patient has right to be informed, and patient's understanding of each medication improves adherence to drug therapy.
9 Position patient supine, drape, and provide for privacy.	Respects patient's dignity.

STEP	RATIONALE
10 Initiate CSQI:	
a Be sure patient is comfortable, sitting or lying down.	Eases pain associated with insertion of needle.
b Select appropriate injection site free of irritation and away from bony prominences and waistline. Most common sites used are subclavicular and abdominal.	Ensures proper medication absorption.
c ✂ Apply clean gloves.	
d Cleanse injection site with alcohol using a circular motion, followed by antiseptic, using straight cleansing strokes. Allow both agents to dry.	Reduces risk for infection at insertion site.
e Hold needle in dominant hand, and remove needle guard.	Prepares needle for insertion.
f Gently pinch or lift up skin with nondominant hand.	Ensures needle will enter subcutaneous tissue.
g Gently and firmly insert needle at a 45- to 90-degree angle (Fig. 17-1).	Decreases pain related to insertion of needle.
h Release skinfold, and apply tape over "wings" of needle.	Secures needle.

SAFETY ALERT Some cannulas have a sharp needle covered with a plastic catheter. In this case, remove the needle and leave the plastic catheter in the skin.

i Place occlusive, transparent dressing over insertion site (Fig. 17-2).	Protects site from infection and allows you to assess site during medication infusion.

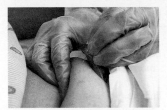

Fig. 17-1 Insertion of butterfly needle into subcutaneous tissue of abdomen.

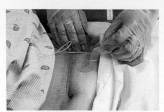

Fig. 17-2 Securing insertion site.

STEP	RATIONALE
j Attach tubing from needle to tubing from infusion pump, and turn pump on.	Allows you to administer medication.
k Dispose of any sharps in appropriate leak- and puncture-proof container. Discard used supplies, remove gloves, and perform hand hygiene.	Prevents accidental needlestick injuries and follows Centers for Disease Control and Prevention (CDC) guidelines for disposal of sharps (Occupational Safety and Health Administration [OSHA], 2012).
11 Discontinue CSQI:	
a Verify order, and establish alternative method for medication administration if applicable.	If medication will be required after discontinuing CSQI, a different medication and/ or route is often necessary to continue to manage patient's illness or pain.
b Stop infusion pump.	Prevents medication from spilling.
c Perform hand hygiene, and put on clean gloves.	Follows CDC recommendations to prevent accidental exposure to blood and body fluids (OSHA, 2012).
d Remove dressing without dislodging or removing the needle. Discard properly.	Exposes needle.

STEP	RATIONALE
e Remove tape from the wings of needle, and pull needle out at the same angle it was inserted.	Minimizes patient discomfort.
f Apply gentle pressure at site until no fluid leaks out of skin.	Dressing will adhere to site if skin remains dry.
g Apply small sterile gauze dressing or adhesive bandage to site.	Prevents bacterial entry into puncture site.
12 Complete postprocedure protocol.	

Recording and Reporting

- After initiating CSQI, immediately chart medication, dose, route, site, time, date, and type of medication pump in patient's medical record. Use initials or signature.
- If medication is an opioid, follow agency policy to document waste.
- Record patient's response to medication and appearance of site every 4 hours or according to agency policy in nurses' notes and electronic health record (EHR).
- Report any adverse effects from medication or infection at insertion site to patient's health care provider, and document according to agency policy. Patient's condition often indicates need for additional medical therapy.

UNEXPECTED OUTCOMES	RELATED INTERVENTIONS
1 Patient complains of localized pain or burning at insertion site, or site appears red or swollen or is leaking, indicating potential infection or needle dislodgment.	• Remove needle, and place new needle in a different site. • Continue to monitor original site for signs of infection, and notify health care provider if you suspect infection.

Continued

UNEXPECTED OUTCOMES	RELATED INTERVENTIONS
2 Patient displays signs of allergic reaction to medication.	• Stop delivering medication immediately, and follow agency policy or guidelines for appropriate response to allergic reaction (e.g., administration of antihistamine such as diphenhydramine [Benadryl] or epinephrine) and reporting of adverse drug reactions. • Notify patient's health care provider of adverse effects immediately. • Add allergy information to patient's medical record per agency policy.
3 CSQI becomes dislodged.	• Stop the infusion, apply pressure at the site until no fluid leaks out of skin, cover site with a gauze dressing or adhesive bandage, and initiate a new site. • Assess patient to determine effects of not receiving medication (e.g., assess patient's pain level using age-appropriate pain scale; obtain blood glucose level).

Dressings:
Dry and Moist-to-Dry

Dry dressings are commonly used for abrasions and nondraining postoperative incisions. Dry dressings are not appropriate for debriding wounds. Moist-to-dry dressings (also called *wet-to-dry* or *damp-to-dry*) are gauze moistened with an appropriate solution. The primary purpose is to mechanically debride wounds, specifically full-thickness wounds healing by secondary intention and wounds with necrotic tissue. A moist-to-dry dressing has a moist contact dressing layer that touches the wound surface. The moistened gauze increases the absorptive ability of the dressing to collect exudate and wound debris. This layer dries and adheres to dead cells, thus debriding the wound when removed. Use a sterile isotonic solution such as normal saline or lactated Ringer's to moisten dressings. The outer absorbent layer is a dry dressing that protects the wound from invasive organisms.

Delegation Considerations

The skill of applying dry and moist-to-dry dressings may sometimes be delegated to nursing assistive personnel (NAP) if the wound is chronic (see agency policy and state Nurse Practice Act). All wound assessments, care of acute new wounds, and wound care requiring sterile technique cannot be delegated. The nurse directs the NAP about:

- Any unique modifications of the dressing change, such as the need for use of special tape or taping techniques to secure the dressing.
- Reporting pain, fever, bleeding, or wound drainage to the nurse immediately.

Equipment

- Clean gloves
- Sterile gloves
- Sterile dressing set (scissors, forceps) (may be *optional*—check agency policy)
- Sterile drape *(optional)*
- Sterile dressings: fine-mesh gauze, 4 × 4–inch gauze, abdominal (ABD) pads
- Sterile basin *(optional)*
- Antiseptic ointment (as prescribed)
- Wound cleanser (as prescribed)

- Sterile normal saline or prescribed solution
- Debriding gel as ordered
- Tape, Montgomery ties, or bandage as needed (include nonallergenic tape if necessary)
- Skin barrier (optional if using Montgomery ties)
- Protective waterproof underpad
- Waterproof bag
- Adhesive remover *(optional)*
- Measurement device *(optional):* cotton-tipped applicator, measuring guide, camera *(optional)*
- Protective gown, mask, goggles (used when splashing from wound is a risk)
- Additional lighting if needed (e.g., flashlight, treatment light)

Implementation

STEP	RATIONALE
1 Complete preprocedure protocol.	
2 Ask patient to rate his or her level of pain using a pain scale of 0 to 10, and assess character of pain. Administer prescribed analgesic as needed 30 minutes before dressing change.	Superficial wounds with multiple exposed nerves may be intensely painful, whereas deeper wounds with destruction of dermis should be less painful (Krasner, 2012). A comfortable patient will be less likely to move suddenly, causing wound or supply contamination.
3 Identify patient using two identifiers (e.g., name and birthday or name and account number) according to agency policy.	Ensures correct patient. Complies with The Joint Commission requirements for patient safety (TJC, 2014).
4 Position patient comfortably, and drape to expose only wound site. Instruct patient not to touch wound or sterile supplies.	Draping provides access to the wound yet minimizes unnecessary exposure. Prevents contamination of the wound or sterile supplies.

STEP	RATIONALE
5 Place disposable waterproof bag within reach of work area. Fold top of bag to make cuff. Apply gown, goggles, and mask if risk for splashing exists.	Ensures easy disposal of soiled dressings. Prevents contamination of bag's outer surface. Use of personal protective equipment reduces transmission of microorganisms.
6 Apply clean gloves. Gently remove tape, bandages, or ties: use nondominant hand to support dressing, and with your dominant hand, pull tape parallel to skin and toward dressing. If dressing is over hairy area, remove in direction of hair growth. Get patient permission to clip or shave area (check agency policy). Remove any adhesive from skin.	Pulling tape toward dressing reduces stress on suture line or wound edges and reduces irritation and discomfort.
7 With gloved hand or forceps, remove dressing one layer at a time, observing appearance and drainage on dressing. Carefully remove outer secondary dressing first, and then remove inner primary dressing that is in contact with the wound bed. If drains are present, slowly and carefully remove dressings and avoid tension on any drainage devices. Keep soiled undersurface from patient's sight:	The purpose of the primary dressing is to remove necrotic tissue and exudate. Appearance of drainage may be upsetting to patient. Avoids accidental removal of drain.
a If moist-to-dry dressing adheres to wound, gently free dressing and alert patient of discomfort.	Moist-to-dry dressing should debride wound. Do not wet the dressing; it should be dry.

STEP	RATIONALE
b If dry dressing adheres to wound that is not to be debrided, moisten with normal saline and remove.	Prevents injury to wound surface and periwound during dressing removal.
8 Inspect wound and periwound for appearance, color, size (length, width, and depth), drainage, edema, presence and condition of drains, approximation (i.e., whether wound edges are together), granulation tissue, and odor. Use measuring guide or ruler to measure size of wound. Gently palpate wound edges for bogginess or patient report of increased pain.	Assesses condition of wound and periwound condition. Indicates status of healing.
9 Fold dressing with drainage contained inside, and remove gloves inside out. With small dressings, remove gloves inside out over the dressing. Dispose of gloves and soiled dressing according to agency policy. Cover wound lightly with sterile gauze pad, and perform hand hygiene.	Contains soiled dressings, prevents contact of nurse's hands with drainage, and reduces cross-contamination.
10 Describe the appearance of the wound and any indicators of wound healing to the patient.	Wounds may appear unsettling to patients; it is helpful for the patient to know that the wound appearance is as expected and that healing is taking place.
11 Create sterile field with a sterile dressing tray or individually wrapped sterile supplies on over-bed table.	Sterile dressings remain sterile while on or within sterile surface. Preparation of all supplies prevents break in technique during dressing change.

STEP	RATIONALE
12 Cleanse wound:	
a Perform hand hygiene, and apply clean gloves. Use gauze or cotton ball moistened in saline or antiseptic swab (per health care provider order) for each cleansing stroke, or spray wound surface with wound cleanser.	Prevents transfer of microorganisms from previously cleaned area.
b Clean from least contaminated area to most contaminated.	Cleansing in this direction prevents introduction of organisms into wound.
c Cleanse around the drain (if present), using circular stroke starting near drain and moving outward and away from the insertion site.	Correct aseptic technique in cleansing to prevent contamination.
13 Use sterile dry gauze to blot in same manner as in Step 12 to dry wound.	Drying reduces excess moisture, which could eventually harbor microorganisms.
14 Apply antiseptic ointment (if ordered) with sterile cotton-tipped swab or gauze, using same technique to apply as for cleaning. Dispose of gloves. Perform hand hygiene.	Helps reduce growth of microorganisms.
15 Apply dressing:	
a **Dry sterile dressing:**	
(1) Apply clean gloves (see agency policy).	Some agencies or condition of wounds may require **sterile gloves.**
(2) Apply loosely woven gauze as contact layer.	Promotes proper absorption of drainage.

STEP	RATIONALE
(3) If drain is present, apply a precut 4 × 4–inch gauze flat around drain.	Secures drain and promotes drainage absorption at site.
(4) Apply additional layers of gauze as needed.	Ensures proper coverage and optimal absorption.
(5) Apply thicker woven pad (e.g., Surgipad, abdominal dressing).	This type of dressing is often used on postoperative wounds with excessive drainage.
b Moist-to-dry dressing:	
(1) Apply **sterile gloves.**	
(2) Place fine-mesh or loose 4 × 4–inch gauze in container of prescribed sterile solution. Wring out excess solution.	Moist gauze absorbs drainage and, when allowed to dry, traps debris.

SAFETY ALERT If a "packing strip" is used to pack the wound, use sterile scissors to cut the amount of dressing that you will use to pack the wound. Do not let packing strip touch the side of the bottle. Pour prescribed solution over the packing gauze or strip to moisten it.

(3) Apply moist fine-mesh, open-weave gauze as a single layer directly onto wound surface. If wound is deep, gently pack gauze into wound with sterile gloved hand or forceps until all wound surfaces are in contact with moist gauze including dead spaces from sinus tracts, tunnels, and undermining. Be sure gauze does not touch periwound skin (Fig. 18-1, A).	Inner gauze should be moist, not dripping wet, to absorb drainage and adhere to debris. Wound is loosely packed to facilitate wicking of drainage into absorbent outer layer of dressing. Moisture that escapes the dressing often macerates the periwound area.

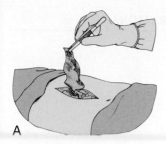

Fig. 18-1 **A,** Packing wound.
B, Wound packed loosely.

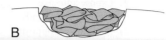

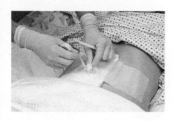

Fig. 18-2 Securing Montgomery ties.

STEP	RATIONALE

SAFETY ALERT If wound is deep, gently lay moistened woven gauze over wound surface with forceps until all surfaces are in contact with moist gauze and the wound is loosely filled. Fill the wound, but avoid packing the wound too tightly or having the gauze extend beyond the top of the wound (Fig. 18-1, B).

STEP	RATIONALE
(4) Apply dry sterile 4 × 4–inch gauze over wet gauze.	Dry layer pulls moisture from wound.
(5) Cover with an ABD pad, Surgipad, or gauze.	Protects wound from entrance of microorganisms.
16 Secure dressing:	
a *Tape:* Apply tape 2.5 to 5 cm (1 to 2 inches) beyond dressing. Use nonallergenic tape when necessary.	Supports wound and ensures placement and stability of dressing.
b *Montgomery ties* (Fig. 18-2):	Ties allow for repeated dressing changes without removal of tape.

STEP	RATIONALE
(1) Be sure that skin is clean. Application of skin barrier is recommended.	
(2) Expose adhesive surface of tape ends.	
(3) Place ties on opposite sides of dressing over skin or skin barrier.	
(4) Secure dressing by lacing ties across dressing snugly enough to hold it secure but without placing pressure on skin.	
c For dressing an extremity, secure with roll gauze (Fig. 18-3) or elastic net.	
17 Complete postprocedure protocol.	
18 Observe appearance of wound for healing, including size of wound; amount, color, and type of drainage; and periwound erythema or swelling.	Determines rate of healing.
19 Ask patient to rate pain using a scale of 0 to 10.	Increased pain is often an indication of wound complications, such as infection, or a result of dressing pulling tissue.

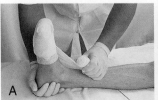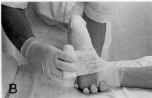

Fig. 18-3 Application of roll gauze.

STEP	RATIONALE
20 Inspect condition of dressing at least every shift.	Determines status of wound drainage.
21 Ask patient and/or family caregiver to describe steps and techniques of dressing change.	Evaluates patient's learning.

Recording and Reporting

- Record appearance and size of wound, characteristics of drainage, presence of necrotic tissue, type of dressing applied, patient's response to dressing change, and level of comfort in nurses' notes and electronic health record (EHR).
- Report any unexpected appearance of wound drainage, accidental removal of drain, bright red bleeding, or evidence of wound dehiscence or evisceration.

UNEXPECTED OUTCOMES	RELATED INTERVENTIONS
1 Wound appears inflamed and tender, drainage is evident, and/or an odor is present.	• Monitor patient for signs of infection. • Notify health care provider. • Obtain wound culture. • If there is yellow, tan, or brown necrotic tissue, refer to health care provider to determine need for debridement.
2 Wound bleeds during dressing change.	• Observe color and amount of drainage. If excessive, apply pressure dressing. • Inspect area along dressing and directly underneath patient to determine the amount of bleeding. • Obtain vital signs as needed. • Notify health care provider.

Continued

UNEXPECTED OUTCOMES	RELATED INTERVENTIONS
3 Patient reports sensation that "something has given way under the dressing."	• Observe wound for increased drainage or dehiscence (partial or total separation of wound layers) or evisceration (total separation of wound layers and protrusion of viscera through wound opening). • Protect wound. Cover with sterile moist dressing. • Instruct patient to lie still. • Remain with patient to monitor vital signs. • Notify health care provider.

Dressings:
Hydrocolloid, Hydrogel, Foam, or Alginate

Hydrocolloid dressings are a formulation of elastomeric, adhesive, and gelling agents. They are indicated as primary dressings for minimally to moderately exudative partial- and full-thickness wounds. Hydrocolloids are used as secondary dressings over fillers such as hydrocolloid powders and pastes (Rolstad, Bryant, and Nix, 2011). International pressure ulcer guidelines recommend use of hydrocolloids for clean stage II and noninfected shallow stage III pressure ulcers in anatomic locations where the product does not roll or melt (National Pressure Ulcer Advisory Panel [NPUAP] and European Pressure Ulcer Advisory Panel [EPUAP], 2009).

Hydrogel dressings are glycerin- or water-based dressings designed to hydrate a wound (Rolstad, Bryant, and Nix, 2011). They are a good choice for painful wounds since they do not adhere to a wound base. In addition, international pressure ulcer guidelines recommend hydrogels for dry to minimally exudative pressure ulcers that are noninfected and granulating in anatomic locations that are not at risk for dressing migration (NPUAP and EPUAP, 2009). They absorb exudate and encourage healing by maintaining a moist wound healing environment. The gel dressings must be covered with a secondary dressing to hold them in place. Because of their "cooling" and soothing properties, they are also used with burns and to soothe radiation burns.

Polyurethane foam dressings are sheets of foamed polymers that contain small open cells capable of holding wound exudate away from a wound bed (Rolstad, Bryant, and Nix, 2011). Foam dressings are used as primary or secondary dressings to absorb moderate to heavy exudates. They are indicated to treat superficial or deep wounds, protect friable periwound skin, pad and protect high-trauma areas, and treat infected wounds following appropriate intervention and close monitoring of wound healing. International pressure ulcer guidelines recommend considering foam for use on exudative stage II and shallow stage III pressure ulcers (NPUAP and EPUAP, 2009). Foam dressings are not appropriate when there is wound tunneling because the dressing expands, which can enlarge the tunnels.

Alginate dressings create a moist environment and thus promote autolysis, granulation, and epithelialization (Rolstad, Bryant, and Nix,

2011). These dressings are appropriate for full-thickness wounds with moderate to high amounts of drainage. You can safely pack deep tracking wounds with calcium-sodium alginate preparation, which allows easy removal with little risk for retained dressing deep in the wound cavity.

Delegation Considerations

The skill of applying a hydrocolloid, hydrogel, foam, or alginate dressing cannot be delegated to nursing assistive personnel (NAP). The nurse directs the NAP about:

- Approach to assist in positioning patient during dressing application.
- What to observe (e.g., leakage of drainage, slippage of dressing) and report back to nurse.

Equipment

- Sterile gloves (optional)
- Clean gloves

Dressing Set *(optional)*

- Sterile scissors
- Sterile drape (optional)
- Necessary primary dressings: gauze, hydrocolloid, hydrogel, foam, or alginate
- Secondary dressing of choice
- Sterile 4 × 4–inch gauze pads
- Sterile saline or other cleansing solution (as ordered)
- Skin barrier wipe
- Tape (nonallergenic paper or adhesive), ties as needed
- Measuring guide (tape measure, tracing paper, camera as needed)
- Adhesive remover
- Waterproof bag
- Debriding gel (as ordered)
- Irrigation solution if indicated
- Protective gown, goggles, and mask (used when splashing from wound is a risk)

Implementation

STEP	RATIONALE
1 Complete preprocedure protocol.	Allows nurse to determine supplies and assistance needed.

STEP	RATIONALE
2 Review health care provider's orders for frequency and type of dressing change. *Do not use alginate or absorptive dressings on nonexudative wounds.*	Health care provider orders mode of therapy. Dressings are designed to absorb moderate to large amounts of wound drainage and should not be used in wounds with minimal or no drainage (Rolstad, Bryant, and Nix, 2011).
3 Expose wound site, and drape patient. Instruct patient not to touch wound or sterile supplies.	Draping provides access to wound while minimizing patient exposure.
	Dressing supplies become contaminated when touched by patient's hand.
4 Cuff top of disposable waterproof bag, and place within reach of work area.	Prevents accidental contamination of top of outer bag. Nurse should not reach across sterile field.
5 ![hand icon] Perform hand hygiene, and put on clean disposable gloves. Don moisture-proof gown, mask, and goggles if there is a risk for splashing.	Reduces transmission of microorganisms.
6 Remove old dressing one layer at a time. Note amount and character of drainage. Use caution to avoid tension on any drains.	Reduces irritation and possible injury to skin.
7 Dispose of soiled dressings in waterproof bag. Remove disposable gloves by pulling them inside out, and dispose of them in waterproof bag. Perform hand hygiene.	Reduces transmission of microorganisms.
8 Prepare sterile field with sterile dressing kit or individually wrapped sterile supplies on over-bed table.	Creates sterile work area.

STEP	RATIONALE
9 Pour saline or prescribed solution over 4 × 4–inch sterile gauze pads, or open spray wound cleanser.	
Option: For hydrocolloid, alginate, or foam dressings, prepare an irrigation solution if needed.	Hydrocolloid forms viscous, colloidal gel that is easily irrigated out of wound bed (Rolstad, Bryant, and Nix, 2011).
10 Apply sterile or clean gloves (check agency policy) or use no-touch technique with sterile forceps to clean wound. Remove gauze covering wound.	Allows nurse to handle dressings.
11 Cleanse wound:	Reduces introduction of organisms into wound.
a Cleanse area gently with moist 4 × 4–inch sterile gauze pads, swabbing exudate away from wound, or spray with wound cleanser or irrigate wound bed.	Cleansing effectively removes any residual dressing gel without injuring newly formed delicate granulation tissue formed in the healing wound bed.
b Clean around any drain, using a circular stroke starting near drain and moving outward away from insertion site.	
12 Use sterile dry 4 × 4–inch gauze pads to blot dry excess saline or cleanser in wound bed and on skin around wound.	Dressing will not adhere to damp surface. Periwound maceration can enlarge wound and impede healing.
13 Inspect appearance and condition of wound. Measure wound size and depth.	Appearance and measurement indicate state of wound healing.
14 Remove gloves, and perform hand hygiene. Apply dressing according to manufacturer's directions.	Ensures proper application of dressing. Different brands of dressings require different application techniques.

STEP	RATIONALE
a **Hydrocolloid dressings:**	
(1) Select proper size wafer, allowing dressing to extend onto intact periwound skin at least 2.5 cm (1 inch) (Rolstad, Bryant, and Nix, 2011).	Hydrocolloid design prevents shear and friction from loosening edges and circumvents need for tape along dressing borders (Rolstad, Bryant, and Nix, 2011).
(2) In the case of a deep wound, apply hydrocolloid granules, impregnated gauze, or paste before the wafer.	Functions as filler material to ensure contact with all wound surfaces.
(3) Remove paper backing from adhesive side and place over wound. Do not stretch dressing, and avoid wrinkles or tenting. Mold wafer to affected body part.	
(4) If cut from larger piece, tape edges with nonallergenic tape to avoid rolling or adherence to clothing (Rolstad, Bryant, and Nix, 2011).	
(5) Hold dressing in place for 30 to 60 seconds.	Hydrocolloids are most effective at body temperature (Rolstad, Bryant, and Nix, 2011).
(6) Use nonallergenic tape to secure.	Prevents edges of dressing from rolling or adhering to sheets and clothing.

STEP	RATIONALE
b **Hydrogel dressings:**	
(1) Apply skin barrier wipe to surrounding skin that will come in contact with any adhesive or gel.	Protects periwound skin. Because of high water content of gels, care must be taken to protect periwound skin through use of skin barrier (Rolstad, Bryant, and Nix, 2011).
(2) Apply gel or gel-impregnated gauze directly into wound, spreading evenly over wound bed. Fill wound cavity with gel about one-half to one-third full, or pack gauze loosely, including any undermined or tunneled areas. Cover with moisture-retentive dressing or hydrocolloid wafer. *Option:* Hydrogel sheets composed of water should be cut to size of wound *only*.	Hydrogels hydrate and facilitate autolytic debridement of wounds. Filling wound cavity partially full allows for expansion with absorption of exudate. Avoids overlapping and maceration of periwound (Rolstad, Bryant, and Nix, 2011).
(3) Cut hydrogel sheet containing glycerin so it extends 2.5 cm (1 inch) out onto intact periwound skin. Cover with secondary moisture-retentive dressing if needed.	Protects skin around wound from maceration.
(4) Secure dressing with nonallergenic tape if secondary dressing is not self-adhering.	

STEP	RATIONALE
c Foam dressings:	
(1) Know removal and application characteristics of specific brand of foam dressing.	Used with absorptive dressings to accommodate highly draining wounds.
(2) Apply skin barrier wipe to surrounding skin that will come in contact with thin foam dressing adhesive. **NOTE:** Traditional-thickness nonadhesive may not have adhesive border.	Protects periwound skin from maceration or irritation from adhesive.
(3) Cut foam sheet to extend 2.5 cm (1 inch) out onto intact periwound skin. (Verify which side of foam dressing should be placed toward wound bed and which side should be facing away from wound bed; check product instructions.)	Ensures proper absorption and keeps wound exudate away from wound bed (Rolstad, Bryant, and Nix, 2011).
(4) Some brands of foam dressings need to be covered with a secondary dressing (Rolstad, Bryant, and Nix, 2011).	Protects wound.
(5) Cut foam to fit around drain or tube.	

STEP	RATIONALE
d **Alginate dressings:**	
(1) Cut sheet or rope to fit size of wound or loosely pack into wound space, filling one-half to two-thirds full.	Highly absorptive product expands with absorption of serous fluid or exudate (Rolstad, Bryant, and Nix, 2011).
(2) Apply secondary dressing such as transparent film, foam, or hydrocolloid.	Secondary dressing prohibits drainage on bedclothes and clothing.
15 Complete postprocedure protocol.	Reduces transfer of microorganisms.

Recording and Reporting

- Record appearance of wound, color, size, characteristics of drainage, response to dressing change, condition of periwound skin, and patient's level of comfort in nurses' notes and electronic health record (EHR).
- Graph wound surface area or volume if wound is chronic.
- Write date, time, and nurse's initials in ink (not marker) on the dressing.
- Report signs of infection, necrosis, or deteriorating wound status to health care provider immediately.

UNEXPECTED OUTCOMES	RELATED INTERVENTIONS
1 Wound develops more necrotic tissue and increases in size.	• In rare instances, some wounds will not tolerate hypoxia induced by hydrocolloid dressings. In these patients, discontinue use.
	• Evaluate appropriateness of wound care protocol.
	• Evaluate patient for other impediments to wound healing.

UNEXPECTED OUTCOMES	RELATED INTERVENTIONS
2 Dressing does not stay in place.	• Evaluate size of dressing used for adequate margin (2.5 to 3.75 cm [1 to $1\frac{1}{2}$ inches]), or dry skin more thoroughly before reapplication.
	• Consider custom shapes for difficult body parts. "Picture frame" the edges of the hydrocolloid dressing using tape.
	• Dressing may be secured with roll gauze, tape, transparent dressing, or dressing sheet.
3 Periwound skin is macerated.	• Assess moisture-control property of dressing or application technique. May need new type of dressing.

Dressings: Transparent

A transparent film dressing is a clear, adherent, nonabsorptive, polyurethane sheet. Once it is applied, a moist exudate forms over the wound surface, which prevents tissue dehydration and allows for rapid, effective healing by speeding epithelial cell growth. The adhesive is inactivated by moisture and does not adhere to a moist surface. A transparent film has no absorbent capacity and is impermeable to fluids and bacteria (Rolstad, Bryant, and Nix, 2011). The dressings are appropriate for prophylaxis on high-risk intact skin (e.g., high-friction areas), superficial wounds with minimal or no exudate, and eschar-covered wounds when autolysis is indicated and safe (National Pressure Ulcer Advisory Panel [NPUAP] and European Pressure Ulcer Advisory Panel [EPUAP], 2009). Clinicians commonly use transparent dressings as the dressing of choice over an IV catheter insertion site.

Delegation Considerations

The skill of applying a transparent dressing for select wounds can be delegated to nursing assistive personnel (NAP) (refer to agency policy). The assessment of the wound and care of sterile or new acute wounds cannot be delegated to NAP. The nurse directs the NAP about:

- Explaining how to adapt the skill for a specific patient.
- Reporting any signs of bleeding, drainage, infection, or poor wound healing immediately to the nurse.

Equipment

- Sterile gloves (optional)
- Dressing set (optional)
- Sterile saline or other agent (as ordered)
- Clean gloves
- Cotton swabs
- Waterproof bag for disposal
- Transparent dressing (size as needed)
- Sterile gauze pads (4 × 4 inches)
- Skin preparation materials (optional)
- Moisture-proof gown, mask, goggles (used when spray from wound is a risk)

Implementation

STEP	RATIONALE
1 Complete preprocedure protocol.	
2 Identify patient using two identifiers (e.g., name and birthday or name and account number) according to agency policy.	Ensures correct patient. Complies with The Joint Commission requirements for patient safety (TJC, 2014).
3 Position patient to allow access to dressing site.	Facilitates application of dressing.
4 Close door or cubicle curtains; keep sheet or gown draped over body parts not requiring exposure.	Provides privacy and decreases transfer of microorganisms.
5 Expose wound site, minimizing exposure. Instruct patient not to touch wound or sterile supplies.	Dressing supplies become contaminated when touched by patient's hand.
6 Cuff top of disposable waterproof bag, and place within reach of work area.	Cuff prevents accidental contamination of tip of outer bag.
7 ⤳ Perform hand hygiene, and apply gloves. Don personal protective equipment (gown, mask, goggles as needed).	Reduces transmission of infectious organisms from soiled dressings to nurse's hands.
8 Remove old dressing by stretching film in direction parallel to wound rather than pulling.	Stretching action gently breaks dressing seal (Rolstad, Bryant, and Nix, 2011). Reduces excoriation, tearing, or irritation of skin after dressing removal.
9 Dispose of soiled dressings in waterproof bag, remove gloves by pulling them inside out, dispose of them in waterproof bag, and perform hand hygiene.	Reduces transmission of microorganisms.
10 Prepare dressing supplies. Use sterile supplies for new wounds.	Reduces risk for break in sterile technique.

STEP	RATIONALE
11 Pour saline or prescribed solution over 4 × 4–inch sterile gauze pads.	Maintains sterility of dressing.
12 ✈ Apply clean or sterile gloves (check agency policy).	Allows nurse to handle dressings.
13 Clean wound and periwound area gently with 4 × 4–inch sterile gauze pads moistened in sterile saline, or spray with wound cleanser. Clean from least to most contaminated area.	Reduces introduction of organisms into wound.
14 Pat-dry skin around wound thoroughly with dry 4 × 4–inch sterile gauze pads.	Transparent dressing with adhesive backing does not adhere to damp surface (Rolstad, Bryant, and Nix, 2011).
15 Inspect wound for tissue type, color, odor, and drainage; measure if indicated.	Provides a baseline for monitoring wound healing.
16 Remove gloves, and perform hand hygiene.	Reduces transmission of microorganisms.

SAFETY ALERT If wound has a large amount of drainage, choose another dressing that can absorb drainage.

17 ✈ Apply clean gloves. Apply transparent dressing according to manufacturer's directions. Do not stretch film during application, and avoid wrinkles.	Wrinkles provide tunnel for exudate drainage.
a Remove paper backing, taking care not to allow adhesive areas to touch each other.	
b Place film smoothly over wound without stretching (Fig. 20-1).	Ensures coverage of wound. Prevents shearing of skin from dressing that is too tight. Stretching can also break wound seal.

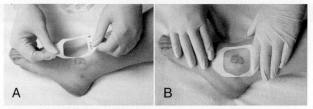

Fig. 20-1 **A,** Transparent dressing placed over small wound on ankle. **B,** Place film smoothly without stretching.

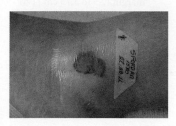

Fig. 20-2 Transparent dressing correctly labeled.

STEP	RATIONALE
c Use your fingers to smooth and adhere dressing. d Mark dressing with date, your initials, and time of dressing change on outer edge of dressing (Fig. 20-2). **18** Complete postprocedure protocol.	

Recording and Reporting

- Record appearance of wound, presence and characteristics of drainage, and presence of odor. Note patient response to dressing change.
- Report any signs of infection to the health care provider

UNEXPECTED OUTCOMES	RELATED INTERVENTIONS
1 Wound is inflamed, tender; drainage, necrosis, and/or an odor is present.	• Remove dressing, and obtain wound culture according to agency policy. • Different type of dressing may be required. • Notify health care provider.
2 Dressing does not stay in place.	• Evaluate size of dressing used for adequate wound margin (2.5 to 3.75 cm [1 to 1½ inches]). • Dry patient's skin thoroughly before reapplication.
3 Outer layer of patient's skin tears on removal of dressing.	• Adhesive backing may be too strong for fragile skin. • Consider other, non–adhesive-backed transparent dressing.

Ear Drop Administration

When administering ear medications, be aware of certain safety precautions. Internal ear structures are very sensitive to temperature extremes; administer ear drops at room temperature. Instilling cold drops can cause vertigo (severe dizziness) or nausea and debilitate a patient for several minutes. Although structures of the outer ear are not sterile, use sterile drops and solutions in case the eardrum is ruptured. A final safety precaution is to avoid forcing any solution into the ear. Do not occlude the ear canal with a medicine dropper because this can cause pressure within the canal during instillation and subsequent injury to the eardrum. If you follow these precautions, instillation of ear drops is a safe and effective therapy.

Delegation Considerations

The skill of administering ear medications cannot be delegated to nursing assistive personnel (NAP). The nurse directs the NAP about:

- Potential side effects of medications and reporting their occurrence to the nurse.

Equipment

- Medication bottle with dropper
- Cotton-tipped applicator, cotton balls *(optional)*
- Clean gloves
- Medication administration record (MAR)

Implementation

STEP	RATIONALE
1 Complete preprocedure protocol.	
2 Check accuracy and completeness of each MAR with prescriber's written medication order. Check patient's name, drug name and dosage, route of administration, number of drops to instill, ear (right, left, or both) to receive medication, and time for administration. Clarify	Ensures patient receives correct medication.

STEP	RATIONALE
incomplete or unclear orders with the prescriber before implementation.	
3 Identify patient using two identifiers (e.g., name and birthday or name and account number) according to agency policy. Compare identifiers with information on patient's MAR or medical record.	Ensures correct patient. Complies with The Joint Commission requirements for patient safety (TJC, 2014). Some agencies are now using a bar-code system to help with patient identification.
4 Discuss the purpose of each medication, action, and possible adverse effects. Allow patient to ask any questions about the drugs.	Patient has right to be informed, and patient's understanding of each medication improves adherence to drug therapy.
5 ![hand] Perform hand hygiene. Apply clean gloves (only if drainage is present).	Reduces transmission of microorganisms.
6 Warm medication to room temperature by running warm water over bottle (make sure not to damage label or allow water to enter bottle).	Ear structures are very sensitive to temperature extremes. Cold may cause vertigo and nausea.
7 Position patient on side (if not contraindicated) with ear to be treated facing up, or patient may sit in chair or at bedside. Stabilize patient's head with his or her own hand.	Facilitates distribution of medication into ear.
8 Straighten ear canal by pulling pinna up and back to 10 o'clock position (child older than age 3) or down and back to 6 to 9 o'clock position (child younger than age 3) (Fig. 21-1).	Straightening of ear canal provides direct access to deeper external ear structures. Anatomical differences in younger children and infants necessitate different methods of medication administration (Hockenberry and Wilson, 2011).

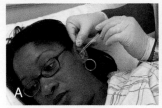 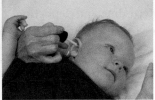

Fig. 21-1 **A,** Pull the pinna up and back for children older than 3 years.
B, Pull the pinna down and back for children 3 years of age or younger.

STEP	RATIONALE
9 If cerumen or drainage occludes outermost portion of ear canal, wipe out gently with cotton-tipped applicator. Do not use the cotton-tipped applicator to clean the ear canal. Take care not to force cerumen into ear canal.	Cerumen and drainage harbor microorganisms and can block distribution of medication into canal. Occlusion blocks sound transmission.
10 Instill prescribed drops holding dropper 1 cm ($\frac{1}{2}$ inch) above ear canal.	Avoiding contact prevents contamination of dropper, which could contaminate medication in container.
11 Ask the patient to remain in side-lying position for a few minutes. Apply gentle massage or pressure to tragus of ear with finger.	Allows complete distribution of medication. Pressure and massage move medication inward.
12 If ordered, gently insert portion of cotton ball into outermost part of canal. Do not press cotton into canal.	Prevents escape of medication when patient sits or stands.
13 Remove cotton after 15 minutes.	Allows for drug distribution and absorption.
14 Dispose of soiled supplies in proper receptacle, remove and dispose of gloves, and perform hand hygiene.	Reduces spread of microorganisms.

Recording and Reporting

- Record drug, concentration, dose or strength, number of drops, site of application (left, right, or both ears), and time of administration on MAR immediately after administration, not before. Include initials or signature. Record patient teaching and validation of understanding in the nurse's notes and electronic health record (EHR).
- Record objective data related to tissues involved (e.g., redness, drainage, irritation), any subjective data (e.g., pain, itching, altered hearing), and patient's response to medications. Note any side effects experienced in the nurses' notes and EHR.
- Report adverse effects/patient response and/or withheld drugs to nurse in charge or health care provider. Depending on medication, immediate health care provider notification may be required.

UNEXPECTED OUTCOMES	RELATED INTERVENTIONS
1 Ear canal remains inflamed, swollen, tender to palpation. Drainage is present.	• Notify health care provider for possible adjustment in medication type and dosage.
2 Patient's hearing acuity continues to be reduced.	• Notify health care provider. • Cerumen may be impacted, requiring ear irrigation.
3 Patient is unable to explain drug information and steps for drug instillation.	• Repeat instructions and include family caregiver as appropriate. Include return demonstration.

Ear Irrigations

The common indications for irrigation of the external ear are presence of foreign bodies, local inflammation, and buildup of cerumen in the ear canal. The procedure is not without potential hazards. Usually irrigations are performed with liquid warmed to body temperature to avoid vertigo or nausea in patients. The greatest danger during ear irrigation is rupture of the tympanic membrane by forcing irrigant into the canal under pressure.

Delegation Considerations

The skill of administering ear irrigation cannot be delegated to nursing assistive personnel (NAP). The nurse directs the NAP to:

- Immediately report any potential side effects of ear irrigation (e.g., pain, drainage, dizziness).
- Help a patient when ambulating because some light-headedness may be present, which increases the patient's risk for falling.

Equipment

- Clean gloves
- Irrigation syringe
- Basin for irrigation solution (use a sterile basin if a sterile irrigating solution is used)
- Emesis basis for drainage or irrigating solution exiting the ear
- Towel
- Cotton balls or 4×4–inch gauze
- Prescribed irrigation solution warmed to body temperature, or mineral oil, or over-the-counter softener
- Medication administration record (MAR)
- Otoscope *(optional)*

Implementation

STEP	RATIONALE
1 Complete preprocedure protocol.	
2 Review health care provider's medication order, including solution to be instilled and affected ear(s) (right, left, or both) to receive irrigation.	Ensures safe and correct administration of medication.

STEP	RATIONALE
3 Identify patient using two identifiers (e.g., name and birthday or name and account number) according to agency policy. Compare identifiers with information on patient's MAR or medical record.	Ensures correct patient. Complies with The Joint Commission requirements for patient safety (TJC, 2014).
4 Perform hand hygiene; arrange supplies at bedside.	Reduces transfer of microorganisms; helps nurse to perform procedure smoothly.
5 Close curtain or room door.	Maintains privacy.
6 Help patient to a sitting or lying position with head turned toward unaffected ear. Place towel under patient's head and shoulder, and have patient, if able, hold emesis basin under affected ear.	Position minimizes leakage of fluids around neck and facial area. Solution will flow from ear canal to basin.
7 Pour irrigating solution into basin. Check temperature of solution by pouring small drop on your inner forearm. NOTE: If a sterile irrigating solution is used, a sterile basin is required.	
8 ✋ Apply clean gloves. Gently clean auricle and outer ear canal with gauze or cotton balls. Do *not* force drainage or cerumen into the ear canal.	Prevents infected material from reentering ear canal. Forceful instillation of solution into occluded canal can cause injury to eardrum.
9 Fill irrigating syringe with solution (approximately 50 mL).	Enough fluid is needed to provide a steady irrigating stream.

STEP	RATIONALE
10 For adults and children older than age 3, gently pull pinna up and back; in children age 3 or younger, pull the pinna down and back (Hockenberry and Wilson, 2011).	Pulling pinna straightens external ear canal. Prevents obstruction of canal with device, which can lead to increased pressure on tympanic membrane.
11 Slowly instill irrigating solution by holding tip of syringe 1 cm ($\frac{1}{2}$ inch) above opening to ear canal. Direct the fluid toward the superior aspect of ear canal. Allow it to drain into basin during instillation. Continue until canal is cleansed or solution is used (Fig. 22-1).	Slow instillation prevents buildup of pressure in ear canal and ensures contact of solution with all canal surfaces.
12 Dry outer ear canal with cotton ball. Leave cotton loosely in place for 5 to 10 minutes.	Drying prevents buildup of moisture that can lead to otitis externa.
13 Help patient to a sitting position.	Maintains comfort.
14 Remove gloves, dispose of supplies, and perform hand hygiene.	Reduces transmission of infection.

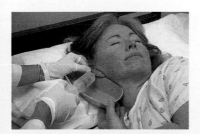

Fig. 22-1 **Tip of syringe does not occlude ear canal during irrigation.**

Recording and Reporting

- Record in the nurses' notes, electronic health record (EHR), and/ or MAR the procedure, amount of solution instilled, time of administration, and ear receiving irrigation.
- Record appearance of external ear and patient's hearing acuity in the nurses' notes and EHR.
- Report adverse effects/patient response and/or withheld drugs to nurse in charge or health care provider.

UNEXPECTED OUTCOMES	RELATED INTERVENTIONS
1 Patient complains of increased ear pain during irrigation.	• Rupture of eardrum may have occurred. Stop irrigations immediately, and notify health care provider immediately.
2 Ear canal remains occluded with cerumen.	• Repeat irrigation.
3 Foreign body remains in ear canal.	• Refer patient to an otolaryngologist if a foreign object remains after irrigation.
4 Patient is unable to explain ear care practices.	• Reinstruction is necessary. • Include family members or caregivers if possible.

Enemas

An enema is the instillation of a solution into the rectum and sigmoid colon to promote defecation by stimulating peristalsis. Cleansing enemas promote complete evacuation of feces from the colon. They act by stimulating peristalsis through infusion of large volumes of solution. Oil-retention enemas act by lubricating the rectum and colon, allowing feces to absorb oil and become softer and easier to pass. Medicated enemas contain pharmacological therapeutic agents. Some are pre-scribed to reduce dangerously high serum potassium levels (e.g., sodium polystyrene sulfonate [Kayexalate] enema) or to reduce bacteria in the colon before bowel surgery (e.g., neomycin enema).

Delegation Considerations

The skill of enema administration can be delegated to nursing assistive personnel (NAP) unless medication is instilled via an enema. The nurse directs the NAP about:

- Properly positioning patients who have mobility restrictions or therapeutic equipment such as drains, IV catheters, or traction.
- Informing nurse about patient's new abdominal pain (*exception:* a patient reports abdominal cramping) or rectal bleeding.
- Informing the nurse immediately about the presence of blood in the stool or around the rectal area, or about any change in the patient's vital signs.

Equipment

- Clean gloves
- Water-soluble lubricant
- Waterproof, absorbent pads
- Toilet tissue
- Bedpan, bedside commode, or access to toilet
- Basin, washcloths, towel, and soap
- IV pole
- Stethoscope

Enema Bag Administration

- Enema container with tubing and clamp
- Appropriate-size rectal tube (adult: 22 to 30 Fr; child: 12 to 18 Fr)
- Correct volume of warmed (tepid) solution (adult: 750 to 1000 mL; adolescent: 500 to 700 mL; school-age child: 300 to 500 mL; toddler: 250 to 350 mL; infant: 150 to 250 mL)

Prepackaged Enema

- Prepackaged enema container with lubricated rectal tip

Implementation

STEP	RATIONALE
1 Complete preprocedure protocol.	

SAFETY ALERT "Enemas until clear" order means that you repeat enemas until patient passes fluid that is clear of fecal matter. Check agency policy, but usually patient should receive only three consecutive enemas to avoid disruption of fluid and electrolyte balance. It is essential to observe contents of solution passed.

2 Help patient turn onto left side-lying (Sims') position with right knee flexed. Encourage him or her to remain in position until procedure is complete. Children are placed in dorsal recumbent position.	Allows enema solution to flow downward by gravity along natural curve of sigmoid colon and rectum, thus improving retention of solution.

SAFETY ALERT Patients with poor sphincter control require placement of a bedpan under the buttocks. Administering enema with patient sitting on toilet is unsafe because curved rectal tubing can abrade rectal wall.

3 Lower side rail on working side and place waterproof pad, absorbent side up, under hips and buttocks. Cover patient with bath blanket, exposing only rectal area, clearly visualizing anus.	Pad prevents soiling of linen. Blanket provides warmth, reduces exposure of body parts, and allows patient to feel more relaxed and comfortable.
4 Separate buttocks, and examine perianal region for abnormalities, including hemorrhoids, anal fissure, and rectal prolapse.	Findings influence approach for inserting enema tip. Prolapse contraindicates enema.
5 Administer enema:	
a Administer prepackaged disposable enema:	
(1) Remove plastic cap from tip of container.	Lubrication provides for smooth insertion of rectal tube without

STEP	RATIONALE
Tip may be already lubricated. Apply more water-soluble lubricant as needed.	causing rectal irritation or trauma. With presence of hemorrhoids, extra lubricant provides added comfort.
(2) Gently separate buttocks, and locate anus. Instruct patient to relax by breathing out slowly through mouth.	Breathing out promotes relaxation of external rectal sphincter.
(3) Expel any air from the enema container.	Introducing air into colon causes further distention and discomfort.
(4) Insert lubricated tip of container gently into anal canal toward the umbilicus (Fig. 23-1). *Adult:* 7.5 to 10 cm (3 to 4 inches) *Adolescent:* 7.5 to 10 cm (3 to 4 inches) *Child:* 5 to 7.5 cm (2 to 3 inches) *Infant:* 2.5 to 3.75 cm (1 to 1½ inches)	Gentle insertion prevents trauma to rectal mucosa.

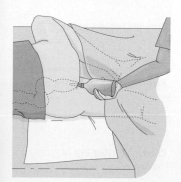

Fig. 23-1 With patient in left lateral Sims' position, insert tip of commercial enema into rectum. (From Sorrentino SA: *Mosby's textbook for nursing assistants,* ed 7, St Louis, 2009, Mosby.)

STEP	RATIONALE

SAFETY ALERT If pain occurs or you feel resistance at any time during procedure, stop and discuss with health care provider. Do not force insertion.

(5) Roll plastic bottle from bottom to tip until all of solution has entered rectum. Instruct patient to retain solution until urge to defecate occurs, usually 2 to 5 minutes.	Prevents instillation of air into colon and ensures all content enters rectum. Hypertonic solutions require only small volumes to stimulate defecation.
b Administer enema using enema bag:	
(1) Add warmed solution to enema bag: Warm tap water as it flows from faucet, place saline container in basin of warm water before adding saline to enema bag, and check temperature of solution by pouring small amount of solution over inner wrist.	Hot water burns intestinal mucosa. Cold water causes abdominal cramping and is difficult to retain.
(2) If soap suds enema (SSE) is ordered, add castile soap after water.	Prevents bubbles in bag.
(3) Raise container, release clamp, and allow solution to flow long enough to fill tubing.	Removes air from tubing.
(4) Reclamp tubing.	Prevents further loss of solution.

STEP	RATIONALE
(5) Lubricate 6 to 8 cm (2½ to 3 inches) of tip of rectal tube with lubricant.	Allows smooth insertion of rectal tube without risk for irritation or trauma to mucosa.
(6) Gently separate buttocks, and locate anus. Instruct patient to relax by breathing out slowly through mouth. Touch patient's skin next to anus with tip of rectal tube.	Breathing out and touching skin with the tube promote relaxation of external anal sphincter.
(7) Insert tip of rectal tube slowly by pointing it in direction of patient's umbilicus. Length of insertion varies: *Adult:* 7.5 to 10 cm (3 to 4 inches) *Adolescent:* 7.5 to 10 cm (3 to 4 inches) *Child:* 5 to 7.5 cm (2 to 3 inches) *Infant:* 2.5 to 3.75 cm (1 to 1½ inches)	Careful insertion prevents trauma to rectal mucosa from accidental lodging of tube against rectal wall. Insertion beyond proper limit causes bowel perforation.

SAFETY ALERT If tube does not pass easily, do not force. Consider allowing a small amount of fluid to infuse, and then try to reinsert the tube slowly. The instillation of liquid relaxes the sphincter and provides additional lubrication. Remove an impaction before administering the enema.

(8) Hold tubing in rectum constantly until end of fluid instillation.	Prevents expulsion of rectal tube during bowel contractions.
(9) Open regulating clamp and allow solution to enter	Rapid instillation stimulates evacuation of tubing and can cause cramping.

STEP	RATIONALE
slowly with container at patient's hip level.	
(10) Raise height of enema container slowly to appropriate level above anus: 30 to 45 cm (12 to 18 inches) for high enema, 30 cm (12 inches) for regular enema, 7.5 cm (3 inches) for low enema. Instillation time varies with volume of solution administered (e.g., 1 L/10 min) (Fig. 23-2). You may use an IV pole to hold an enema bag once you get a slow flow of fluid established.	Allows for continuous, slow instillation of solution. Raising container too high causes rapid instillation and possible painful distention of colon. High pressure causes rupture of bowel in infant.

SAFETY ALERT Temporary cessation of infusion minimizes cramping and promotes ability to retain solution. Lower container or clamp tubing if patient complains of cramping or if fluid escapes around rectal tube.

STEP	RATIONALE
(11) Instill all solution and clamp tubing. Tell patient that procedure is completed and that you will be removing tubing.	Prevents entrance of air into rectum. Patients may misinterpret sensation of removing tube as loss of control.
6 Place layers of toilet tissue around tube at anus and gently withdraw rectal tube and tip.	Provides for patient's comfort and cleanliness.

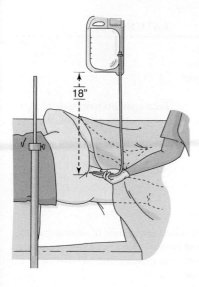

Fig. 23-2 Enema is given in Sims' position. IV pole is positioned so that enema bag is 18 inches above anus.

18"

STEP	RATIONALE
7 Explain to patient that some distention and abdominal cramping are normal. Ask patient to retain solution as long as possible until urge to defecate occurs. This usually takes a few minutes. Stay at bedside. Have patient lie quietly in bed if possible. (For infant or young child, gently hold buttocks together for few minutes.)	Solution distends bowel. Length of retention varies with type of enema and patient's ability to contract rectal sphincter. Longer retention promotes stimulation of peristalsis and defecation.
8 Discard enema container and tubing in proper receptacle.	Reduces transmission and growth of microorganisms.
9 Help patient to bathroom or commode if possible. If using bedpan, help to as near normal position for evacuation as possible.	Normal squatting position promotes defecation.

STEP	RATIONALE
10 Observe characteristics of stool and solution. (Caution patient against flushing toilet before inspection.)	
11 Help patient as needed to wash anal area with warm soap and water (if nurse administers perineal care, use gloves).	Fecal contents irritate skin. Hygiene promotes patient's comfort.
12 Complete postprocedure protocol.	

Recording and Reporting

- Record type and volume of enema given, time of administration, characteristics of results, and patient's tolerance of the procedure.
- Report the failure of the patient to defecate and any adverse effects to health care provider.

UNEXPECTED OUTCOMES	RELATED INTERVENTIONS
1 Severe abdominal cramping, bleeding, or sudden abdominal pain develops and is unrelieved by temporarily stopping or slowing flow of solution.	• Stop enema. • Notify health care provider.
2 Patient is unable to hold enema solution.	• If this occurs during installation, slow rate of infusion.

Enteral Nutrition via a Gastrostomy or Jejunostomy Tube

Feeding tubes can be placed directly into the gastrointestinal (GI) tract through the abdominal wall in patients who cannot tolerate nasoenteric feeding tubes or require long-term enteral nutrition. The stomach (gastrostomy tube) and jejunum (jejunostomy tube) are the most common sites for long-term feeding tubes. Feedings delivered via a gastrostomy tube are relatively safe to administer, provided the patient has normal gastric emptying. Gastrostomy tubes are often called *G tubes* but are also referred to as percutaneous endoscopic gastrostomy *(PEG)* tubes. Gastrostomy tubes range in size from 16 Fr to 28 Fr and exit through an incision in the upper left quadrant of the abdomen, where an internal bumper or balloon and an external bumper or disk hold the tube in place (Fig. 24-1).

Jejunostomy tubes are indicated when the risk of regurgitation and aspiration is especially high. Jejunostomy tubes can be placed into the small intestine in a surgical procedure or threaded through the stomach into the jejunum under fluoroscopy. The percutaneous endoscopic jejunostomy (PEJ) tube is passed through the PEG and advanced into the jejunum (Fig. 24-2).

Delegation Considerations

The skill of administration of nasoenteral tube feeding can be delegated to nursing assistive personnel (NAP). However, a registered nurse (RN) or licensed practical nurse (LPN) must first verify tube placement and patency. The nurse directs the NAP to:

- Elevate the head of bed to a minimum of 30 degrees (preferably 45 degrees) or sit the patient up in bed or a chair.
- Not adjust feeding rate; infuse the feeding as ordered.
- Report any difficulty infusing the feeding or any discomfort voiced by the patient.
- Report any gagging, paroxysms of coughing, or choking.

Equipment

- Disposable feeding bag, tubing, or ready-to-hang system
- 60-mL or larger catheter-tip syringe
- Stethoscope

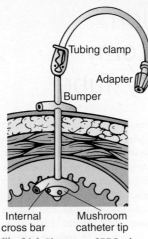

Internal cross bar   Mushroom catheter tip

Fig. 24-1 Placement of PEG tube into stomach.

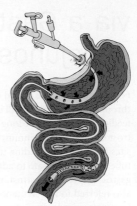

Fig. 24-2 Endoscopic insertion of jejunostomy tube.

- Enteral infusion pump
- pH indicator strip (scale 0.0 to 11.0)
- Prescribed enteral formula
- Clean gloves
- Equipment to obtain blood glucose level by fingerstick, if ordered

Implementation

STEP	RATIONALE
1 Complete preprocedure protocol.	
2 Perform hand hygiene. Apply clean gloves (Bankhead et al., 2009).	Reduces transmission of microorganisms and potential contamination of enteral formula.
3 Obtain formula to administer:	
a Verify correct formula and check expiration date; note condition of container.	Ensures that correct therapy is administered and checks integrity of formula.
b Provide formula at room temperature.	Cold formula causes gastric cramping and discomfort because liquid is not warmed by mouth and esophagus.

STEP	RATIONALE
4 Prepare formula for administration:	
a Use aseptic technique when manipulating components of feeding system (e.g., formula, administration set, connections).	Bag, connections, and tubing must be free of contamination to prevent bacterial growth (Bankhead et al., 2009).
b Shake formula container well. Clean top of canned formula with alcohol swab before opening it (Bankhead et al., 2009).	Ensures integrity of formula; prevents transmission of microorganisms.
c For closed systems, connect administration tubing to container. If using open system, pour formula from brick pack or can into administration bag.	Formulas are available in closed-system containers that contain a 24- to 48-hour supply of formula or in an open system, in which formula must be transferred from brick packs or cans to a bag before administration.
5 Open roller clamp and allow administration tubing to fill. Clamp off tubing with roller clamp. Hang container on intravenous (IV) pole.	Prevents introduction of air into stomach once feeding begins.
6 Place patient in high-Fowler's position or elevate head of bed at least 30 degrees (preferably 45 degrees). For patient forced to remain supine, place in reverse Trendelenburg's position.	Elevated head helps prevent pulmonary aspiration.
7 Verify tube placement (see Skill 43). Observe appearance of aspirate and note pH measurement.	Verifies if tip of tube is in stomach or intestine based on pH value.

STEP	RATIONALE
8 Check gastric residual volume (GRV) before each feeding (for bolus and intermittent feedings) and every 4 to 6 hours (for continuous feedings) (Metheny et al., 2008; Bankhead et al., 2009).	GRV determines if gastric emptying is delayed. Intestinal residual is usually very small. If residual volume is greater than 10 mL, displacement of tube into stomach may have occurred.
a Draw up 10 to 30 mL of air into syringe and connect to end of feeding tube.	
b Inject air into tube. Pull back slowly and aspirate total amount of gastric contents.	
c Return aspirated contents to stomach unless volume exceeds 250 mL (see agency policy) (Metheny, 2010).	Prevents loss of nutrients and electrolytes in discarded fluid. Some questions exist regarding safety of returning high volumes of fluid into stomach (Metheny, 2010).
d Do not administer feeding when a single GRV measurement exceeds 500 mL or when two measurements taken 1 hour apart each exceed 250 mL (Bankhead et al., 2009) (check agency policy).	Some controversy exists regarding ability of elevated GRVs to identify risk for pulmonary aspiration. However, frequent interruptions of feeding based on GRV levels is a well-recognized reason for failure to meet nutritional goals (Bankhead et al., 2009; DeLegge, 2011; Metheny et al., 2008).
e Flush feeding tube with 30 mL water (see Skill 43).	Prevents clogging of tubing.
9 Before attaching feeding administration set to feeding tube, trace tube to its point of origin. Label administration set "Tube Feeding Only."	Avoids misconnections between feeding set and IV systems or other medical tubing or devices (Bankhead et al., 2009; Simmons et al., 2011).

STEP	RATIONALE
10 Intermittent gravity drip:	
a Pinch proximal end of feeding tube, and remove cap. Connect distal end of administration set tubing to feeding tube and release tubing.	Prevents excessive air from entering patient's stomach and leakage of gastric contents.
b Set rate by adjusting roller clamp on tubing or placing on a feeding pump. Allow bag to empty gradually over 30 to 45 minutes. Label bag with tube-feeding type, strength, and amount. Include date, time, and initials.	Gradual emptying of tube feeding by gravity from feeding bag reduces risk for abdominal discomfort, vomiting, or diarrhea induced by bolus or too-rapid infusion of tube feedings.
c Change bag every 24 hours.	Decreases risk for bacterial colonization.
11 Continuous drip method:	Continuous feeding method is designed to deliver prescribed hourly rate of feeding. This method reduces risk for abdominal discomfort.
a Connect distal end of administration set tubing to proximal end of feeding tube as in Step 10a.	
b Thread tubing through feeding pump; set rate on pump and turn on (see Skill 25).	Delivers continuous feeding at a steady rate and pressure. Feeding pump alarms for increased resistance.

SAFETY ALERT Maximum hang time for formula is 12 hours in an open system, and 24 to 48 hours in a closed, ready-to-hang system (if it remains closed). Refer to manufacturer's guidelines.

SAFETY ALERT Use pumps designated for tube feeding (not intravenous fluids).

| 12 Advance rate of tube feeding gradually, as ordered. | Tube feeding can usually begin with full-strength formula. |

STEP	RATIONALE
	Gradual advancement to goal rates helps to prevent diarrhea and gastric intolerance to formula (Bankhead et al., 2009).
13 Flush tubing with 30 mL of water every 4 hours during continuous feeding (see agency policy), before and after an intermittent feeding. Have registered dietitian recommend total free water requirement per day and obtain health care provider's order.	Provides patient with source of water to help maintain fluid and electrolyte balance. Clears tubing of formula.
14 When patient is receiving intermittent tube feeding, cap or clamp end of feeding tube when not being used.	Prevents air from entering stomach between feedings and limits microbial contamination of system.
15 Rinse bag and tubing with warm water whenever feedings are interrupted. Use a new administration set every 24 hours.	Rinsing bag and tubing with warm water clears old tube feedings and reduces bacterial growth.
16 Complete postprocedure protocol.	

Recording and Reporting

- Record and report amount and type of feeding, method of infusion, patient's response to tube feeding (e.g., GRV, cramping), patency of tube, condition of skin at tube site.
- Record volume of formula and any additional water on intake and output form.
- Report type of feeding, status of feeding tube, patient's tolerance, and adverse outcomes.

UNEXPECTED OUTCOMES	RELATED INTERVENTIONS
1 Feeding tube becomes clogged.	• Attempt to flush tube with water. • Special products are available for unclogging

UNEXPECTED OUTCOMES	RELATED INTERVENTIONS
	feeding tubes; do not use soda and juice.
	• Hold feeding and notify health care provider.
	• Maintain patient in semi-Fowler's position
2 GRV exceeds 250 mL or cutoff per agency policy.	• Recheck residual in 1 hour (see agency policy).
	• Notify health care provider if GRV remains high (typically hold feeding if residual >250 mL two consecutive checks).
3 The patient develops large amount of diarrhea (more than three loose stools in less than 24 hours).	• Notify health care provider. Consult dietitian about need to change formula.
	• Consider other causes such as *Clostridium difficile* infection or bacterial contamination of feeding (Bankhead et al., 2009).
	• Determine if patient is receiving medications (e.g., containing sorbitol) that induce diarrhea (Btaiche et al., 2010).
	• Provide perineal skin care after each stool.
4 Patient develops nausea and vomiting, which may indicate paralytic ileus	• Withhold tube feeding, and notify health care provider.
5 Aspirated fluid has foul odor or unusual appearance.	• Notify the health care provider.
	• Do not return aspirated material of unusual odor or appearance without first consulting health care provider.
6 Skin around gastrostomy or jejunostomy site deteriorates.	• Institute skin care.
	• Use pressure-relief measures around tube.
	• Provide wound care.

Enteral Nutrition via a Nasoenteric Feeding Tube

Enteral nutrition, or tube feeding, is a method for providing nutrients to patients who are not able to meet their nutritional requirements orally. As a rule, candidates for enteral nutrition must have a sufficiently functional gastrointestinal (GI) tract to absorb nutrients. Examples of indications for enteral feeding include the following:

- Situations in which normal eating is not safe because of high risk for aspiration.
- Clinical conditions that interfere with normal ingestion or absorption of nutrients or create hypermetabolic states: surgical resection of oropharynx, proximal intestinal obstruction or fistula, pancreatitis, burns, and severe pressure ulcers.
- Conditions in which disease or treatment-related symptoms reduce oral intake: anorexia, nausea, pain, fatigue, shortness of breath, or depression.

Gastric feedings are the most common type of enteral nutrition, allowing tube-feeding formulas to enter the stomach and then pass gradually through the intestinal tract to ensure absorption. In contrast, small bowel feeding occurs beyond the pyloric sphincter of the stomach, which theoretically reduces the risk for pulmonary aspiration, provided that feedings do not reflux into the stomach (Metheny et al., 2011).

Delegation Considerations

The skill of administration of nasoenteric tube feeding can be delegated to nursing assistive personnel (NAP). However, a registered nurse (RN) or licensed practical nurse (LPN) must first verify tube placement and patency. The nurse directs the NAP to:

- Elevate the head of bed to a minimum of 30 degrees (preferably 45 degrees) or sit the patient up in bed or a chair.
- Not adjust feeding rate; infuse the feeding as ordered.
- Report any difficulty infusing the feeding or any discomfort voiced by the patient.
- Report any gagging, paroxysms of coughing, or choking.
- Provide frequent oral hygiene.

Equipment

- Disposable feeding bag, tubing, and formula or ready-to-hang system
- 60-mL or larger catheter-tip syringe
- Stethoscope
- Enteral infusion pump for continuous feedings
- pH indicator strip (scale 0.0 to 11.0)
- Prescribed enteral formula
- Clean gloves

Implementation

STEP	RATIONALE
1 Complete preprocedure protocol.	
2 Obtain formula to administer:	
a Verify correct formula and check expiration date; note condition of container.	Ensures that correct therapy is administered and checks integrity of formula.
b Provide formula at room temperature.	Cold formula causes gastric cramping and discomfort because liquid is not warmed by mouth and esophagus.
3 Prepare formula for administration:	
a Use aseptic technique when manipulating components of feeding system (e.g., formula, administration set, connections).	Bag, connections, and tubing must be free of contamination to prevent bacterial growth (Bankhead et al., 2009).
b Shake formula container well. Clean top of canned formula with alcohol swab before opening it (Bankhead et al., 2009).	Ensures integrity of formula; prevents transmission of microorganisms.
c For closed systems, connect administration tubing to container. If using open system,	Formulas are available in closed-system containers that contain a 24- to 48-hour supply of formula or in an

STEP	RATIONALE
pour formula from brick pack or can into administration bag.	open system, in which formula must be transferred from brick packs or cans to a bag before administration.
4 Open roller clamp and allow administration tubing to fill. Clamp off tubing with roller clamp. Hang container on intravenous (IV) pole.	Prevents introduction of air into stomach once feeding begins.
5 Place patient in high-Fowler's position or elevate head of bed at least 30 degrees (preferably 45 degrees). For patient forced to remain supine, place in reverse Trendelenburg's position.	Elevated head helps prevent pulmonary aspiration.
6 Verify placement of tube. Observe appearance of aspirate and note pH measurement.	Verifies if tip of tube is in stomach or intestine based on pH value.
7 Check gastric residual volume (GRV) before each feeding (for bolus and intermittent feedings) or every 4 to 6 hours (for continuous feedings) (Fig. 25-1) (Metheny et al., 2008; Bankhead et al., 2009).	GRV determines if gastric emptying is delayed. Intestinal residual is usually very small. If residual volume is greater than 10 mL, displacement of tube into stomach may have occurred.

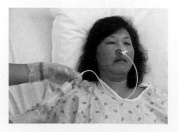

Fig. 25-1 Check for gastric residual volume (GRV).

STEP	RATIONALE
a Draw up 10 to 30 mL of air into syringe and connect to end of feeding tube.	
b Inject air into tube. Pull back slowly and aspirate total amount of gastric contents.	
c Return aspirated contents to stomach unless volume exceeds 250 mL (see agency policy) (Metheny, 2010).	Prevents loss of nutrients and electrolytes in discarded fluid. Some questions exist regarding safety of returning high volumes of fluid into stomach (Metheny, 2010).
d Do not administer feeding when a single GRV measurement exceeds 500 mL or when two measurements taken 1 hour apart each exceed 250 mL (Bankhead et al., 2009) (check agency policy).	Some controversy exists regarding ability of elevated GRVs to identify risk for pulmonary aspiration. However, frequent interruptions of feeding based on GRV levels is a well-recognized reason for failure to meet nutritional goals (Bankhead et al., 2009; DeLegge, 2011; Metheny et al., 2008).
e Flush feeding tube with 30 mL of water.	Prevents clogging of tubing.
8 Before attaching feeding administration set to feeding tube, trace tube to its point of origin. Label administration set "Tube Feeding Only."	Avoids misconnections between feeding set and IV systems or other medical tubing or devices (Bankhead et al., 2009; Simmons et al., 2011).
9 Intermittent gravity drip:	
a Pinch proximal end of feeding tube and remove cap. Connect distal end of administration set tubing to feeding tube and release tubing.	Prevents excessive air from entering patient's stomach and leakage of gastric contents.

STEP	RATIONALE
b Set rate by adjusting roller clamp on tubing, or attach tubing to feeding pump. Allow bag to empty gradually over 30 to 45 minutes. Label bag with tube-feeding type, strength, and amount. Include date, time, and initials.	Gradual emptying of tube feeding reduces risk for abdominal discomfort, vomiting, or diarrhea induced by bolus or extremely rapid infusion of tube feedings.
c Change bag every 24 hours.	Decreases risk for bacterial colonization.
10 Continuous drip method:	Continuous feeding method is designed to deliver prescribed hourly rate of feeding and reduce risk for abdominal discomfort.
a Connect distal end of administration set tubing to feeding tube as in Step 9a.	
b Thread tubing through feeding pump; set rate on pump and turn on (Fig. 25-2).	Delivers continuous feeding at steady rate and pressure. Feeding pump alarms for increased resistance.

SAFETY ALERT Maximum hang time for formula is 12 hours in an open system; 24 to 48 hours in a closed, ready-to-hang system (if it remains closed). Refer to manufacturer's guidelines.

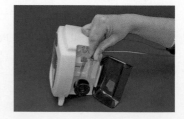

Fig. 25-2 Connect tubing through infusion pump. (Image used with permission of Covidien. All rights reserved.)

STEP	RATIONALE
11 Advance rate of tube feeding gradually, as ordered.	Tube feeding can usually begin with full-strength formula. Gradual advancement to goal rates helps to prevent diarrhea and gastric intolerance to formula (Bankhead et al., 2009).
12 Flush tubing with 30 mL of water every 4 hours during continuous feeding (see agency policy) and before and after an intermittent feeding. Have registered dietitian recommend total free water requirement per day and obtain health care provider's order.	Provides patient with source of water to help maintain fluid and electrolyte balance. Clears tubing of formula.
13 When patient is receiving intermittent tube feeding, cap or clamp end of feeding tube when not being used.	Prevents air from entering stomach between feedings and limits microbial contamination of system.
14 Rinse bag and tubing with warm water whenever feedings are interrupted. Use new administration set every 24 hours.	Rinsing bag and tubing with warm water clears old tube feedings and reduces bacterial growth.
15 Complete postprocedure protocol.	

Recording and Reporting

- Record and report amount and type of feeding, method of infusion, response of patient to tube feeding, patency of tube, and condition of skin at tube site.
- Record volume of formula and any additional water on intake and output form.
- Report type of feeding, status of feeding tube, tolerance of patient, and adverse outcomes.

UNEXPECTED OUTCOMES	RELATED INTERVENTIONS
1 The feeding tube becomes clogged.	• Attempt to flush the tube with water.
	• Special products are available for unclogging feeding tubes; do not use soda and juice.
	• Hold feeding and notify health care provider.
	• Maintain patient in semi-Fowler's position.
2 Gastric residual volume is excessive.	• Recheck residual in 1 hour (see agency policy). Notify health care provider if GRV remains high (typically hold feeding if residual >250 mL for two consecutive checks).
3 Patient aspirates formula.	• See interventions following Skill 43.
4 The patient develops a large amount of diarrhea (more than three loose stools in less than 24 hours).	• Notify health care provider, and consult dietitian about need to change formula.
	• Consider other causes such as *Clostridium difficile* infection or bacterial contamination of feeding (Bankhead et al., 2009).
	• Provide perianal skin care after each stool.
	• Determine if patient is receiving medications (e.g., containing sorbitol) that induce diarrhea (Btaiche et al., 2010).
5 Patient develops nausea and vomiting, which may indicate paralytic ileus.	• Withhold tube feeding, and notify health care provider.
	• Ensure tubing is patent; aspirate for residual.

UNEXPECTED OUTCOMES	RELATED INTERVENTIONS
6 Aspirated fluid has foul odor or unusual appearance.	• Notify the health care provider. • Do not return aspirated material of unusual odor or appearance without first consulting health care provider.
7 Skin around gastrostomy or jejunostomy site breaks down.	• Notify health care provider. • Institute skin care.

Epidural Analgesia

Administration of analgesics into the epidural space is an efficient intervention to manage acute pain (D'Arcy, 2011). The epidural space is a potential space that contains a network of vessels, nerves, and fat located between the vertebral column and the dura mater, the outermost meninges covering the spinal cord (Fig. 26-1). Analgesics delivered into this space are distributed by (1) diffusion through the dura mater into the cerebrospinal fluid (CSF), where they act directly on the receptors in the dorsal horn of the spinal cord; (2) circulation of blood vessels in the epidural space, from which they are delivered systemically; and/or (3) absorption by fat in the epidural space, creating a depot where the analgesia is slowly released systemically.

Opioids and local anesthetics, separately or in combination, are often used in epidural analgesia. Opioids are delivered close to their site of action (central nervous system) and thus require much smaller doses to achieve the same degree of pain relief (D'Arcy, 2009; D'Arcy, 2011). Common opioids administered epidurally include morphine, hydromorphone (Dilaudid), fentanyl, and sufentanil.

A patient should be placed in the lateral side-lying or sitting position with the shoulders and hips in alignment and the hips and head flexed during insertion of an epidural catheter. An anesthesia provider places a catheter into the epidural space below the second lumbar vertebra, where the spinal cord ends (Fig. 26-2). However, epidurals may also be placed at the thoracic level of the spinal cord. Catheters intended for temporary or short-term use are not sutured in place and exit from the insertion site on the back. A catheter intended for permanent or long-term use is "tunneled" subcutaneously and exits on the side of the body (Fig. 26-3) or on the abdomen. Tunneling reduces the risk for infection and catheter dislodgement. A sterile occlusive dressing covers the catheter exit site and is secured to the patient. An x-ray film is the only way to confirm epidural catheter placement.

The use of epidural opioids requires astute nursing observation and care. The catheter poses a threat to patient safety because of its anatomical location, its potential for migration through the dura, and its proximity to spinal nerves and vessels (Pasero and McCaffery, 2011). Catheter migration into the subarachnoid space can produce dangerously high medication levels. Monitor a patient's motor and sensory function, including any onset of urinary retention. You should not administer other supplemental opioids or sedatives when patients have been administered an epidural because the combined effect may cause respiratory depression. In many health care agencies anesthesiologists

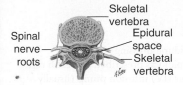

Spinal nerve roots — Skeletal vertebra — Epidural space — Skeletal vertebra

Fig. 26-1 Anatomical drawing of epidural space. (Reprinted from www.netterimages.com Elsevier, Inc. All rights reserved.)

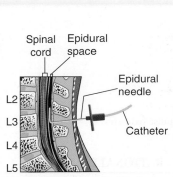

Fig. 26-2 Placement of epidural catheter.

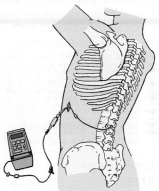

Fig. 26-3 Epidural catheter attached to ambulatory infusion pump. (Image courtesy Astra Zeneca Pharmaceuticals, Wilmington, Del. All rights reserved.)

and nurse anesthetists are the only health care providers who may initiate epidural opioid infusions or administer a medication bolus.

Delegation Considerations

The skill of epidural analgesia administration cannot be delegated to nursing assistive personnel (NAP). The nurse directs the NAP to:

- Pay particular attention to the insertion site when repositioning or ambulating patients to prevent catheter disruption.
- Avoid pulling the patient up in bed while he or she is lying flat on the back, which can dislodge the epidural catheter.
- Immediately report to the nurse any change in level of consciousness.
- Report any catheter disconnection immediately.
- Immediately report to the nurse any change in patient status or comfort level.

Equipment

- Clean gloves
- Sterile gloves (if removing epidural dressing)
- Prediluted preservative-free opioid as prescribed by health care provider for use in intravenous (IV) infusion pump (usually prepared by pharmacy)
- Infusion pump and compatible tubing (Do not use Y-ports for continuous infusion; some infusion pumps have color-coded tubing for intraspinal use.)
- 20-gauge needleless adapter
- Filter needle (per agency policy)
- Syringe
- Antiseptic swab
- Sterile gauze pad
- Tape
- Label (for injection port)
- Equipment for vital signs and pulse oximetry

Implementation

STEP	RATIONALE
1 Complete preprocedure protocol.	
2 Verify that catheter is secured to patient's skin from the back or front.	Prevents dislodging or migration of catheter.
3 Assess catheter insertion site for redness, warmth, tenderness, swelling, and drainage. Apply sterile gloves when removing occlusive dressing.	Catheter sites are at risk for local infections. Purulent drainage is a sign of infection. Clear drainage may indicate CSF leakage from punctured dura. Bloody drainage may indicate that catheter entered blood vessel.
4 Verify health care provider's order against medication administration record (MAR) for name of medication, dosage, route, infusion method (bolus, continuous, or demand), and lockout settings.	Ensures that right drug is administered to patient. *This is the first check for accuracy.*

STEP	RATIONALE
5 For continuous infusion check patency of IV tubing and check infusion pump for proper calibration and operation. Keep IV line patent for 24 hours after epidural analgesia is completed.	Kinked or clamped tubing will interrupt analgesic infusion; may cause clotting at end of IV catheter and require replacement. Patent IV line allows IV access in case medications are needed to counteract adverse reactions.
6 Prepare analgesia, following "six rights" of medication administration. NOTE: Pharmacy prepares medication for pump. In the case of a bolus injection, draw up prediluted, preservative-free opioid solution through the filter needle into syringe.	Ensures safe and appropriate medication administration. *This is the second check for accuracy.*
7 Identify patient using two identifiers (e.g., name and birthday or name and account number) according to agency policy. Compare identifiers with information on patient's MAR or medical record.	Ensures correct patient. Complies with The Joint Commission requirements for patient safety (TJC, 2014).
8 Attach "epidural line" label to the epidural infusion tubing. Be sure that there are *no Y-ports* for continuous or demand infusions.	Labeling helps to ensure that analgesic medication is administered into correct line and epidural space. Labeling of high-risk catheters prevents connection with an inappropriate tube or catheter (TJC, 2014). Using tubing without Y-ports prevents accidental injection or infusion of other medications.
9 At bedside compare the MAR or computer printout with the name of medication on the drug container.	*This is the third check for accuracy* and ensures that the right patient receives the right medication.

STEP	RATIONALE
10 ![icon] Perform hand hygiene, and apply clean gloves.	
11 Administer continuous infusion:	
a Attach container of diluted, preservative-free medication to infusion pump tubing, and prime tubing (see Skill 55).	Tubing should be filled with solution and free of air bubbles to avoid air embolus.
b Insert tubing into infusion pump; then attach distal end of tubing to epidural catheter.	Infusion pumps propel fluid through tubing.
c Check infusion pump for proper calibration and operation. Many institutions have two nurses check settings.	Ensures patient is receiving proper dose and pain relief.
d Tape all connections. Give ordered bolus, or start infusion.	Taping maintains a secure, closed system to help prevent infection. Sometimes a filter is necessary in the tubing (see agency policy).
12 Administer bolus dose of medication:	
a Take prepared syringe, and change filter needle to regular 20-gauge needleless adapter.	Prevents infusion of microscopic glass particles and allows medication to be injected.
b Clean injection cap of epidural catheter with antiinfective according to agency policy. (Do not use alcohol.)	Cleaning agent prevents introduction of microorganisms into the central nervous system. Alcohol causes pain and is toxic to neural tissue.
c Dry injection cap with sterile gauze.	Reduces possible injection of antiseptic.
d Insert needleless adapter of syringe into injection cap. Aspirate.	Aspiration determines position of catheter. Should aspirate less than 1 mL of clear fluid.

STEP	RATIONALE

SAFETY ALERT Aspiration of more than 1 mL of clear fluid or bloody return means catheter may have migrated into subarachnoid space or into a vessel. Do not inject drug. Notify anesthesia care provider.

STEP	RATIONALE
e Inject opioid at a rate of 1 mL over 30 seconds.	Slow injection prevents discomfort by lowering the pressure exerted by fluid as it enters the epidural space.
f Remove syringe from injection cap. There is no need to flush with saline.	The catheter is in a space, not a blood vessel; thus flushing with saline is not required (Pasero and McCaffery, 2011).
g Dispose of syringe in sharps container.	Prevents possible exposure to blood.
13 Complete postprocedure protocol.	

Recording and Reporting

- Record drug, dose, method (bolus, demand, or continuous), and time given (if injection) or time begun and ended (if demand or continuous) on appropriate medication record. Specify concentration and diluent.
- With continuous or demand infusion, obtain and record pump readout hourly for first 24 hours after infusion begins and then every 4 hours. Review pump settings and usage together with staff starting the next shift.
- Record regular periodic assessments of patient's status in nurses' notes, in electronic health record (EHR), and/or on appropriate flow sheet, including vital signs, pulse oximetry, intake and output (I&O), sedation level, pain severity score, neurological status, appearance of epidural site, presence or absence of adverse reactions to medication, and presence or absence of complications resulting from placement and maintenance of epidural catheter (Pasero and McCaffery, 2011).
- Report any adverse reactions or complications to health care provider immediately.

UNEXPECTED OUTCOMES	RELATED INTERVENTIONS
1 Patient states pain is still present or has increased. Primary causes are insufficient drug dose or catheter blockage, breakage, or improper position.	• Check all tubing, connections, medication doses, and pump settings. • Report to health care provider adequacy of medication dose.
2 Patient is sedated or not easily arousable.	• Stop epidural infusion and elevate patient's head of bed 30 degrees (unless contraindicated). • Prepare to administer opioid-reversing agent per health care provider's order. • Monitor all vital signs, pulse oximetry, and sedation level continuously until patient is easily aroused.
3 Patient experiences periods of apnea or respirations are less than 8 breaths per minute, shallow, or irregular.	• Instruct patient to take deep breaths. • Notify health care provider. • Prepare to administer opioid-reversing agent, such as naloxone (Narcan), per health care provider's order. (Agency manual may have protocol.) • Monitor at least every 30 minutes until respirations are 8 breaths or more per minute and of adequate depth for 2 hours.
4 Patient reports sudden headache. Clear drainage is present on epidural dressing or more than 1 mL of fluid is aspirated from catheter. Possible indication that catheter has migrated into the subarachnoid space.	• Stop infusion. • Notify health care provider.

UNEXPECTED OUTCOMES	RELATED INTERVENTIONS
5 Blood is present on epidural dressing or aspirated from the catheter. Probable indication that catheter has punctured a blood vessel.	• Stop infusion. • Notify health care provider.
6 Redness, warmth, tenderness, swelling, or exudate is noted at catheter insertion site. These are signs and symptoms of infection.	• Notify health care provider.
7 Patient experiences minimal urinary output, urinary frequency or urgency, bladder distention, pruritus, or nausea and vomiting.	• Consult with health care provider about reducing the dose of opioid, and discuss treatment for side effects.

Eye Irrigation

Eye irrigation effectively flushes out exudates, irritating solutions, or foreign bodies from the eye. The procedure is typically used in emergency situations to preserve vision. When a chemical or irritating substance contaminates the eyes, irrigate immediately with copious amounts of cool water for at least 15 minutes to minimize corneal damage (National Library of Medicine, 2011). Users of contact lenses or artificial eyes may need eye irrigation to flush out particles of dust or fibers from the eye or socket.

Delegation Considerations

The skill of eye irrigation cannot be delegated to nursing assistive personnel (NAP). The nurse directs the NAP to:

- Report any patient complaint of discomfort or excess tearing following irrigation.

Equipment

- Prescribed irrigating solution: volume usually 30 to 180 mL at 32° to 38°C (90° to 100°F) (For chemical flushing, use normal saline or lactated Ringer's fluid in large volume to provide continuous irrigation over 15 minutes.)
- Sterile basin or bag of solution
- Curved emesis basin
- Waterproof pad or towel
- 4 × 4–inch gauze pads
- Soft bulb syringe, eyedropper, or intravenous (IV) tubing
- Clean gloves
- Penlight
- Medication administration record (MAR)

Implementation

STEP	RATIONALE
1 Complete preprocedure protocol.	
2 Assess the eye for redness, excessive tearing, discharge, and swelling. Ask the patient about symptoms of itching, burning, pain, blurred vision, or photophobia.	Establishes baseline signs and symptoms.

STEP	RATIONALE
3 Help patient to side-lying position on side of affected eye. Turn head toward affected eye. If both eyes are affected, place patient supine for simultaneous irrigation of both eyes.	Position facilitates flow of solution from inner to outer canthus, preventing contamination of unaffected eye and nasolacrimal duct.
4 ![icon] Perform hand hygiene. Apply clean gloves.	Reduces transmission of microorganisms. Protects hands from chemical irritants.
5 Remove any contact lens if possible. Remove gloves after contact lens is removed. Reapply new gloves.	Prompt removal of lenses is needed to safely and completely irrigate foreign substances from patient's eyes. Removal of gloves after contact lens removal prevents reintroduction of chemical transferred from lens to glove.

SAFETY ALERT In an emergency such as first aid for a chemical burn, do not delay by removing patient's contact lens before irrigation. Do not remove contact lens unless rapid swelling is occurring. Flush eye, from the inner to outer canthus, with cool tap water immediately (National Library of Medicine, 2011). Advise patient to consult prescriber before reusing contact lens.

6 Place towel or waterproof pad under patient's face and curved emesis basin just below patient's cheek on side of affected eye.	Catches irrigation fluid.
7 Explain next steps to patient and encourage relaxation:	
a With gloved finger gently retract upper and lower eyelids to expose conjunctival sacs.	Retraction minimizes blinking and allows irrigation of conjunctiva.
b To hold lids open, apply gentle pressure to lower bony orbit and bony prominence beneath	

STEP	RATIONALE
eyebrow. Do not apply pressure over eye.	
8 Hold irrigating syringe, dropper, or IV tubing approximately 2.5 cm (1 inch) from inner canthus.	Direct contact with irrigation equipment may injure the eye.
9 Ask patient to look toward brow. Gently irrigate with a steady stream toward the lower conjunctival sac, moving from inner to outer canthus (Fig. 27-1).	Minimizes force of stream on cornea. Flushes irritant out of eye and away from other eye and nasolacrimal duct.
10 Reinforce the importance of the procedure, and encourage patient using calm, confident, soft voice.	Reduces anxiety.
11 Allow patient to blink periodically.	Moves irritant from upper conjunctival sac.
12 Continue irrigation with prescribed solution volume or time or until secretions have been cleared. (**NOTE:** An irrigation of 15 minutes or more is needed to flush chemicals.)	Ensures complete removal of irritant. Assessment of eye secretion pH may be necessary if eye was exposed to an acidic or basic solution during injury (National Library of Medicine, 2011).

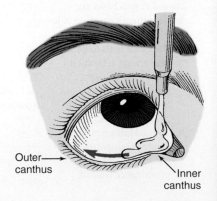

Fig. 27-1 Irrigation of eye from inner to outer canthus.

Outer canthus

Inner canthus

STEP	RATIONALE
13 Blot excess moisture from eyelids and face with gauze or towel.	Removes moisture that may contain microbes or irritant. Promotes patient comfort.
14 Compete postprocedure protocol.	

Recording and Reporting

- Record in nurses' notes and electronic health record (EHR) condition of eye and patient's report of pain and visual symptoms. Record amount and type of irrigation on patient's MAR.
- Report continuing symptoms of pain or blurred vision.

UNEXPECTED OUTCOMES	RELATED INTERVENTIONS
1 Anxiety.	• Reinforce rationale for irrigation. • Allow patient to close eye periodically during irrigation. • Instruct patient to take slow, deep breaths.
2 Patient complains of photophobia, excessive tearing, pain, or foreign body sensation in eye following irrigation.	• Advise patient to close eye and avoid eye movement. • Immediately notify health care provider or eye care practitioner.

Eye Medications:
Drops and Ointment

The eye is the most sensitive organ to which you apply medications. The cornea is richly supplied with sensitive nerve fibers. Care must be taken to prevent instilling medication directly onto the cornea. The conjunctival sac is much less sensitive and thus a more appropriate site for medication instillation.

Any patient receiving topical eye medications should learn correct self-administration of the medication, especially patients with glaucoma, who must often undergo lifelong medication administration for control of their disease. Nurses can easily instruct patients while administering medications. Family caregivers may need to administer eye medications when a patient is unable to manipulate an applicator, when a patient has recently undergone eye surgery, or when a patient's vision is so impaired that it is difficult to assemble needed supplies and handle applicators correctly.

Delegation Considerations

The skill of administering eye medications cannot be delegated to nursing assistive personnel (NAP). The nurse directs the NAP about:

- Potential side effects of medications and when to report their occurrence.
- The potential for temporary visual impairment after administration of eye medications.

Equipment

- Appropriate medication (eyedrops with sterile eyedropper, ointment tube, or medicated intraocular disk)
- Clean gloves
- Medication administration record (MAR) (electronic or printed)
- Cotton ball or tissue
- Wash basin filled with warm water and washcloth
- Eye patch and tape (*optional*)

Implementation

STEP	RATIONALE
1 Complete preprocedure protocol.	

STEP	RATIONALE
2 Check accuracy and completeness of each MAR with prescriber's written medication order. Check patient's name, drug name and dosage, route (eye[s]), and time of administration. Clarify incomplete or unclear orders with health care provider before administration.	The health care provider's order is the most reliable source and only legal record of drugs the patient should receive. Ensures that patient receives correct medication. Handwritten MARs are a source of medication errors (ISMP, 2010; Jones and Treiber, 2010).
3 Identify patient using two identifiers (e.g., name and birthday or name and account number) according to agency policy. Compare identifiers with information on patient's MAR or medical record.	Ensures correct patient. Complies with The Joint Commission requirements for patient safety (TJC, 2014). Some agencies are now using a bar-code system to help with patient identification.
4 Discuss purpose of each medication, action, and possible adverse effects. Allow patient to ask any questions about the drugs. Patients who self-instill medications may be allowed to give drops under nurse's supervision (check agency policy). Tell patients receiving eyedrops (mydriatics) that vision will be blurred temporarily and sensitivity to light may occur.	Patient has right to be informed, and patient's understanding of each medication improves adherence to drug therapy.
5 ![icon] Apply clean gloves. Ask patient to lie supine or to sit back in chair with head slightly hyperextended, looking up.	Position provides easy access to eye for medication instillation and minimizes drainage of medication into tear duct.
6 If drainage or crusting is present along eyelid margins or inner canthus, gently wash	Soaking allows easy removal of crusts without applying pressure to eye. Cleaning from

STEP	RATIONALE
away. Soak any dried crusts with warm, damp washcloth or cotton ball applied over eye for several minutes. Always wipe clean from inner to outer canthus (Fig. 28-1). Remove gloves and perform hand hygiene.	inner to outer canthus avoids entrance of microorganisms into lacrimal duct (Lilley et al., 2011).

SAFETY ALERT Do not hyperextend the neck of a patient with cervical spine injury.

a Instill eyedrops:	
(1) 🖐 Apply clean gloves. Hold cotton ball or clean tissue in nondominant hand on patient's cheekbone just below lower eyelid.	Cotton or tissue absorbs medication that escapes eye.
(2) With tissue or cotton resting below lower lid, gently press downward with thumb or forefinger against bony orbit, exposing conjunctival sac. Never press directly against patient's eyeball.	Prevents pressure and trauma to eyeball and prevents fingers from touching eye.
(3) Ask patient to look at ceiling. Rest dominant hand on patient's forehead; hold filled medication eyedropper approximately 1 to 2 cm ($\frac{1}{2}$ to $\frac{3}{4}$ inches) above conjunctival sac.	Action moves cornea up and away from conjunctival sac and reduces blink reflex. Prevents accidental contact of eyedropper with eye and reduces risk of injury and transfer of microorganisms to dropper (ophthalmic medications are sterile).
(4) Drop prescribed number of drops into conjunctival sac (Fig. 28-2).	Conjunctival sac normally holds 1 or 2 drops. Provides even distribution of medication across eye.

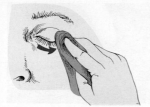

Fig. 28-1 Cleanse eye, washing from inner to outer canthus before administering drops or ointment.

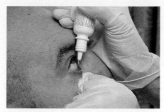

Fig. 28-2 Eyedropper held above conjunctival sac.

STEP	RATIONALE
(5) If patient blinks or closes eye, causing drops to land on outer lid margins, repeat procedure.	Therapeutic effect of drug is obtained only when drops enter conjunctival sac.
(6) When administering drops that may cause systemic effects, apply gentle pressure to patient's nasolacrimal duct with clean tissue for 30 to 60 seconds over each eye, one at a time. Avoid pressure directly against patient's eyeball.	Prevents overflow of medication into nasal and pharyngeal passages. Prevents absorption into systemic circulation.
(7) After instilling drops, ask patient to close eyes gently.	Helps distribute medication. Squinting or squeezing eyelids forces medication from conjunctival sac.
b Instill eye ointment:	
(1) Holding applicator above lower lid margin, apply thin ribbon of ointment evenly along inner edge of lower eyelid on conjunctiva (Fig. 28-3) from inner to outer canthus.	Distributes medication evenly across eye and lid margin.

Fig. 28-3 Nurse applies ointment along the lower eyelid from the inner to outer canthus.

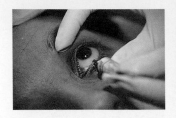

STEP	RATIONALE
(2) Have patient close eye and rub lid lightly in circular motion with cotton ball, if rubbing is not contraindicated. Avoid placing pressure directly against patient's eyeball.	Further distributes medication without traumatizing eye.
(3) If excess medication is on eyelid, gently wipe it from inner to outer canthus.	Promotes comfort and prevents trauma to eye.
(4) If patient needs an eye patch, apply clean one by placing it over affected eye so entire eye is covered. Tape securely without applying pressure to eye.	Clean eye patch reduces risk of infection.
c Apply intraocular disk:	
(1) Open package containing the disk. Gently press your fingertip against the disk so that it adheres to your finger. It may be necessary to moisten gloved finger with sterile saline. Position the convex side of the disk on your fingertip.	Allows nurse to inspect disk for damage or deformity.

STEP	RATIONALE
(2) With your other hand, gently pull the patient's lower eyelid away from the eye. Ask patient to look up.	Prepares conjunctival sac for receiving medicated disk and moves sensitive cornea away.
(3) Place the disk in the conjunctival sac, so that it floats on the sclera between the iris and lower eyelid (Fig. 28-4).	Ensures delivery of medication.
(4) Pull the patient's lower eyelid out and over the disk (Fig. 28-5).	Ensures accurate medication delivery.
d Remove intraocular disk:	Intraocular disks may remain in place for up to 1 week (duration varies).
(1) ✈ Perform hand hygiene and apply clean gloves. Gently pull on the patient's lower eyelid to expose the disk.	Exposes disk.
(2) Using your forefinger and thumb of your dominant hand, pinch the disk, and lift it out of the patient's eye (Fig. 28-6).	
7 Complete postprocedure protocol.	

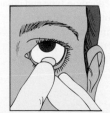

Fig. 28-4 Place intraocular disk in the conjunctival sac between the iris and the lower eyelid.

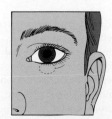

Fig. 28-5 Gently pull the patient's lower eyelid over the disk.

Fig. 28-6 Carefully pinch the disk to remove it from the patient's eye.

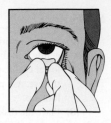

Recording and Reporting

- Record drug, concentration, dose or strength, number of drops, site of application (left, right, or both eyes), and time of administration on MAR immediately after administration, not before. Include initials or signature. Record patient teaching and validation of understanding in nurses' notes and electronic health record (EHR).
- Record objective data related to tissues involved (e.g., redness, drainage, irritation), any subjective data (e.g., pain, itching, altered vision), and patient's response to medications. Note any side effects experienced in nurses' notes and EHR.
- Report adverse effects/patient response and/or withheld drugs to nurse in charge or health care provider. Depending on medication, immediate health care provider notification may be required.

UNEXPECTED OUTCOMES	RELATED INTERVENTIONS
1 Patient complains of burning or pain or experiences local side effects (e.g., headache, bloodshot eyes, local eye irritation).	• Eyedrops may have been instilled onto cornea, or dropper touched surface of eye. • Notify health care provider for possible adjustment in medication type and dosage.
2 Patient experiences systemic effects from drops (e.g., increased heart rate and blood pressure from epinephrine, decreased heart rate and blood pressure from timolol).	• Notify prescriber immediately. • Remain with patient. • Withhold further doses.

Fall Prevention in a Health Care Facility

Patient falls are the most common type of inpatient accident (Oliver, Healey, and Haines, 2010). Between 1% and 3% of these falls result in fractures. Risk factors for falls among inpatients include a history of falling, muscle weakness, agitation and confusion, urinary incontinence or frequency, postural hypotension, and use of high-risk medications (e.g., benzodiazepines, opioids, antihistamines, and sedative-hypnotics) (Chang et al., 2011; Oliver et al., 2010).

A fall-reduction program includes a fall risk assessment of every patient, which is usually conducted on admission to a hospital and then routinely (see agency policy) until the patient's discharge.

Remember that patient situations change. Preventing falls and fall-related injuries requires diligent ongoing nursing assessment and engagement of the entire health care team in the implementation of patient-specific interventions (ICSI, 2010).

A full set of raised side rails (two to a bed or four to a bed) is a physical restraint. Raising only one of two, or three of four, side rails gives patients room to exit a bed safely and move around within the bed. It is also important to keep a bed in low position with wheels locked when stationary.

Electronic bed and chair alarms warn nursing staff when patients try to leave the bed or chair on their own. Additional devices to use at a patient's bedside are a gait belt, a bedside commode, a nonskid floor mat, an overhead trapeze, and a ceiling lift.

Delegation Considerations

Assessment of a patient's risk for falling cannot be delegated to nursing assistive personnel (NAP). However, the skills necessary to prevent falls can be delegated. The nurse directs NAP by:

- Explaining a patient's mobility limitations and specific measures needed to minimize risks.
- Teaching specific environmental safety precautions to use (e.g., bed locked in low position, nonskid footwear).
- Explaining patient behaviors (e.g., disorientation, wandering, anxiousness) that are precursors to falls and that should be reported immediately.

Equipment

- Fall risk assessment tool for falls
- Hospital bed with side rails
- Wedge cushion
- Call light
- Seat belt
- Gait belt
- Wheelchair
- Bed alarm

Implementation

STEP	RATIONALE
1 Assess patient's fall risks using an agency fall risk assessment tool (Kojima et al., 2011; Viera, Freund-Heritage, and da Costa, 2011).	Certain physiological factors predispose patients to fall (e.g., incontinence or urgency and the attempt to rush to a bathroom or find a urinal).
2 Determine if patient has a history of recent falls (TJC, 2012a) or other injuries within the home. Assess previous falls; be specific and follow the acronym SPLATT (Meiner, 2011): • *Symptoms* at time of fall • *Previous* fall • *Location* of fall • *Activity* at time of fall • *Time* of fall • *Trauma* after fall	Key symptoms are often helpful in identifying cause for falls. Onset, location, and activity associated with a fall provide further details on causative factors and how to prevent future falls.
3 Review patient's medication history, including over-the-counter (OTC) medications and herbal products, antidepressants, anticonvulsants, antihypertensives, antihistamines, anti-Parkinson drugs, antipsychotics, anxiolytics,	Certain medications have been associated with patient falls (Chang et al., 2011; Gribbin et al., 2010; Kojima et al., 2011; Viera et al., 2011). Use of multiple medications (polypharmacy) is also associated with falls, especially in older adults (Beer et al., 2011).

STEP	RATIONALE
corticosteroids, diuretics, histamine (H_2) receptors, hypnotics (especially benzodiazepines), hypoglycemics, and muscle relaxants.	
4 Assess patient for fear of falling (Boyd and Stevens, 2009).	Fear and/or anxiety, as well as the fear of falling are interrelated problems; each is a risk factor for the other (Scheffer et al., 2008).
5 Assess risk factors in health care agency (e.g., being attached to equipment such as sequential compression hose or intravenous [IV] or oxygen tubing, improperly lighted room, obstructed walkway to bathroom, clutter of supplies and equipment).	Environmental barriers pose risk for falls.
6 Assess condition of equipment.	Equipment in poor repair (e.g., uneven legs on bedside commode) increases fall risk.
7 Perform the timed "get up and go" (TGUG) test if patient is able to ambulate: • Have patient rise from sitting position without using arms for support. • Instruct patient to walk 10 feet (3 m), turn around, and walk back to the chair. • Return to chair, and sit down without using arms for support. • Look for unsteadiness in patient's gait.	Examination easily incorporated into clinical encounters with patient is a measure of physical performance, with low scores associated with risk for falling (Khazzani et al., 2009). Patient taking less than 20 seconds to complete test is adequate for independent mobility. Patient who takes longer than 30 seconds is dependent and at risk for fall.
8 Assess patient for osteoporosis, anticoagulant therapy, history of previous	Factors increase likelihood of injury from a fall.

STEP	RATIONALE
fracture, and recent chest or abdominal surgery.	
9 Use patient-centered approach, and determine what patient knows about risks for falling and steps the patient can take to prevent falls.	Patient's own knowledge of risks influences ability to take necessary precautions in reducing falls.
10 After assessment apply color-coded wristband (e.g., yellow) for patients at risk for falling. Some organizations institute fall risk signs on doors and special yellow labels on patient charts and assignment boards.	Color-coded bands are easily recognizable. National efforts in a majority of states have resulted in the standardization of yellow as a color for fall risk wristbands.
11 Complete preprocedure protocol.	
12 Adjust bed to low position with wheels locked. Place padded mats on floor at side of bed.	Allows for proper body mechanics. Height of bed allows ambulatory patient to easily get in and out of bed safely. Pads provide nonslippery surface on which to stand.
13 Encourage patient to wear properly fitted skidproof footwear. *Option:* Place nonslip padded floor mat on exit side of bed.	Prevents falls caused by slipping on floor.
14 Orient patient to surroundings and call light/ bed control system:	
a Provide patient's hearing aid and glasses.	Enables patient to remain alert to conditions in environment.
b Explain and demonstrate how to turn call light/ intercom system on and off at bedside and in bathroom.	Knowledge of location and use of call light is essential to patient safety.

STEP	RATIONALE
c Explain to patient and family when and why to use call system (e.g., report pain, get out of bed, go to bathroom).	Increases likelihood of nurse's being able to respond.
d Consistently secure call light/bed control system to an accessible location within patient's reach.	Ensures patient is able to reach device immediately when needed.
15 Use of hospital side rails (acute care):	
a Explain to patient and family the main reason for using side rails: moving and turning self in bed.	Promotes patient and family cooperation.
b Check agency policies regarding side rail use.	Side rails are a restraint device if they immobilize or reduce ability of patient to move arms, legs, body, or head freely (CMS, 2008).
(1) Dependent, less mobile patients: In a two–side rail bed, keep both rails up. (NOTE: Rails on newer hospital beds allow for room at foot of bed for patient to safely exit bed.) In a four–side rail bed, leave two upper rails up.	
(2) Patient able to get out of bed independently: In a four–side rail bed, leave only one upper side rail up. In a two–	Allows for safe exit out of bed.

STEP	RATIONALE
side rail bed, keep only one rail up.	

SAFETY ALERT Assess for excessive gaps and openings between mattress, bedframe, and side rails.

STEP	RATIONALE
16 Provide environmental interventions:	
a Remove excess equipment, supplies, and furniture from rooms and halls.	Reduces likelihood of falls from tripping.
b Keep floors, particularly path to bathroom, free of clutter and obstacles. Coil and secure excess electrical, telephone, and other cords or tubing.	Reduces likelihood of falls from tripping.
c Clean all spills promptly. Post sign indicating wet floor. Remove sign when floor is dry.	Reduces falls from slipping on wet surface.
d Ensure adequate glare-free lighting: use night-light at night.	Reduces fall risk since glare is a problem for older adults because of normal visual changes.
e Have assistive devices (e.g., walker, cane, bedside commodes) located on exit side of bed.	Provides added support when transferring out of bed. Commode eliminates need to get up to walk to bathroom.
f Arrange necessary items (e.g., water pitcher, eyeglasses, dentures, telephone) within patient's easy reach.	Prevents patient from reaching and allows patient to perform self-care activities safely.
g Secure locks on beds, stretchers, and wheelchairs.	Prevents accidental movement of devices during patient transfer
17 Additional interventions for patients at high risk (based on fall risk assessment):	Level of risk defined by fall risk assessment tool.

STEP	RATIONALE
a Prioritize call-light responses to patients at high risk, using a team approach.	Ensures rapid response to calls from patients.
b Monitor and assist patients in following daily schedules.	Patients are less likely to try an activity on their own when they have a defined schedule.
c Establish elimination schedule, using bedside commode when appropriate.	Proactive toileting keeps patients from being unattended with sudden urge to use toilet.
d Stay with patient during toileting.	
e Place patients in geri chair or wheelchair with wedge cushion. Use wheelchair only for transport, not for sitting an extended time.	Designed to maintain alignment and comfort and makes it difficult to exit chair.
f Use low bed that has low height above floor and floor mats.	Reduces fall-related injuries.
g Activate bed alarm for patient.	
18 When ambulating a patient, have patient wear a gait belt, and walk along patient's side.	Gait belt gives nurse a secure hold on patient during ambulation.
19 Explain to patient that hourly rounds will be conducted to reassess for fall risks, provide toileting needs, and attend to symptom management.	Use of hourly rounds has been shown to reduce incidence of falls (Halm, 2009).
20 Explain to patient specific safety measures used to prevent falls (e.g., wear well-fitting, flat footwear with nonskid soles; dangle feet for a few minutes before standing; walk slowly; ask for help if dizzy or weak).	Promotes patient understanding and cooperation. Dangling provides adjustment to orthostatic hypotension, allowing blood pressure to stabilize before ambulation.

STEP	RATIONALE
21 Consult with physical therapist about the possibility of gait training and muscle-strengthening exercise.	There is evidence that implementation of sustained exercise programs may reduce falls (Oliver et al., 2010).
22 Discuss with health care provider and pharmacist possibility of adjusting patient's medications to reduce side effects and interactions.	Evidence shows that medication assessment with modification (e.g., eliminating unnecessary medications, adjusting dosages) can reduce incidence of falls in home setting (Costello and Edelstein, 2008). Drug interactions can also have effects that place patients at risk in an acute care setting.

Recording and Reporting

- Record fall risk assessment findings and specific interventions, including instructions, used to prevent falls in nurses' notes, electronic health record (EHR), and/or care plan.
- Report to health care personnel specific risks to patient's safety and measures taken to minimize risks.
- If patient suffers a fall, inform primary health care provider. Document what occurred, including description of the fall as given by patient or witness. Be sure to include baseline assessment, any injuries noted, tests or treatments given, follow-up care, and additional safety precautions taken after fall.

UNEXPECTED OUTCOMES	RELATED INTERVENTIONS
1 Patient is unable to identify safety risks.	• Reinforce identified risks with patient, or review needed safety measures with family.
2 Patient starts to fall while ambulating with a caregiver.	• Put both arms around patient's waist, or grasp gait belt.
	• Stand with feet apart to provide broad base of support.

UNEXPECTED OUTCOMES	RELATED INTERVENTIONS
	• Extend one leg, and let patient slide against it to the floor.
	• Bend knees to lower body as patient slides to floor.
3 Patient found after suffering a fall.	• Call for assistance.
	• Assess patient for injury, and stay with patient until assistance arrives.
	• Notify health care provider.
	• Follow institution's incident/ occurrence reporting policy.
	• Evaluate patient and environment; determine if fall could have been prevented.
	• Reinforce identified risks with patient and measures recommended to prevent recurrent fall.
	• Monitor patient closely after fall to assess for possible injury.

Fecal Impaction:
Removing Digitally

Fecal impaction is the inability to pass a collection of hard stool. This condition occurs in all age-groups. Physically and mentally incapacitated persons and institutionalized older adult patients are at greatest risk. Symptoms of fecal impaction include constipation, rectal discomfort, anorexia, nausea, vomiting, abdominal pain, diarrhea (leaking around the impacted stool), and urinary frequency. Digital removal of an impaction is very uncomfortable and embarrassing for the patient. Excessive rectal manipulation causes irritation to the mucosa and subsequent bleeding or vagus nerve stimulation, which can cause a reflex slowing of the heart rate.

Delegation Considerations

The skill of removing a fecal impaction digitally cannot be delegated to nursing assistive personnel (NAP). The nurse directs the NAP to:

- Help the nurse position the patient for the procedure.
- Observe the stool for color, consistency, rectal bleeding, or bloody mucus and report immediately to the nurse.
- Provide perineal care following each bowel movement.

Equipment

- Clean gloves
- Water-soluble local anesthetic lubricant (**NOTE:** Some agencies require use of water-soluble lubricant without anesthetic when nurse performs procedure.)
- Waterproof, absorbent pads
- Bedpan
- Bedpan cover *(optional)*
- Bath blanket
- Wash basin, washcloths, towels, and soap
- Vital signs equipment

Implementation

STEP	RATIONALE
1 Complete preprocedure protocol.	

STEP	RATIONALE

SAFETY ALERT Because of the potential to stimulate the sacral branch of the vagus nerve, patients with a history of dysrhythmias or heart disease have a greater risk for changes in heart rhythm. Be sure to monitor patient's pulse before and during procedure. This procedure is often contraindicated in patients who have cardiac abnormalities: if in doubt, verify with the health care provider.

STEP	RATIONALE
2 Check patient's record for health care provider's order for digital removal of impaction and use of anesthetic lubricant.	Obtain written order before performing procedure, because this procedure involves excessive stimulation of vagus nerve.
3 Identify patient using two identifiers (e.g., name and birthday or name and account number) according to agency policy. Compare identifiers with information on patient's MAR or medical record.	Ensures correct patient. Complies with The Joint Commission requirements for patient safety (TJC, 2014).
4 Obtain assistance to help change patient's position if necessary. Raise bed horizontally to comfortable working height.	Promotes patient safety and use of good body mechanics.
5 Pull curtains around bed, or close door to room.	
6 Lower side rail on patient's right side. Keeping the far side rail raised, help patient to left side-lying position with knees flexed.	Promotes patient safety. Provides access to rectum.
7 Drape patient's trunk and lower extremities with bath blanket, and place waterproof pad under patient's buttocks.	Maintains patient's sense of privacy and prevents unnecessary exposure of body parts.
8 Place bedpan next to patient.	

STEP	RATIONALE
9 🗽 Perform hand hygiene and apply clean gloves. Lubricate gloved index finger and middle finger of dominant hand with anesthetic lubricant.	Prevents transmission of microorganisms. Reduces discomfort and permits smooth insertion of finger into anus and rectum.
10 Instruct patient to take slow, deep breaths during procedure. Gradually and gently insert gloved index finger, and feel anus relax around the finger. Insert middle finger.	Slow, deep breaths help to relax patient. Gradual insertion of index finger helps to dilate anal sphincter.
11 Gradually advance fingers slowly along rectal wall toward umbilicus.	Allows you to reach impacted stool high in rectum.
12 Gently loosen fecal mass by moving fingers in scissors motion to fragment the fecal mass. Work fingers into hardened mass.	Loosening and penetrating mass allow for removal of stool in small pieces, resulting in less discomfort to patient.
13 Work stool downward toward end of rectum. Remove small sections of feces, and discard into bedpan.	Prevents need to force finger up into rectum and minimizes trauma to mucosa.
14 Observe patient's response and periodically assess heart rate. Look for signs of fatigue.	Vagal stimulation slows heart rate and causes dysrhythmias. Procedure often exhausts patient.

SAFETY ALERT Stop procedure if heart rate drops or rhythm changes from patient's baseline, or if patient has dyspnea or complaints of palpitations.

15 Continue to clear rectum of feces, and allow patient to rest at intervals.	Rest improves patient's tolerance of procedure, allowing heart rate to return to normal.
16 After removal of impaction, perform perineal hygiene.	Promotes patient's sense of comfort and cleanliness.

STEP	RATIONALE
17 Remove bedpan, and inspect feces for color and consistency. Dispose of feces in toilet.	Reduces transmission of microorganisms.
18 If needed, help patient to toilet or clean bedpan. (Procedure may be followed with enema or cathartic.)	Removal of impaction stimulates defecation reflex.
19 Remove gloves by turning inside out and discarding in proper receptacle. Perform hand hygiene.	Reduces transmission of microorganisms.
20 Complete postprocedure protocol.	

Recording and Reporting

- Record patient's tolerance to procedure, amount and consistency of stool removed, vital signs, and adverse effects.
- Report any changes in vital signs and adverse effects to health care provider.

UNEXPECTED OUTCOMES	RELATED INTERVENTIONS
1 Patient experiences trauma to rectal mucosa as evidenced by rectal bleeding.	• Assess anal and perianal region for source of bleeding. • Stop procedure if bleeding is excessive.
2 Patient experiences bradycardia, decrease in blood pressure, and decrease in level of consciousness as result of vagus nerve stimulation.	• Stop procedure, and measure vital signs. • Notify health care provider and remain with patient.
3 Patient has seepage of liquid stool after procedure complete.	• Assess patient for continuing impaction. • Notify health care provider for possible suppository or enema. • Increase patient's fluid intake and dietary fiber.

Hypothermia and Hyperthermia Blankets

A hypothermia-hyperthermia blanket raises, lowers, or maintains body temperature through conductive heat or cold transfer between the blanket and the patient. When placed on top of a patient, the blanket helps to raise or lower the patient's body temperature (Fig. 31-1). When operated manually, the unit maintains a preset temperature regardless of the patient's temperature. When operating in the automatic setting, the unit continually monitors a patient's temperature with a thermistor probe (rectal, skin, or esophageal). The system increases or decreases the temperature of the circulating water in response to the preset target temperature and actual measured patient temperature.

Recent research shows that induced hypothermia prevents or moderates neurological outcomes after neurosurgery or during traumatic brain injury and acute stroke (Fox et al., 2010; Linares and Mayer, 2009; Polderman, 2008; Polderman and Herold, 2009). Mild hypothermia (32° to 34°C [89.6° to 93.2°F]) in the first hours after an ischemic event and for 72 hours or until stabilization occurs helps prevent permanent damage (Fox et al., 2010).

Delegation Considerations

The skill of applying a hypothermia or hyperthermia blanket can be delegated to nursing assistive personnel (NAP) (see agency policy). The nurse is responsible for assessing and evaluating treatment and related patient education. If the patient is unstable and at risk for complications, this skill is not delegated. The nurse directs the NAP to:

- Maintain proper temperature of the application throughout the treatment and discontinue the application as specified in the health care provider's order.
- Inform the nurse of any unexpected patient outcomes (e.g., shivering or redness to the skin).
- Report when treatment is complete so an evaluation of the patient's response can be made.

Equipment

- Hypothermia or hyperthermia blanket with control panel and rectal probe
- Sheet or thin bath blanket

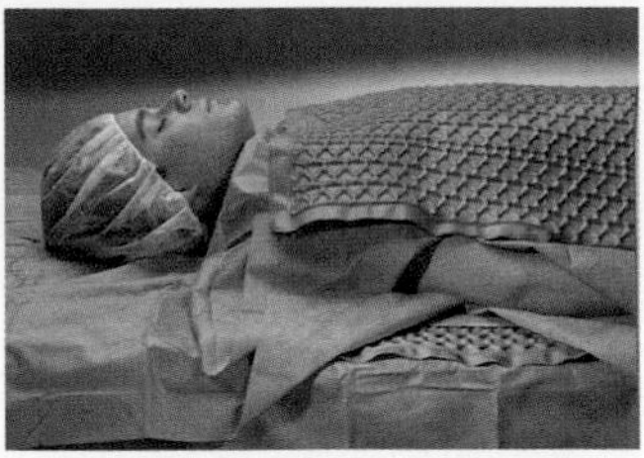

Fig. 31-1 Hypothermia cooling blanket is applied over paper sheet before additional top sheet is applied to bed. (Courtesy Cincinnati Sub-Zero Maxi-Therm Hyper-Hypothermia Blanket.)

- Distilled water to fill the units if necessary
- Disposable gloves
- Rectal thermometer

Implementation

STEP	RATIONALE
1 Complete preprocedure protocol.	

SAFETY ALERT Antipyretic therapy may be used in combination with a cooling blanket. Temperatures greater than 41° C (105.8° F) have detrimental effects in the patient with neurological disease. As a result some neurological injuries and their sequelae are permanent. A 1° C (1.8° F) rise in body temperature results in a 10% increase in the metabolic demands of the body (Kiekkas et al., 2008, 2011).

STEP	RATIONALE
2 Prepare blanket according to agency policy and manufacturer's instructions.	Agencies have specific policies on maintaining equipment in functional order.
3 Perform hand hygiene, and apply clean gloves.	Reduces transmission of microorganisms.
4 Apply lanolin or a mixture of lanolin and cold cream to patient's skin where it will touch blanket.	Helps protect skin from heat and cold sensations.
5 Turn on blanket, and observe that cool or warm light is on. Precool or prewarm blanket, setting pad temperature to desired level.	Verifies that blanket is correctly set to help decrease (cool) or increase (warm) patient's body temperature. Prepares blanket for prescribed therapy.
6 Verify that pad temperature limits are set at desired safety ranges.	Safety ranges prevent excessive cooling or warming. The blanket automatically shuts off

STEP	RATIONALE
	when preset body temperature is achieved.
7 Cover the hypothermia or hyperthermia blanket with a thin paper or cloth sheet or bath blanket.	Injuries from hot or cold therapies are preventable events (NQF, 2011). Thin sheet protects patient's skin from direct contact with blanket, thus reducing risk for injury to skin.
8 Position hypothermia or hyperthermia blanket on top of patient.	Provides wide distribution of blanket against patient's skin.
a Wrap patient's hands and feet in gauze.	Reduces risk for thermal injury to body's distal areas.
b Wrap scrotum with towels.	Protects sensitive tissue from direct contact with cold.
9 Lubricate rectal probe, and insert into patient's rectum.	When using hypothermia or hyperthermia blanket, it is imperative that you continuously monitor patient's core interior (rectal) temperature.
10 Turn and position patient regularly to protect from pressure ulcer development and impaired body alignment (see Skill 59). Keep linens free of perspiration and condensation.	Patient has an increased risk for pressure ulcer development because of skin moisture created by blanket and patient's body temperature.
11 Double-check fluid thermometer on control panel of blanket before leaving room.	Verifies that pad temperature is maintained at desired level.
12 Complete postprocedure protocol.	

Recording and Reporting

- Record baseline data: vital signs, neurological and mental status, status of peripheral circulation and skin integrity when therapy was initiated.

- Note type of hyperthermia-hypothermia unit used; control settings (manual or automatic, and temperature settings); date, time, duration, and patient's tolerance of treatment.
- Chart on temperature graphic repeated measurements of vital signs to document response to therapy.
- Report any unexpected outcome to health care provider. Further treatment may be required.

UNEXPECTED OUTCOMES	RELATED INTERVENTIONS
1 Patient's core body temperature decreases or increases rapidly.	• Adjust blanket temperature no more than 1°F (0.6°C) every 15 minutes to avoid complications.
2 Patient's core temperature remains unchanged.	• Patient may need hypothermic or hyperthermic treatment of additional sites, such as axilla, groin, and neck, in addition to those covered by blanket.
	• Discuss use of an antipyretic with health care provider.
3 Patient begins to shiver.	• Adjust temperature to more comfortable range, and assess if shivering decreases.
	• If shivering continues, stop treatment and notify health care provider.
4 Skin breaks down, indicating that patient's skin may have received thermal injury (frostbite or burn) from blanket.	• Stop treatment.
	• Notify physician.

Incentive Spirometry

Incentive spirometry helps a patient deep breathe. An incentive spirometer (IS) is most often used following abdominal or thoracic surgery to reduce the incidence of postoperative pulmonary atelectasis. The use of IS is especially important in patients with underlying pulmonary diseases because of their risk for postoperative pneumonia.

Delegation Considerations

The skill of assisting a patient to use incentive spirometry can be delegated to nursing assistive personnel (NAP). The nurse is responsible for assessing, monitoring, and evaluating the patient's response. The nurse directs the NAP by:

- Informing about the patient's target goal for incentive spirometry.
- Informing to immediately notify the nurse about any unexpected outcomes such as chest pain, excessive sputum production, and fever.

Equipment

- Flow or volume-oriented IS

Implementation

STEP	RATIONALE
1 Complete preprocedure protocol.	
2 🐾 Perform hand hygiene.	Reduces transmission of microorganisms.
3 Position patient in the most erect position (e.g., high-Fowler's position if tolerated) (Smeltzer et al., 2009).	Promotes optimal lung expansion during respiratory maneuver.
4 Instruct patient to exhale completely through mouth and place lips tightly around the mouthpiece.	Showing patient how to correctly place mouthpiece is reliable technique for teaching psychomotor skill and enables patient to ask questions.
5 Instruct patient to take a slow, deep breath and maintain a constant flow, like pulling through a straw. When the patient cannot inhale any	Maintains maximal inspiration; reduces risk for progressive collapse of individual alveoli.

STEP	RATIONALE
more, he or she has reached maximal inspiration. Have patient hold breath for at least 3 seconds and then exhale normally.	

SAFETY ALERT Some patients with chronic obstructive pulmonary disease (COPD) are able to hold their breath for only 2 to 3 seconds. Encourage them to do their best and to try to extend the duration of breath holding. Allow patients to rest between IS breaths to prevent hyperventilation and fatigue.

6 Have patient repeat the maneuver, encouraging patient to reach prescribed goal.	Ensures correct use of the spirometer and patient's understanding of use.
7 Complete postprocedure protocol.	

Recording and Reporting

- Record lung sounds before and after incentive spirometry, the frequency of use, the volumes achieved, and any adverse effects.
- Report any changes in respiratory assessment or inability of patient to use IS to health care provider.

UNEXPECTED OUTCOMES	RELATED INTERVENTIONS
1 Patient is unable to achieve incentive spirometry target volume.	• Encourage patient to attempt incentive spirometry more frequently, followed by rest periods. • Teach cough-control exercises. • Teach patient how to splint and protect incision sites during deep breathing. • Administer ordered analgesic if acute pain is inhibiting use of IS.
2 Patient has decreased lung expansion and/or abnormal breath sounds.	• Teach patient cough-control exercises. • Provide assistance with suctioning if patient cannot effectively expel secretions.

Intradermal Injections

You typically give intradermal (ID) injections for skin testing (e.g., tuberculosis screening and allergy tests). Because such medications are potent, you inject them into the dermis, where blood supply is reduced and drug absorption occurs slowly. A patient may have an anaphylactic reaction if the medications enter the circulation too rapidly. Skin testing often requires you to visually inspect the test site; therefore make sure that the ID sites are free of lesions and injuries and relatively hairless. The inner forearm and upper back are ideal locations. To administer an ID injection, use a tuberculin (TB) or small syringe with a short (⅜ to ⅝ inch), fine-gauge (25 to 27) needle. The angle of insertion for an intradermal injection is 5 to 15 degrees (Fig. 33-1). Inject only small amounts of medication (0.01 to 0.1 mL) intradermally.

Delegation Considerations

The skill of administering ID injections cannot be delegated to nursing assistive personnel (NAP). The nurse directs the NAP about:

- Potential medication side effects and reporting their occurrence to the nurse.
- Reporting any change in the patient's condition to the nurse.

Equipment

- Syringe: 1-mL tuberculin syringe with preattached 25- or 27-gauge needle, ⅜ to ⅝ inch
- Small gauze pad
- Alcohol swab
- Vial or ampule of medication
- Clean gloves
- Medication administration record (MAR) or computer printout
- Puncture-proof container

Implementation

STEP	RATIONALE
1 Complete preprocedure protocol.	
2 Check accuracy and completeness of the MAR or computer printout with prescriber's original medication order. Check	The prescriber's order is the most reliable source and legal record of the patient's medications. Ensures patient receives the correct medication.

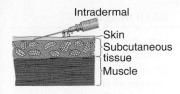
Intradermal

Skin
Subcutaneous tissue
Muscle

Fig. 33-1 Intradermal needle tip inserted into dermis.

STEP	RATIONALE
patient's name, medication name and dosage, route of administration, and time of administration.	
3 Prepare medications for one patient at a time using aseptic technique and avoiding distractions. Check label of medication carefully with MAR or computer printout 2 times when preparing medication.	Ensures that medication is sterile. Preventing distractions reduces medication preparation errors (LePorte et al., 2009; Nguyen et al., 2010). *These are the first and second checks for accuracy* and ensure that the correct medication is administered.
4 Take medication(s) to patient at correct time. Medications that require exact timing include STAT, first-time or loading doses, and one-time doses. Give time-critical scheduled medications (e.g., antibiotics, anticoagulants, insulin, anticonvulsants, immunosuppressive agents) at exact time ordered (no later than 30 minutes before or after scheduled dose). Give non–time-critical scheduled medications within a range of 1 or 2 hours of scheduled dose (ISMP, 2011). During administration, apply	Hospitals must adopt medication administration policy and procedure for timing of medication administration that considers nature of the prescribed medication, specific clinical application, and patient needs (CMS, 2011; ISMP, 2011). Time-critical scheduled medications are those for which early or delayed administration of maintenance doses of greater than 30 minutes before or after the scheduled dose may cause harm or result in substantial suboptimal therapy or pharmacological effect. Non–time-critical medications are those for which early or delayed administration within a

STEP	RATIONALE
six rights of medication administration.	specified range of either 1 or 2 hours should not cause harm or result in substantial suboptimal therapy or pharmacological effect (CMS, 2011; ISMP, 2011).
5 Identify patient using two identifiers (e.g., name and birthday or name and account number) according to agency policy. Compare identifiers with information on patient's MAR or medical record.	Ensures correct patient. Complies with The Joint Commission requirements for patient safety (TJC, 2014). Some agencies are now using a bar-code system to help with patient identification.
6 At patient's bedside again compare MAR or computer printout with names of medications on medication labels and patient name. Ask patient if he or she has allergies.	*This is the third check for accuracy* and ensures that patient receives correct medication. Confirms patient's allergy history.
7 Discuss purpose of each medication, action, and possible adverse effects. Allow patient to ask any questions. Tell patient that injection will cause a slight burning or sting.	Patient has right to be informed, and patient's understanding of each medication improves adherence to drug therapy. Helps minimize patient's anxiety.
8 ✦ Perform hand hygiene and apply clean gloves. Keep sheet or gown draped over body parts not requiring exposure.	Reduces transfer of infection.
9 Select appropriate site. Note lesions or discolorations of skin. If possible, select site three to four finger widths below antecubital space and one hand width above wrist. If you cannot use forearm, inspect the	Intradermal injection site should be free of discoloration or hair so you can see results of skin test and interpret them correctly (CDC, 2011).

STEP	RATIONALE
upper back. If necessary, use sites appropriate for subcutaneous injections (see Skill 71).	
10 Help patient to comfortable position. Have patient extend elbow and support it and forearm on flat surface.	Stabilizes injection site for easiest accessibility.
11 Clean site with an antiseptic swab. Apply swab at center of site and rotate outward in a circular direction for about 5 cm (2 inches). *Option:* Use vapocoolant spray (e.g., ethyl chloride) before injection.	Mechanical action of swab removes secretions containing microorganisms. Decreases pain at injection site.
12 Hold swab or gauze between third and fourth fingers of nondominant hand.	Gauze or swab remains readily accessible when withdrawing needle.
13 Remove needle cap from needle by pulling it straight off.	Preventing needle from touching sides of cap prevents contamination.
14 Hold syringe between thumb and forefinger of dominant hand with bevel of needle pointing up.	Smooth injection requires proper manipulation of syringe parts. With bevel up, you are less likely to deposit medication into tissues below dermis.
15 With nondominant hand, stretch skin over site with forefinger or thumb.	Needle pierces tight skin more easily.
16 With needle almost against patient's skin, insert it slowly at 5- to 15-degree angle until resistance is felt. Then advance needle through epidermis to approximately 3 mm ($\frac{1}{8}$ inch) below skin surface. You will see bulge of needle tip through skin.	Ensures that needle tip is in dermis. Inaccurate results will be obtained if needle is not injected at correct angle and depth (CDC, 2011).

STEP	RATIONALE
17 Inject medication slowly. Normally you feel resistance. If not, needle is too deep; remove and begin again.	Slow injection minimizes discomfort at site. Dermal layer is tight and does not expand easily when you inject solution.

SAFETY ALERT It is not necessary to aspirate because dermis is relatively avascular.

18 While injecting medication, note that small bleb (approximately 6 mm [$\frac{1}{4}$ inch]) resembling mosquito bite appears on skin surface (Fig. 33-2).	Bleb indicates you deposited medication in dermis.
19 After withdrawing needle, apply alcohol swab or gauze gently over site.	Do not massage site. Apply bandage if needed.
20 Complete postprocedure protocol.	
21 Inspect bleb. *Optional:* Use skin pencil and draw circle around perimeter of injection site. Read TB test site at 48 to 72 hours; look for induration (hard, dense, raised area) of skin around injection site of: • 15 mm or more in patients with no known risk factors for tuberculosis. • 10 mm or more in patients who are recent immigrants; injection drug users; residents and employees of high-risk settings; patients with certain chronic illnesses; children less than 4 years of age; and infants, children, and adolescents exposed to high-risk adults.	Determines if reaction to antigen occurs; indication positive for TB or tested allergens. Degree of reaction varies based on patient condition. Site must be read at various intervals to determine test results. Pencil marks make site easy to find. You determine the results of skin testing at various times, based on type of medication used or type of skin testing completed. Manufacturer's directions determine when to read test results.

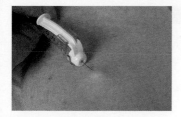

Fig. 33-2 Injection creates small bleb.

Recording and Reporting

- Record drug, dose, route, site, time, and date on MAR immediately after administration, not before. Correctly sign MAR according to agency policy.
- Record area of ID injection and appearance of skin in your notes.
- Report any undesirable effects from medication to patient's health care provider, and document adverse effects according to agency policy.
- Record patient teaching, validation of patient understanding, and patient's response to medication.

UNEXPECTED OUTCOMES	RELATED INTERVENTIONS
1 Patient complains of localized pain or continued burning at injection site, indicating potential injury to nerve or vessels.	• Assess injection site. • Notify patient's health care provider.
2 Raised, reddened, or hard zone (induration) forms around ID test site.	• Notify patient's health care provider. • Document sensitivity to injected allergen or positive test if tuberculin skin testing was completed.
3 Patient has adverse reaction with signs of urticaria, pruritus, wheezing, and dyspnea.	• Notify patient's health care provider. • Follow agency policy for appropriate response to drug reactions (e.g., administration of antihistamine such as diphenhydramine [Benadryl] or epinephrine).

Continued

UNEXPECTED OUTCOMES	RELATED INTERVENTIONS
	• Add allergy information to patient's record.
4 Patient is unable to explain purpose or signs of skin testing.	• Provide further teaching to patient or family caregiver.
	• Recognize patient is unable to learn at this time.

Intramuscular Injections

The intramuscular (IM) injection route deposits medication into deep muscle tissue, which has a rich blood supply, allowing medication to absorb faster than with the subcutaneous route. However, there is an increased risk for injecting drugs directly into blood vessels. Any factor that interferes with local tissue blood flow affects the rate and extent of drug absorption.

Determine needle gauge by the medication to be administered. For example, administer immunizations and parenteral medications in aqueous solutions with a 20- to 25-gauge needle. Give viscous or oil-based solution with an 18- to 21-gauge needle. Use a small-gauge (22 to 25) needle for children. The current recommendations for needle length from the Centers for Disease Control and Prevention (2011a) are based on patient weight and body mass index (BMI). An adult patient who is thin requires a needle length of $\frac{5}{8}$ to 1 inch, whereas an average patient requires a 1-inch needle; patients weighing more than 70 kg require a 1- to $1\frac{1}{2}$-inch needle; and patients weighing more than 90 kg require a $1\frac{1}{2}$-inch needle (CDC, 2011a). Evidence-based practice recommends needle lengths for adults based on site selection: vastus lateralis, 16 to 25 mm ($\frac{5}{8}$ to 1 inch); ventrogluteal, 38 mm ($1\frac{1}{2}$ inches); and deltoid, 25 to 38 mm (1 to $1\frac{1}{2}$ inches) (Nicholl and Hesby, 2002). Recommendations for needle length include 25 mm (1 inch) for infants, 25 to 32 mm (1 to $1\frac{1}{4}$ inches) in toddlers, and 38 to 51 mm ($1\frac{1}{2}$ to 2 inches) in older children (Hockenberry and Wilson, 2011). Preterm and small, emaciated infants may require a shorter needle based on weight and muscle mass. Obese children may require a longer needle up to 38 mm ($1\frac{1}{2}$ inches) (Middleman et al., 2010). Based on the evidence, the recommendation for pediatric IM injection sites includes use of the anterolateral thigh for infants up to 12 months of age, deltoid in children 18 months and older, and ventrogluteal for children of all ages (Hockenberry and Wilson, 2011).

When selecting an IM site, determine that the site is free of pain, infection, necrosis, bruising, and abrasions. Also consider the location of underlying bones, nerves, and blood vessels and the volume of medication you will administer. To locate the ventrogluteal muscle, place the heel of your hand over the greater trochanter of the patient's hip with the wrist almost perpendicular to the femur. Use your right hand for the left hip, and your left hand for the right hip. Point the thumb toward the patient's groin; point the index finger toward the anterior superior iliac spine; and extend the middle finger back along the iliac crest toward the buttock. The index finger, the middle finger, and the iliac crest form a V-shaped triangle. The injection site is the center of the triangle (Fig. 34-1, *A*).

The vastus lateralis muscle is another injection site used in adults and is the preferred site for administration of biologicals (e.g., immunizations) to infants, toddlers, and children (Hockenberry and Wilson, 2011). It extends in an adult from a hand breadth above the knee to a hand breadth below the greater trochanter of the femur (Fig. 34-1, *B*). Use the middle third of the muscle for injection.

Locate the deltoid muscle by fully exposing the patient's upper arm and shoulder and asking him or her to relax the arm at the side, or by supporting the patient's arm and flexing the elbow. Do not roll up any tight-fitting sleeve. Allow the patient to sit, stand, or lie down. Palpate the lower edge of the acromion process, which forms the base of a triangle in line with the midpoint of the lateral aspect of the upper arm.

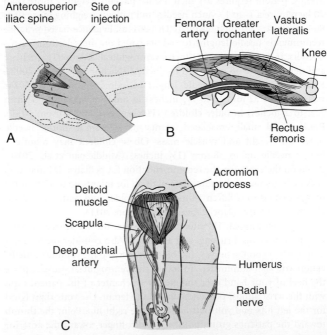

Fig. 34-1 **A,** Anatomical site for ventrogluteal injection. **B,** Anatomical site for vastus lateralis injection. **C,** Anatomical site for deltoid injection.

The injection site is in the center of the triangle, about 3 to 5 cm (1 to 2 inches) below the acromion process (Fig. 34-1, *C*).

The Z-track method, a technique for pulling the skin during an injection, is recommended for IM injections (Nicholl and Hesby, 2002). It prevents leakage of medication into subcutaneous tissues, seals medication in the muscle, and minimizes irritation. To use the Z-track method, apply the appropriate-size needle to the syringe and select an IM site, preferably in a large, deep muscle such as the ventrogluteal. Pull the overlying skin and subcutaneous tissues approximately 2.5 to 3.5 cm (1 to 1½ inches) laterally to the side with the ulnar side of the nondominant hand. Hold the skin in this position until you have administered the injection (Fig. 34-2). After cleaning a site, inject the needle deeply into the muscle. To reduce injection site discomfort, there is no longer any need to aspirate after the needle is injected when *administering vaccines* (CDC, 2011a). It is the nurse's responsibility to follow agency policy for aspirating after injecting the needle. Keep the needle inserted for 10 seconds to allow the medication to disperse evenly. Release the skin after withdrawing the needle. This leaves a zigzag path that seals the needle track wherever tissue planes slide across one another (Fig. 34-3). The medication is sealed in the muscle tissue.

Delegation Considerations

The skill of administering intramuscular injections cannot be delegated to nursing assistive personnel (NAP). The nurse instructs the NAP about:

- Potential medication side effects and to report their occurrence to the nurse.
- Reporting any change in the patient's condition to the nurse.

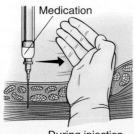

During injection

Fig. 34-2 Pulling on overlying skin during IM injection moves tissue to prevent later tracking.

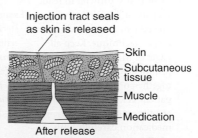

Injection tract seals as skin is released

- Skin
- Subcutaneous tissue
- Muscle
- Medication

After release

Fig. 34-3 The Z-track left after injection prevents the deposit of medication from leaking through sensitive tissue.

Equipment

- Proper-size syringe and needle:
  - 2 to 3 mL for adults
  - 0.5 to 1 mL for infants and small children
  - Needle length corresponds to site of injection and age of patient
  - Needle gauge often depends on length of needle; administer biological and medication in aqueous solution with a 20- to 25-gauge needle
- Alcohol swab
- Small gauze pad
- Vial or ampule of medication
- Clean gloves
- Medication administration record (MAR) or computer printout
- Puncture-proof container

Implementation

STEP	RATIONALE
1 Complete preprocedure protocol.	
2 Check accuracy and completeness of the MAR or computer printout with prescriber's written medication order. Check patient's name, medication name and dosage, route of administration, and time of administration. Recopy or reprint any portion of the MAR that is difficult to read.	The prescriber's order is the most reliable source and legal record of patient's medications. Ensures patient receives the correct medication. Illegible MARs are a source of medication errors.
3 Prepare medications for one patient at a time using aseptic technique. Keep all pages of MARs or computer printouts for one patient together, or look at only one patient's electronic MAR at a time. Check label of medication carefully with MAR or computer printout 2 times when preparing medication.	Ensures that medication is sterile. Preventing distractions reduces medication preparation errors (LePorte et al., 2009; Nguyen et al., 2010). *These are the first and second checks for accuracy* and ensure that correct medication is administered.

STEP	RATIONALE
4 Take medication to patient at right time.	Hospitals must adopt medication administration policy and procedure for timing of medication administration that considers nature of the prescribed medication, specific clinical application, and patient needs (DHHS, 2011; ISMP, 2011).
5 Identify patient using two identifiers (e.g., name and birthday or name and account number) according to agency policy. Compare identifiers with information on patient's MAR or medical record.	Ensures correct patient. Complies with The Joint Commission requirements for patient safety (TJC, 2014). Some agencies are now using a bar-code system to help with patient identification.
6 At patient's bedside again compare MAR or computer printout with names of medications on medication labels and patient name. Ask patient if he or she has allergies.	*This is the third check for accuracy* and ensures that patient receives correct medication. Confirms patient's allergy history.
7 Discuss purpose of each medication, action, and possible adverse effects. Allow patient to ask any questions. Tell patient that injection will cause a slight burning or sting.	Patient has right to be informed, and patient's understanding of each medication improves adherence to drug therapy. Helps minimize patient's anxiety.
8 ⬛ Perform hand hygiene and apply clean gloves. Keep sheet or gown draped over body parts not requiring exposure.	Reduces transmission of infection. Respects patient's dignity while exposing injection site.
9 Select appropriate site. Note integrity and size of muscle. Palpate for tenderness or	Ventrogluteal is preferred injection site for adults. It is also preferred site for children

STEP	RATIONALE
hardness. Avoid these areas. If patient receives frequent injections, rotate sites. Use ventrogluteal if possible.	of all ages (Hockenberry and Wilson, 2011; Hunt, 2008; Zimmerman, 2010).
10 Help patient to comfortable position. Position patient depending on chosen site (e.g., sit, lie flat, on side, or prone).	Reduces strain on muscle and minimizes injection discomfort.
11 Relocate site using anatomical landmarks.	Injection into correct anatomical site prevents injury to nerves, bone, and blood vessels.
12 Cleanse site with antiseptic swab. Apply swab at center of site, and rotate outward in circular direction for about 5 cm (2 inches). *Option:* Apply EMLA cream on injection site at least 1 hour before IM injection, or use vapocoolant spray (e.g., ethyl chloride) just before injection.	Mechanical action of swab removes secretions containing microorganisms. Decreases pain at injection site.
13 Hold swab or gauze between third and fourth fingers of nondominant hand.	Swab or gauze remains readily accessible when withdrawing needle.
14 Remove needle cap by pulling it straight off.	Preventing needle from touching sides of cap prevents contamination.
15 Hold syringe between thumb and forefinger of dominant hand; hold as dart, palm down (Fig. 34-4).	Quick, smooth injection requires proper manipulation of syringe parts.
16 Administer injection.	
a Position ulnar side of nondominant hand just below site, and pull skin laterally approximately 2.5 to 3.5 cm (1 to 1½ inches). Hold position	Z-track creates zigzag path through tissues that seals needle track to avoid tracking medication. A quick dartlike injection reduces discomfort. Z-track injections can be used

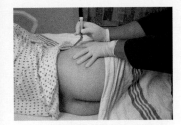

Fig. 34-4 Injection at the ventrogluteal site avoids major nerves and blood vessels.

STEP	RATIONALE
until medication is injected. With dominant hand, inject needle quickly at 90-degree angle into muscle.	for all IM injections (Hunter, 2008a; Nicholl and Hesby, 2002).
b *Option:* If patient's muscle mass is small, grasp body of muscle between thumb and forefingers.	Ensures that the medication reaches muscle mass (CDC, 2011a; Hockenberry and Wilson, 2011).
c After needle pierces skin, still pulling on skin with nondominant hand, grasp lower end of syringe barrel with fingers of nondominant hand to stabilize it. Move dominant hand to end of plunger. Avoid moving syringe.	Smooth manipulation of syringe reduces discomfort from needle movement. Skin remains pulled until after medication is injected to ensure Z-track administration.
d Pull back on plunger 5 to 10 seconds. If no blood appears, inject medication slowly at a rate of 10 sec/mL (Nicholl and Hesby, 2002).	Aspiration of blood into syringe indicates possible placement into a vein. Slow injection reduces pain and tissue trauma. The CDC no longer recommends aspiration for blood after administering vaccine (CDC, 2011a).

SAFETY ALERT If blood appears in syringe, remove needle, dispose of medication and syringe properly, and prepare another dose of medication for injection.

STEP	RATIONALE
e Wait 10 seconds, then smoothly and steadily withdraw needle, release skin, and apply alcohol swab or gauze gently over site.	Allows time for medication to absorb into muscle before syringe is removed. Dry gauze minimizes discomfort associated with alcohol on nonintact skin.
17 Apply gentle pressure to site. Do not massage site. Apply bandage if needed.	Massage damages underlying tissue.
18 Discard uncapped needle or needle enclosed in safety shield and attached syringe into a puncture-proof and leak-proof receptacle.	Prevents injury to patients and health care personnel. Recapping needles increases risk for a needlestick injury (OSHA, 2012).
19 Complete postprocedure protocol.	
20 Return to room in 15 to 30 minutes, and ask if patient feels any acute pain, burning, numbness, or tingling at injection site.	Continued discomfort may indicate injury to underlying bones or nerves.

Recording and Reporting

- Immediately after administration, record medication dose, route, site, time, and date given on MAR. Correctly sign MAR according to institutional policy.
- Record patient teaching, validation of understanding, and patient's response to medication in nurses' notes and electronic health record (EHR).
- Report any undesirable effects from medication to patient's health care provider, and document adverse effects in record.

UNEXPECTED OUTCOMES	RELATED INTERVENTIONS
1 Patient complains of localized pain or continued burning at injection site, indicating potential injury to nerve or vessels.	• Assess injection site. • Notify patient's health care provider.

UNEXPECTED OUTCOMES	RELATED INTERVENTIONS
2 During injection, blood is aspirated.	• Immediately stop injection, and remove needle. • Prepare new syringe of medication for administration.
3 Patient displays adverse reaction with signs of urticaria, eczema, pruritus, wheezing, and dyspnea.	• Follow institutional policy or guidelines for appropriate response to allergic reactions (e.g., administration of antihistamine such as diphenhydramine [Benadryl] or epinephrine). • Notify patient's health care provider immediately. • Add allergy information to patient's record.

Intravenous Medications:
Intermittent Infusion Sets and Mini-Infusion Pumps

One method of administering intravenous (IV) medications uses small volumes (25 to 250 mL) of compatible IV fluids infused over a desired period of time. This method reduces the risk for rapid dose infusion and provides independence for patients. Patients must have an established IV line that is kept patent either by continuous infusion or by intermittent flushes of normal saline. You can administer intermittent infusion of medication with any of the following methods: piggyback, volume-control administration (Volutrol, Buretrol, or Pediatrol), or mini-infusion pump.

Delegation Considerations

The skill of administering IV medications by piggyback, intermittent infusion sets, and mini-infusion pumps cannot be delegated to nursing assistive personnel (NAP). The nurse directs the NAP about:

- Potential medication side effects and to report their occurrence to the nurse.
- Reporting any patient complaint of moisture or discomfort around the IV insertion site.
- Reporting any change in the patient's condition or vital signs to the nurse.

Equipment

- Adhesive tape *(optional)*
- Antiseptic swab
- Clean gloves
- IV pole or rack
- Medication administration record (MAR) or computer printout
- Puncture-proof container

Piggyback or Mini-Infusion Pump

- Medication prepared in 50- to 250-mL labeled infusion bag or syringe
- Prefilled syringe of normal saline flush solution (for saline lock only)

- Short microdrip, macrodrip, or mini-infusion IV tubing set with blunt-ended (needleless) cannula attachment
- Needleless device
- Mini-infusion pump if indicated

Volume-Control Administration Set

- Volutrol or Buretrol
- Infusion tubing with needleless system attachment
- Syringe (1 to 20 mL)
- Vial or ampule of ordered medication

Implementation

STEP	RATIONALE
1 Complete preprocedure protocol.	

SAFETY ALERT Never administer IV medications through tubing that is infusing blood, blood products, or parenteral nutrition solutions.

STEP	RATIONALE
2 Assess patency of patient's existing IV infusion line or saline lock (see Skill 53).	Do not administer medication if site is edematous or inflamed.

SAFETY ALERT If the patient's IV site is saline locked, cleanse the port with alcohol, and assess the patency of the IV line by flushing it with 2 to 3 mL of sodium chloride.

STEP	RATIONALE
3 Assess patient's symptoms before initiating medication therapy.	Provides information to evaluate the desired effects of medication.
4 Assess patient's knowledge of medication.	Poses implications for patient education.
5 Prepare medications for one patient at a time using aseptic technique. Check label of medication carefully with MAR or computer printout 2 times when preparing medication. Pharmacy prepares piggyback and prefilled syringes. You will prepare medication for Volutrol.	Ensures that medication is sterile. Preventing distractions reduces medication preparation errors (LePorte et al., 2009; Nguyen et al., 2010). *These are the first and second checks for accuracy* and ensure that correct medication is administered.

STEP	RATIONALE
6 Take medication(s) to patient at correct time (see agency policy). Medications that require exact timing include STAT, first-time or loading doses, and one-time doses. Give time-critical scheduled medications (e.g., antibiotics, anticoagulants, insulin, anticonvulsants, immunosuppressive agents) at exact time ordered (no later than 30 minutes before or after scheduled dose). Give non–time-critical scheduled medications within a range of 1 or 2 hours of scheduled dose (ISMP, 2011). During administration, apply six rights of medication administration.	Hospitals must adopt medication administration policy and procedure for timing of medication administration that considers nature of the prescribed medication, specific clinical application, and patient needs (DHHS, 2011; ISMP, 2011).
7 Identify patient using two identifiers (e.g., name and birthday or name and account number) according to agency policy. Compare identifiers with information on patient's MAR or medical record.	Ensures correct patient. Complies with The Joint Commission requirements for patient safety (TJC, 2014). Some agencies are now using a bar-code system to help with patient identification.
8 At patient's bedside again compare MAR or computer printout with names of medications on medication labels and patient name. Ask patient if he or she has allergies.	*This is the third check for accuracy* and ensures that patient receives correct medication. Confirms patient's allergy history.
9 Discuss purpose of each medication, action, and possible adverse effects. Allow patient to ask any	Keeps patient informed of planned therapies, minimizing anxiety. Patients who verbalize pain at IV site help detect IV

STEP	RATIONALE
questions. Explain that you will give medication through existing IV line. Encourage patient to report symptoms of discomfort at site.	infiltrations early, lessening damage to surrounding tissues.
10 Administer infusion:	
a **Piggyback infusion:**	
(1) Connect infusion tubing to medication bag (see Skill 54). Fill tubing by opening regulator flow clamp. Once tubing is full, close clamp, and cap end of tubing.	Filling infusion tubing with solution and freeing air bubbles prevent air embolus.
(2) Hang piggyback medication bag above level of primary fluid bag. (Use hook to lower main bag.)	Height of fluid bag affects rate of flow to patient.
(3) Connect tubing of piggyback to appropriate connector on upper Y-port of primary infusion line:	Connection allows IV medication to enter main IV line.
(a) *Needleless system:* Wipe off needleless port on main IV line with alcohol swab, allow it to dry, and then insert tip of piggyback infusion tubing (Fig. 35-1).	Use needleless connections to prevent accidental needlestick injuries (INS, 2011a; OSHA, 2012).
(4) Regulate flow rate of medication solution by adjusting regulator clamp or IV pump infusion rate. Infusion	Provides slow, safe, intermittent infusion of medication and maintains therapeutic blood levels.

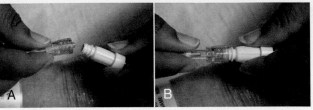

Fig. 35-1 **A,** Needleless lever lock cannula system. **B,** Blunt-ended cannula inserts into ports and locks.

STEP	RATIONALE
times vary. Refer to medication reference or institutional policy for safe flow rate.	
(5) Once medication has infused:	
(a) Continuous infusion: Check flow rate of primary infusion. Primary infusion automatically begins after piggyback solution is empty.	Back-check valve on piggyback prevents flow of primary infusion until medication infuses. Checking flow rate ensures proper administration of IV fluids.
(b) Normal saline lock: Disconnect tubing, clean port with alcohol, and flush IV line with 2 to 3 mL of sterile 0.9% sodium chloride. Maintain sterility of IV tubing between intermittent infusions.	

STEP	RATIONALE
(6) Regulate continuous main infusion line to ordered rate.	Infusion of piggyback sometimes interferes with main line infusion rate.
(7) Leave IV piggyback and tubing in place for future drug administration (see agency policy), or discard in puncture- and leak-proof container.	Establishment of secondary line produces route for microorganisms to enter main line. Repeated changes in tubing increase risk for infection transmission.
b **Volume-control administration set (e.g., Volutrol):**	
(1) Fill Volutrol with desired amount of IV fluid (50 to 100 mL) by opening clamp between Volutrol and main IV bag.	Small volume of fluid dilutes IV medication and reduces risk of fluid infusing too rapidly.
(2) Close clamp, and check to be sure that clamp on air vent Volutrol chamber is open.	Prevents additional leakage of fluid into Volutrol. Air vent allows fluid in Volutrol to exit at regulated rate.
(3) Clean injection port on top of Volutrol with antiseptic swab.	Prevents introduction of microorganisms during needle insertion.
(4) Remove needle cap or sheath, and insert needleless syringe or syringe needle through port and inject medication (Fig. 35-2). Gently rotate Volutrol between hands.	Rotating mixes medication with solution to ensure equal distribution in Volutrol.
(5) Regulate IV infusion rate to allow medication to infuse	For optimal therapeutic effect, medication should infuse in prescribed time interval.

Fig. 35-2 Medication injected into volume-control set.

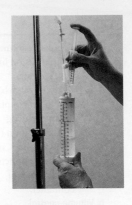

STEP	RATIONALE
in time recommended by agency policy, pharmacist, or medication reference manual.	
(6) Label Volutrol with name of medication, dosage, total volume including diluent, and time of administration following ISMP (2011) safe medication label format.	Alerts nurses to medication being infused. Prevents other medications from being added to Volutrol.
(7) If patient is receiving continuous IV infusion, check infusion rate after Volutrol infusion is complete.	Ensures appropriate rate of administration.
(8) Dispose of uncapped needle or needle enclosed in safety shield and syringe in puncture- and leak-proof container.	Prevents accidental needlesticks (OSHA, 2012). Reduces transmission of microorganisms.

STEP	RATIONALE
Discard supplies in appropriate container. Perform hand hygiene.	
c Mini-infusion administration:	
(1) Connect prefilled syringe to mini-infusion tubing. Remove end cap of tubing.	Special tubing designed to fit syringe delivers medication to main IV line.
(2) Carefully apply pressure to syringe plunger, allowing tubing to fill with medication.	Ensures tubing is free of air bubbles to prevent air embolus.
(3) Place syringe into mini-infusion pump (follow product directions) and hang on IV pole. Be sure syringe is secured (Fig. 35-3).	Secure placement is needed for proper medication administration.
(4) Connect mini-infusion tubing to main IV line or saline lock:	Establishes route for IV medication to enter main IV line.

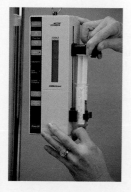

Fig. 35-3 Ensure that syringe is secure after placing it into mini-infusion pump.

STEP	RATIONALE
(a) *Existing IV line:* Wipe off needleless port on main IV line with alcohol swab, allow it to dry, and then insert tip of mini-infusion tubing through center of port.	Needleless connections reduce risk for accidental needlestick injuries (OSHA, 2012).
(b) *Normal saline lock:* Flush and prepare lock. Wipe off port with alcohol swab, allow it to dry, and then insert tip of mini-infusion tubing.	
(5) Set pump to deliver medication within time recommended by agency policy, pharmacist, or medication reference manual. Press button on pump to begin infusion.	Pump automatically delivers medication at safe, constant rate based on volume in syringe.
(6) Once medication has infused:	
(a) *Main IV infusion:* Check flow rate. Infusion automatically begins to flow once pump stops. Regulate infusion to desired rate as needed.	Maintains patent primary IV fluids.

STEP	RATIONALE
(b) *Normal saline lock:* Disconnect tubing, clean port with alcohol, and flush IV line with 2 to 3 mL of sterile 0.9% sodium chloride. Maintain sterility of IV tubing between intermittent infusions.	
(7) Complete postprocedure protocol.	
(8) Stay with patient for several minutes and observe for any allergic reactions.	Dyspnea, wheezing, and circulatory collapse are signs of severe anaphylactic reaction.

Recording and Reporting

- Immediately record medication, dose, route, infusion rate, and date and time administered on MAR or computer printout.
- Record volume of fluid in medication bag or Volutrol on intake and output (I&O) form.
- Report any adverse reactions to patient's health care provider.

UNEXPECTED OUTCOMES	RELATED INTERVENTIONS
1 Patient develops adverse or allergic reaction to medication.	• Stop medication infusion immediately. • Follow agency policy or guidelines for appropriate response to allergic reaction (e.g., administration of antihistamine such as diphenhydramine [Benadryl] or epinephrine) and reporting of adverse medication reactions.

Continued

UNEXPECTED OUTCOMES	RELATED INTERVENTIONS
	• Notify patient's health care provider of adverse effects immediately.
	• Add allergy information to patient record per agency policy.
2 Medication does not infuse over established time frame.	• Determine reason (e.g., improper calculation of flow rate, poor position of IV needle at insertion site, infiltration).
	• Take corrective action as indicated, and resume infusion.
3 Intravenous site shows signs of infiltration or phlebitis (see Skill 54).	• Stop IV infusion and discontinue access device.
	• Treat IV site as indicated by agency policy.
	• Insert new IV catheter if therapy continues.
	• For infiltration, determine how harmful IV medication is to subcutaneous tissue. Provide IV extravasation care (e.g., injecting phentolamine [Regitine] around the IV infiltration site) as indicated by agency policy, or consult pharmacist to determine appropriate follow-up care.

Intravenous Medications:
Intravenous Bolus

An intravenous (IV) bolus introduces a concentrated dose of a medication directly into a vein by way of an existing IV access. An IV bolus, or "push," usually requires small volumes of fluid, which is an advantage for patients who are at risk for fluid overload. The IV bolus is a dangerous method for administering medications because it allows no time for correction of errors. Therefore, be very careful in calculating the correct amount of the medication for administration. In addition, a bolus may cause direct irritation to the lining of blood vessels; thus always confirm placement of the IV catheter or needle. Accidental injection of some medications into tissues surrounding a vein can cause pain, sloughing of tissues, and abscesses.

The Institute for Safe Medication Practices (2011) has identified the following four strategies to reduce harm from rapid IV push medications:

- Make sure that the information regarding rate of administration of IV push medication is readily available.
- Use less-concentrated solutions whenever possible.
- Avoid using terms such as *IV push, IVP,* or *IV bolus* in orders with medications that should be administered over 1 minute or longer. Use more descriptive terms such as *IV over 5 minutes.*
- Consider alternatives such as a syringe pump to administer a medication that has a high risk for adverse effects. If this is not an alternative to IV push, have pharmacy dilute the medication and administer in a piggyback.

Verify the rate of administration of IV push medication using institutional guidelines or a medication reference manual.

Delegation Considerations

The skill of administering intravenous medications by IV bolus cannot be delegated to nursing assistive personnel (NAP). The nurse directs the NAP about:

- Potential actions and side effects of the medications and to report their occurrence to the nurse.
- Reporting any patient complaint of moisture or discomfort around infusion site.
- Obtaining any required vital signs and reporting them to the nurse.

Equipment

- Watch with second hand
- Clean gloves
- Antiseptic swab
- Medication in vial or ampule
- Proper-size syringes for medication and saline flush with needleless device or sharps with engineered sharps injury protection (SESIP) needle (21- to 25-gauge)
- Intravenous lock: Vial of normal saline flush solution (saline recommended [INS, 2011]); if agency continues to use heparin flush, the most common concentration is 10 units/mL; check agency policy
- Medication administration record (MAR) or computer printout
- Puncture-proof container

Implementation

STEP	RATIONALE
1 Complete preprocedure protocol.	
2 Check accuracy and completeness of each MAR or computer printout with prescriber's written medication order. Check patient's name, medication name and dosage, route of administration, and time of administration.	The prescriber's order is the most reliable source and legal record of patient's correct medications. Ensures patient receives the correct medications.
3 Perform hand hygiene. Assess condition of IV needle insertion site for patency and signs of infiltration or phlebitis.	Do not administer medication if site is edematous or inflamed. For medication to reach venous circulation effectively, IV line must be patent, and fluids must infuse easily.

SAFETY ALERT Some IV medications require dilution before administration. Verify with agency policy or pharmacy. If a small amount of medication is given (e.g., less than 1 mL), dilute medication in small amount (e.g., 5 mL) of normal saline or sterile water so the medication does not collect in the "dead spaces" (e.g., Y-site injection port, IV cap) of the IV delivery system.

STEP	RATIONALE
4 Take medication(s) to patient at correct time (see agency policy).	Hospitals must adopt medication administration policy and procedure for timing of medication administration that considers nature of the prescribed medication, specific clinical application, and patient needs (DHHS, 2011; ISMP, 2011). Time-critical scheduled medications are those for which early or delayed administration of maintenance doses of greater than 30 minutes before or after the scheduled dose may cause harm or result in substantial suboptimal therapy or pharmacological effect. Non–time-critical medications are those for which early or delayed administration within a specified range of either 1 or 2 hours should not cause harm or result in substantial suboptimal therapy or pharmacological effect (DHHS, 2011; ISMP, 2011).
5 Identify patient using two identifiers (e.g., name and birthday or name and account number) according to agency policy. Compare identifiers with information on patient's MAR or medical record.	Ensures correct patient. Complies with The Joint Commission requirements for patient safety (TJC, 2014). Some agencies are now using a bar-code system to help with patient identification.
6 At the patient's bedside again compare MAR or computer printout with names of medications on medication labels and patient name. Ask patient if he or she has allergies.	*This is the third check for accuracy* and ensures that patient receives correct medication. Confirms patient's allergy history.

STEP	RATIONALE
7 Discuss purpose of each medication, action, and possible adverse effects. Allow patient to ask any questions. Explain that you will give medication through existing IV line. Encourage patient to report symptoms of discomfort at IV site.	Keep patient informed of planned therapies, minimizing anxiety. Patients who verbalize pain at IV site help detect IV infiltrations early, lessening damage to surrounding tissues.
8 ![hand] Perform hand hygiene and put on clean gloves.	Reduces transmission of infection.
9 Intravenous push (existing line):	
a Select injection port of IV tubing closest to patient. Use needleless injection port.	Follows provisions of the Needle Safety and Prevention Act of 2001 (OSHA, 2012).
b Clean injection port with antiseptic swab. Allow it to dry.	Prevents transfer of microorganisms during blunt cannula insertion.
c Connect syringe to IV line: Insert needleless tip of syringe containing drug through center of port (Fig. 36-1).	Prevents introduction of microorganisms. Prevents damage to port diaphragm and possible leakage from site.
d Occlude IV line by pinching tubing just above injection port (Fig. 36-2). Pull back gently on plunger of syringe to aspirate for blood return.	Final check ensures that medication is being delivered into bloodstream.

SAFETY ALERT In the case of smaller-gauge IV needles, blood return sometimes is not aspirated even if IV is patent. If IV site does not show signs of infiltration and IV fluid is infusing without difficulty, give IV push.

e Release tubing, and inject medication within amount of time recommended by agency policy, pharmacist, or medication reference	Ensures safe medication infusion. Rapid injection of IV drug can be fatal. Allowing IV fluids to infuse while pushing IV drug enables medication

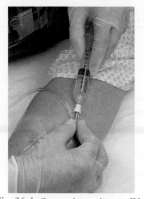

Fig. 36-1 Connecting syringe to IV line with needleless blunt cannula tip.

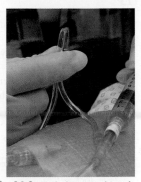

Fig. 36-2 Occluding IV tubing above injection port.

STEP	RATIONALE
manual. Use watch to time administrations. You can pinch IV line while pushing medication and release it when not pushing medication. Allow IV fluids to infuse when not pushing medication.	to be delivered to patient at prescribed rate.
f After injecting medication, withdraw syringe, and recheck IV fluid infusion rate.	Injection of bolus may alter rate of fluid infusion. Rapid fluid infusion can cause circulatory fluid overload.
10 Intravenous push (intravenous lock):	
a Prepare flush solutions according to agency policy.	
(1) *Saline flush method (preferred method):* Prepare two syringes filled with 2 to 3 mL of normal saline (0.9%).	Normal saline is effective in keeping IV locks patent and is compatible with wide range of medications.

STEP	RATIONALE
(2) *Heparin flush method* (not recommended; refer to agency policy).	
b Administer medication:	
(1) Clean injection port with antiseptic swab.	Prevents transfer of microorganisms.
(2) Insert needleless tip of syringe with normal saline 0.9% through center of injection port of IV lock.	
(3) Pull back gently on syringe plunger and check for blood return.	Indicates if needle or catheter is in vein.
(4) Flush IV site with normal saline by pushing slowly on plunger.	Clears needle and reservoir of blood. Flushing without difficulty indicates patent IV.

SAFETY ALERT Carefully observe the area of skin above the IV catheter. Note any puffiness or swelling as the IV site is flushed, which could indicate infiltration into the vein, requiring removal of catheter.

(5) Remove saline-filled syringe.	
(6) Clean injection port with antiseptic swab.	Prevents transmission of microorganisms.
(7) Insert needleless tip of syringe containing prepared medication through injection port of IV lock.	Allows administration of medication.
(8) Inject medication within amount of time recommended by agency policy, pharmacist, or medication reference manual. Use watch to time administration.	Many medication errors are associated with IV pushes being administered too quickly. Following guidelines for IV push rates promotes patient safety.

STEP	RATIONALE
(9) After administering medication, withdraw syringe.	
(10) Clean lock's injection site with antiseptic swab.	Prevents transmission of microorganisms.
(11) Flush injection port.	
(a) Attach syringe with normal saline, and inject flush at the same rate that the medication was delivered.	Flushing IV line with saline prevents occlusion of IV access device and ensures that all medication is delivered. Flushing IV site at same rate as medication ensures that any medication remaining within IV needle is delivered at the correct rate.
11 Dispose of SESIP needles and syringes in puncture- and leak-proof container.	Prevents accidental needlestick injuries and follows CDC guidelines for disposal of sharps (OSHA, 2012).
12 Complete postprocedure protocol.	

Recording and Reporting

- Immediately record medication administration, including drug, dose, route, time instilled, and date and time administered on MAR. Include initials or signature.
- Report any adverse reactions to patient's health care provider. Patient's response sometimes indicates need for additional medical therapy.
- Record patient's medication response in nurses' notes and electronic health record (EHR).

UNEXPECTED OUTCOMES	RELATED INTERVENTIONS
1 Patient develops adverse reaction to medication.	• Stop delivering medication immediately, and follow agency policy or guidelines for appropriate response to allergic reaction

Continued

UNEXPECTED OUTCOMES	RELATED INTERVENTIONS
	(e.g., administration of antihistamine such as diphenhydramine [Benadryl] or epinephrine) and reporting of adverse drug reactions.
	• Notify patient's health care provider of adverse effects immediately.
	• Add allergy information to patient's medical record.
2 IV medication is incompatible with IV fluids (e.g., IV fluid becomes cloudy in tubing) (see agency policy).	• Stop the IV fluids, and clamp the IV line.
	• Flush the IV with 10 mL of 0.9% sodium chloride or sterile water.
	• Give IV bolus over appropriate amount of time.
	• Flush with another 10 mL of 0.9% sodium chloride or sterile water at the same rate as the medication was administered.
	• Restart the IV fluids with new tubing at prescribed rate.
	• If unable to stop IV infusion, start a new IV site, and administer medication using IV push (IV lock) method.
3 Intravenous site shows signs of infiltration or phlebitis.	• Stop IV infusion immediately, or discontinue access device and restart in another site.
	• Determine how much damage IV medication can produce in subcutaneous tissue.
	• Provide IV extravasation care (e.g., injecting

UNEXPECTED OUTCOMES	RELATED INTERVENTIONS
	phentolamine [Regitine] around the IV infiltration site) as indicated by agency policy. Use a medication reference and consult pharmacist to determine appropriate follow-up care.
4 Patient is unable to explain medication information.	• Provide patient with additional information, or acknowledge that patient is unable to learn at this time.

Isolation Precautions

In 2007 the Hospital Infection Control Practices Advisory Committee (HICPAC) of the Centers for Disease Control and Prevention (CDC) published revised guidelines for isolation precautions (Box 37-1). These recommendations were based on current epidemiological information regarding disease transmission in health care settings. Although primarily intended for care of patients in acute care, you can apply the recommendations to patients in subacute care or long-term care facilities. HICPAC recommends that hospitals modify the recommendations according to their needs and as dictated by federal, state, or local regulations (CDC, 2007b).

Standard Precautions are the primary strategies for prevention of infection transmission and apply to contact with blood, body fluids, nonintact skin, and mucous membranes and with equipment or surfaces contaminated with these potentially infectious materials. The strategy of respiratory hygiene/cough etiquette applies to any person with signs of respiratory tract infection, including cough, congestion, rhinorrhea, or increased production of respiratory secretions when entering a health care site. Education of health care staff, patients, and visitors to cover the mouth and nose with a tissue when coughing, dispose properly of used tissues, and perform hand hygiene is among the elements of respiratory hygiene.

The second tier (Table 37-1) includes precautions designed for care of patients who are known or suspected to be infected, or colonized, with microorganisms transmitted by the contact, droplet, or airborne route (Brisko, 2011; CDC, 2007a) or by contact with contaminated surfaces. The three types of transmission-based precautions—airborne, droplet, and contact—may be combined for diseases that have multiple routes of transmission (e.g., chickenpox). They are used either singly or in combination when Standard Precautions are implemented.

Delegation Considerations

The skill of caring for patients on isolation precautions can be delegated to nursing assistive personnel (NAP). However, the nurse must assess the patient's status and isolation indications. The nurse instructs the NAP to:

- Take special precautions regarding individual patient needs such as transportation to diagnostic tests.
- Take precautions about bringing equipment into the patient's room.
- Be aware of high-risk factors for infection transmission that pertain to the assigned patient.

BOX 37-1 CDC Isolation Guidelines: Standard Precautions (Tier 1)* for Use with All Patients

- Standard Precautions apply to blood, blood products, all body fluids, secretions, excretions (except sweat), nonintact skin, and mucous membranes.
- Perform hand hygiene before, after, and between direct contact with patients (e.g., between contact: cleaning hands after a patient care activity, moving to a nonpatient care activity, and cleaning hands again before returning to perform patient contact).
- Perform hand hygiene after contact with blood, body fluids, secretions, and excretions; after contact with surfaces or articles in a patient room; and immediately after gloves are removed.
- When hands are visibly soiled or contaminated with blood or body fluids, wash them with either a nonantimicrobial soap or an antimicrobial soap and water.
- When hands are not visibly soiled or contaminated with blood or body fluids, use an alcohol-based hand rub to perform hand hygiene.
- Wash hands with nonantimicrobial soap and water if contact with spores (e.g., *Clostridium difficile*) is likely to have occurred.
- Do not wear artificial fingernails or extenders if duties include direct contact with patients at high risk for infection and associated adverse outcomes.
- Wear gloves when touching blood, body fluids, secretions, excretions, nonintact skin, mucous membranes, or contaminated items or surfaces is likely. Remove gloves and perform hand hygiene between patient care encounters and when going from a contaminated to a clean body site.
- Wear personal protective equipment when the anticipated patient interaction indicates that contact with blood or body fluids may occur.
- A private room is unnecessary unless the patient's hygiene is unacceptable (e.g., uncontained secretions, excretions, or wound drainage).
- Discard all contaminated sharp instruments and needles in a puncture-resistant container. Health care agencies must make available needleless devices. Any needles should be disposed of uncapped, or a mechanical safety device should be activated for recapping.
- Respiratory hygiene/cough etiquette—Have patients:
  - Cover the nose/mouth when coughing or sneezing.
  - Use tissues to contain respiratory secretions and dispose of them in nearest waste container.
  - Perform hand hygiene after contacting respiratory secretions and contaminated objects/materials.
  - Contain respiratory secretions with procedure or surgical mask.
  - Sit at least 91.4 cm (3 feet) away from others if coughing.

*Formerly universal precautions and body substance isolation.

TABLE 37-1 CDC Isolation Guidelines: Transmission-Based Precautions (Tier 2) for Use With Specific Types of Patients

Category	Disease	Barrier Protection
Airborne Precautions (droplet nuclei smaller than 5 microns)	Measles, chickenpox (varicella), disseminated varicella zoster, pulmonary or laryngeal tuberculosis	Private room, negative-pressure airflow of at least 6 to 12 exchanges per hour via HEPA* filtration; mask or respiratory protection device, N95 respirator required (depending on condition)
Droplet Precautions (droplets larger than 5 microns; being within 3 feet of patient)	Diphtheria (pharyngeal), rubella, streptococcal pharyngitis, pneumonia or scarlet fever in infants and young children, pertussis, mumps, *Mycoplasma* pneumonia, meningococcal pneumonia or sepsis, pneumonic plague	Private room or cohort patients; mask or respirator required (depending on condition) (refer to agency policy)
Contact Precautions (direct patient or environmental contact)	Colonization or infection with multidrug-resistant organisms such as VRE and MRSA, *Clostridium difficile, Shigella,* and other enteric pathogens; major wound infections; herpes simplex; scabies; varicella zoster (disseminated); respiratory syncytial virus in infants, young children, or immunocompromised adults	Private room or cohort patients (see agency policy), gloves, gowns

TABLE 37-1 CDC Isolation Guidelines: Transmission-Based Precautions (Tier 2) for Use With Specific Types of Patients—cont'd

Category	Disease	Barrier Protection
Protective environment	Allogeneic hematopoietic stem cell transplants	Private room; positive airflow with 12 or more air exchanges per hour; HEPA filtration for incoming air; mask to be worn by patient when out of room during times of construction in area

Modified from Centers for Disease Control and Prevention (CDC), Hospital Infection Control Practice Advisory Committee: Guidelines for isolation precautions in hospitals, *MMWR Morb Mortal Wkly Rep* 57(RR-16):39, 2007.

*HEPA, High-efficiency particulate air; *MRSA,* methicillin-resistant *Staphylococcus aureus; VRE,* vancomycin-resistant enterococcus.

Equipment

- Barrier protection determined by type of isolation required, such as clean gloves, mask, eyewear or goggles, face shield, and gown (gowns may be disposable or reusable, depending on agency policy)
- Other patient care equipment (as appropriate) (e.g., hygiene items, medications, dressing supplies, sharps container, disposable blood pressure cuff)
- Soiled linen bag and trash receptacle
- Sign for door indicating type of isolation and, if applicable, directing visitors to nurses' station before entering room

Implementation

STEP	RATIONALE
1 Complete preprocedure protocol.	
2 Review laboratory test results (e.g., wound culture, acid-fast bacillus [AFB] smears, changes in white blood cell [WBC] count).	Reveals type of microorganism for which patient is being isolated, body fluid in which it was identified, and whether patient is immunosuppressed.

STEP	RATIONALE
3 Consider types of care measures that you will perform while in patient's room (e.g., medication administration or dressing change).	Allows you to organize care items for procedures and time spent in patient's room.
4 Perform hand hygiene.	Reduces transmission of microorganisms.
5 Prepare all equipment needed in patient's room.	Prevents you from making more than one trip into room.
6 Prepare for entrance into isolation room. Before applying personal protective equipment (PPE), step into patient's room and stay by door. Introduce yourself and explain the care that you are providing.	Proper preparation ensures nurse is protected from microorganism exposure.
a Apply gown, being sure it covers all outer garments. Pull sleeves down to wrist. Tie securely at neck and waist (Fig. 37-1).	Prevents transmission of infection and protects you when patient has excessive drainage or discharges.

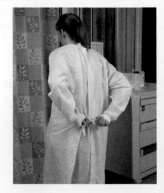

Fig. 37-1 Nurse with protective equipment for contact and droplet infection.

STEP	RATIONALE
b Apply either surgical mask or a fitted respirator around mouth and nose (type and fit-testing will depend on type of isolation and agency policy).	Prevents exposure to airborne microorganisms or exposure to microorganisms that may occur during splashing of fluids.
c If needed, apply eyewear or goggles snugly around face and eyes. If you wear glasses, side shield may be used.	Protects you from exposure to microorganisms that may occur during splashing of fluids.
d 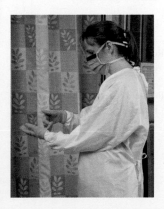 Apply clean gloves. (**NOTE:** Wear unpowdered latex-free gloves if you, the patient, or another health care worker has a latex allergy.) Position glove cuffs over edge of gown sleeves (Fig. 37-2).	Reduces transmission of microorganisms.
7 Enter patient's room. Arrange supplies and equipment.	Prevents extra trips entering and leaving the room.

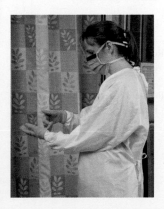

Fig. 37-2 Nurse applies clean gloves.

STEP	RATIONALE
8 Explain purpose of isolation and precautions that should be taken by patient and family. Offer opportunity to ask questions.	Improves patient's and family's ability to participate in care and minimizes anxiety. Identifies opportunity for planning social interaction and diversional activities.
9 Assess vital signs:	
a Reusable equipment brought into the room must be thoroughly disinfected when removed from the room.	Decreases the risk of infection transmission to another patient.
b If stethoscope is to be reused, clean earpieces and diaphragm or bell with 70% alcohol or facility-approved germicide. Set aside on clean surface.	Systematic disinfection of stethoscopes with 70% alcohol or approved germicide minimizes chance of spreading infectious agents between patients (CDC, 2007b).
c Use individual or disposable thermometers and blood pressure cuffs when available.	Prevents cross-contamination.
10 Administer medications:	
a Give oral medication in wrapper or cup.	Handle and discard supplies to minimize transfer of microorganisms.
b Dispose of wrapper or cup in plastic-lined receptacle.	
c Wear gloves when administering an injection.	Reduces the risk for exposure to blood.
d Discard disposable syringe and uncapped or sheathed needle into designated sharps container.	Reduces risk for needlestick injury.

STEP	RATIONALE
e Place reusable plastic syringe (e.g., Carpuject) on clean towel for eventual removal and disinfection.	Prevents added contamination of syringe.
f If you are not wearing gloves and hands contact a contaminated article or body fluids, perform hand hygiene as soon as possible.	Reduces transmission of microorganisms.
11 Administer hygiene, encouraging patient to ask any questions or express concerns about isolation. Provide informal teaching at this time.	Hygiene practices further minimize transfer of microorganisms. Quality time should be spent with patient when in room.
a Avoid allowing isolation gown to become wet; carry wash basin outward away from gown; avoid leaning against wet tabletop.	Moisture allows organisms to travel through gown to uniform.

SAFETY ALERT When there is a risk for excess soiling, wear a gown impervious to moisture.

STEP	RATIONALE
b Help patient remove own gown; discard in leak-proof linen bag.	Reduces transfer of microorganisms.
c Remove linen from bed; avoid contact with isolation gown. Place in leak-proof linen bag.	Handle linen soiled by patient's body fluids to prevent contact with clean items.
d Provide clean bed linen and set of towels.	
e ✋ Remove gloves and perform hand hygiene if gloves become excessively soiled and further care is necessary. Reglove.	

STEP	RATIONALE
12 Collect specimens:	
a Place specimen containers on clean paper towel in patient's bathroom.	Container will be taken out of patient's room; prevents contamination of outer surface.
b Follow agency procedure for collecting specimen of body fluids.	
c Transfer specimen to container without soiling outside of container. Place container in plastic bag and place label on outside of bag or per agency policy. Label specimen in front of patient (TJC, 2014). Perform hand hygiene and reglove if additional procedures are needed.	Specimens of blood and body fluids are placed in well-constructed containers with secure lids to prevent leaks during transport.
d Check label on specimen for accuracy. Send to laboratory (warning labels are often used, depending on hospital policy). Label containers of blood or body fluids with a biohazard sticker.	Ensures that health care providers who transport or handle containers are aware of infectious contents.
13 Dispose of linen, trash, and disposable items:	
a Use single bags that are sturdy and impervious to moisture to contain soiled articles. Use double bag if necessary for heavily soiled linen or heavy wet trash.	Linen or refuse should be totally contained to prevent exposure of personnel to infectious material.
b Tie bags securely at top in knot.	

STEP	RATIONALE
14 Remove all reusable pieces of equipment. Clean any contaminated surfaces with hospital-approved disinfectant (CDC, 2007b) (see agency policy).	All items must be properly cleaned, disinfected, or sterilized for reuse.
15 Resupply room as needed. Have staff colleague hand new supplies to you.	Limiting trips of personnel into and out of room reduces exposure to microorganisms for you and your patient.
16 Leave isolation room. Remember, order of removal of protective barriers depends on what you wear in room. This sequence describes steps to take if all barriers are worn:	
a Remove gloves. Remove one glove by grasping cuff and pulling glove inside out over hand. Hold removed glove in gloved hand. Slide fingers of ungloved hand under remaining glove at wrist. Peel glove off over first glove (Fig. 37-3). Discard gloves in proper container.	Technique prevents contact with contaminated glove's outer surface.
b Remove eyewear, face shield, or goggles. Handle by headband or earpieces. Discard in proper container.	Outside of goggles is contaminated. Hands have not been soiled.
c Untie neck strings, and then untie back strings of gown. Allow gown to fall from shoulders (Fig. 37-4); touch inside of gown only. Remove hands	Hands do not come in contact with soiled front of gown.

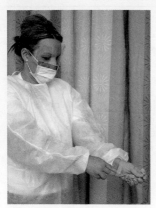

Fig. 37-3 Nurse removes gloves.

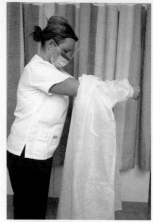

Fig. 37-4 Nurse removes gown.

STEP	RATIONALE
from sleeves without touching outside of gown. Hold gown inside at shoulder seams, and fold inside out into a bundle; discard in laundry bag.	
d Remove mask. If the mask secures over the ears, remove elastic from ears and pull mask away from face. For a tie-on mask, untie *bottom* mask strings and then top strings, pull mask away from face, and drop mask into trash receptacle (do not touch outer surface of mask).	Ungloved hands will not be contaminated by touching only elastic or mask strings. Prevents top part of mask from falling down over nurse's uniform.
e Perform hand hygiene.	Reduces transmission of microorganisms.
f Retrieve wristwatch and stethoscope (unless items must remain in room), and record vital sign values on notepaper.	Clean hands can contact clean items.

STEP	RATIONALE
g Explain to patient when you plan to return to room. Ask whether patient requires any personal care items. Offer books, magazines, audiotapes	Diversions help to minimize boredom and feeling of social isolation.
h Leave room and close door if necessary. Close door if patient is in negative airflow room.	
17 While in room, ask if patient has had sufficient opportunity to discuss health problems, course of treatment, or other topics important to patient.	Measures patient's perception of adequacy of discussions with caregivers.
18 Complete postprocedure protocol.	

Recording and Reporting

- Document procedures performed and patient's response to social isolation. Also document any patient education performed and reinforced.
- Document type of isolation in use and the microorganisms (if known).

UNEXPECTED OUTCOMES	RELATED INTERVENTIONS
1 Patient avoids social and therapeutic discussions.	• Confer with family and/ or significant other, and determine best approach to reduce patient's sense of loneliness and depression.
2 Patient or health care worker may have an allergy to latex gloves.	• Notify physician/employee health department, and treat sensitivity or allergic reaction appropriately.
	• Use latex-free gloves for future care activities.

Mechanical Lifts

One of the major concerns during transfer is the safety of the patient and the nurse. The nurse prevents self-injury by using correct posture, minimal muscle strength, effective body mechanics and lifting techniques, and appropriate lift devices. Consider individual patient problems during transfer. For example, a patient who has been immobile for several days or longer may be weak or dizzy or may develop orthostatic hypotension (a drop in blood pressure) when transferred. If there is any doubt about safe transfer, use a transfer belt and obtain assistance when transferring patients.

Delegation Considerations

The skill of effective transfer techniques can be delegated to nursing assistive personnel (NAP). The nurse directs NAP by:

- Assisting and supervising when moving patients who are transferred for the first time after prolonged bed rest, extensive surgery, critical illness, or spinal cord trauma.
- Informing NAP about the patient's mobility restrictions, changes in blood pressure, or sensory alterations that may affect safe transfer.
- Explaining what to observe and report to the nurse, such as dizziness or the patient's ability to assist.

Equipment

- Nonskid shoes, bath blankets, pillows
- Mechanical/hydraulic lift: Use frame, canvas strips or chains, and hammock or canvas strips; stand-assist lift device

Implementation

STEP	RATIONALE
1 Complete preprocedure protocol.	
2 Assess physiological capacity of a patient to transfer and the need for special adaptive techniques. Assess the following:	Determines patient's ability to tolerate and assist with transfer and whether special adaptive techniques are necessary.
a Muscle strength (legs and upper arms)	Immobile patients have decreased muscle strength,

STEP	RATIONALE
	tone, and mass. Affects ability to bear weight or raise body.
b Joint mobility and contracture formation	Immobility or inflammatory processes (e.g., arthritis) may lead to contracture formation and impaired joint mobility.
c Paralysis or paresis (spastic or flaccid)	Patient with central nervous system (CNS) damage may have bilateral paralysis (requiring transfer by swivel bar, sliding bar, mechanical lift) or unilateral paralysis, which requires belt transfer to strong side. Weakness (paresis) requires stabilization of knee while transferring. Flaccid arm must be supported with sling during transfer.
d Bone continuity (trauma, amputation), or calcium loss from long bones	Patients with trauma to one leg or hip may be non–weight-bearing when transferred. Amputees may use sliding board to transfer. Osteoporosis increases risk for injury.
3 Assess presence of weakness, dizziness, or postural hypotension.	Determines risk for fainting or falling during transfer. The move from a supine to a vertical position redistributes about 500 mL of blood; immobile patients may have decreased autonomic nervous system response to equalize blood supply, resulting in orthostatic hypotension (Lewis et al., 2011).
4 Assess patient's cognitive status.	Determines patient's ability to follow directions and learn transfer techniques.
a Ability to follow verbal instructions	May indicate patients at risk for injury.

STEP	RATIONALE
b Short-term memory	Patients with short-term memory deficits may have difficulty with transfer, initial learning, or consistent performance.
c Recognition of physical deficits and limitations to movement	Patient's knowledge of deficits can help the nurse plan a safe transfer.
5 Determine if a lift device is needed and the number of people needed to assist with transfer. Do not start procedure until all required caregivers are available.	Ensures safe patient transfer.
6 Use mechanical/hydraulic lift to transfer patient from bed to chair:	
a Bring lift to bedside, or lower ceiling lift and position properly.	Ensures safe elevation of patient off bed.
b Position chair near bed, and allow adequate space to maneuver lift.	Prepares environment for safe use of lift and subsequent transfer.
c Raise bed to high position with mattress flat. Lower side rail on side near chair.	Allows you to use proper body mechanics.
d Raise opposite side rail unless a second nurse is assisting.	Maintains patient safety.
e Roll patient on side away from you.	Positions patient for placement of lift sling.
f Place hammock or canvas strips under patient to form sling. With two canvas pieces, lower edge fits under patient's knees (wide piece), and upper edge fits under patient's shoulders (narrow piece).	Two types of seats are supplied with mechanical/hydraulic lift: hammock style is better for patients who are flaccid, weak, and need support; canvas strips can be used for patients with normal muscle tone. Hooks should face away from patient's skin. Place sling under patient's center of gravity and greatest portion of body weight.

STEP	RATIONALE
g Raise bedrail.	Maintains patient safety.
h Go to opposite side of bed, and lower side rail.	
i Roll patient to opposite side, and pull hammock (strips) through.	Completes positioning of patient on mechanical/hydraulic sling.
j Roll patient supine onto canvas hammock.	Sling should extend from shoulders to knees (hammock) to support patient's body weight equally.
k Place lift's horseshoe bar under side of bed (on side with chair).	Positions lift efficiently and promotes smooth transfer.
l Lower horizontal bar to sling level by releasing hydraulic valve. Lock valve if required.	Positions hydraulic lift close to patient. Locking valve prevents injury to patient.
m Attach hooks on strap (chain) to holes in sling. Short chains or straps hook to top holes of sling; longer chains hook to bottom of sling (Fig. 38-1).	Secures hydraulic lift to sling.
n Elevate head of bed.	Positions patient in sitting position.
o Fold patient's arms over chest.	Prevents injury to patient's arms.
p Pump hydraulic handle using long, slow, even strokes until patient is raised off bed. For ceiling lift, turn on control device to move lift.	Ensures safe support of patient during elevation.
q Use steering handle to pull lift from bed and maneuver patient to chair.	Moves patient from bed to chair.
r Roll base around chair.	Positions lift in front of the chair to which patient is to be transferred.

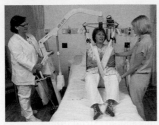

Fig. 38-1 Sling positioned under the patient and attached to the lift.

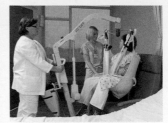

Fig. 38-2 Lowering patient into the chair.

STEP	RATIONALE
s Release check valve slowly (turn to left), and lower patient into chair (Fig. 38-2).	Safely guides patient into back of chair as seat descends.
t Close check valve or turn off control device as soon as patient is down and straps can be released.	If valve is left open or device left on, boom may continue to lower and injure patient.
u Remove straps and mechanical/hydraulic lift.	Prevents damage to skin and underlying tissues from canvas or hooks.
v Check patient's sitting alignment, and correct if necessary.	Prevents injury from poor posture.
7 Complete postprocedure protocol.	

Recording and Reporting

- Record procedure, including pertinent observations: weakness, ability to follow directions, weight-bearing ability, balance, ability to pivot, number of personnel needed to assist, and amount of assistance (muscle strength) required.
- Report transfer ability and assistance needed to next shift or other caregivers. Report progress or remission to rehabilitation staff (physical therapist, occupational therapist).

UNEXPECTED OUTCOMES	RELATED INTERVENTIONS
1 Patient is unable to comprehend and follow directions for transfer.	• Reassess continuity and simplicity of instruction. • Transfers may be difficult when patient is fatigued or in pain; assess before transfer (allow for a rest period before transferring, or medicate for pain if indicated).
2 Patient sustains injury on transfer.	• Evaluate incident that caused injury (e.g., assessment was inadequate, patient status changed, equipment used improperly). • Complete incident report according to agency policy.

Metered-Dose Inhalers

Pressurized metered-dose inhalers (pMDIs), breath-actuated metered-dose inhalers (BAIs), and dry powder inhalers (DPIs) deliver medications that produce local effects such as bronchodilation. Some of these medications are absorbed rapidly through the pulmonary circulation and create systemic side effects (e.g., albuterol [Proventil] may cause palpitations, tremors, and tachycardia). Patients who receive drugs by inhalation frequently suffer from asthma and chronic respiratory disease. Drugs administered by inhalation provide control of airway hyperactivity or constriction. Because patients depend on these medications for disease control, they must understand both how these medications work and how they are safely administered.

Delegation Considerations

The skill of administering MDIs cannot be delegated to nursing assistive personnel (NAP). The nurse directs the NAP about:

- Potential side effects of medications and to report their occurrence to the nurse.
- Reporting breathing difficulty (e.g., paroxysmal coughing, audible wheezing).

Equipment

- Inhaler device with medication canister (MDI or DPI)
- Spacer device such as AeroChamber or InspirEase (*optional*)
- Facial tissues (*optional*)
- Stethoscope
- Medication administration record (MAR) (electronic or printed)
- Pulse oximeter (*optional*)

Implementation

STEP	RATIONALE
1 Complete preprocedure protocol.	
2 Assess patient's ability to hold, manipulate, and depress canister and inhaler.	Any impairment of grasp or presence of hand tremors interferes with patient's ability to depress canister within inhaler. A spacer device is often necessary.

STEP	RATIONALE
3 Assess patient's readiness and ability to learn: asks questions about medication; is alert; participates in own care; is not fatigued, in pain, or in respiratory distress.	Mental or physical limitations affect patient's ability to learn and methods nurse will need to use for instruction.
4 Assess patient's knowledge and understanding of disease and purpose and action of prescribed medications.	Knowledge of disease is essential for patient to realistically understand use of inhaler.
5 Prepare medications for inhalation. Check label of medication against MAR 2 times. Preparation usually involves taking inhaler device out of storage and into patient room. Check expiration date on container.	*These are the first and second checks for accuracy.* Process ensures that right patient receives right medication.
6 Take medication(s) to patient at correct time (see agency policy). Medications that require exact timing include STAT, first-time or loading doses, and one-time doses. Give time-critical scheduled medications (e.g., antibiotics, anticoagulants, insulin, anticonvulsants, immunosuppressive agents) at exact time ordered (no later than 30 minutes before or after scheduled dose). Give non–time-critical scheduled medications within a range of 1 or 2 hours of scheduled dose (ISMP, 2011). During administration, apply six rights of medication administration.	Hospitals must adopt medication administration policy and procedure for timing of medication administration that considers nature of the prescribed medication, specific clinical application, and patient needs (DHHS, 2011; ISMP, 2011).

STEP	RATIONALE
7 Identify patient using two identifiers (e.g., name and birthday or name and account number) according to agency policy. Compare identifiers with information on patient's MAR or medical record.	Ensures correct patient. Complies with The Joint Commission requirements for patient safety (TJC, 2014). Some agencies are now using a bar-code system to help with patient identification.
8 At patient's bedside again compare MAR or computer printout with names of medications on medication labels and patient name. Ask patient if he or she has allergies.	*This is the third check for accuracy* and ensures that patient receives correct medication. Confirms patient's allergy history.
9 Discuss purpose of each medication, action, and possible adverse effects. Allow patient to ask any questions about the drugs. Define metered-dose to patient and explain correct method of administration. Warn about overuse of inhaler and side effects.	Patient has right to be informed, and patient's understanding of each medication improves adherence to drug therapy.
10 Allow adequate time for patient to manipulate inhaler, canister, and spacer device (if provided). Explain and demonstrate how canister fits into inhaler.	Patient must be familiar with how to use equipment.

SAFETY ALERT If using an MDI that is new or has not been used for several days, push a "test spray" into the air to prime the device before using. This ensures that the MDI is patent and the metal canister is positioned properly.

11 Explain steps for administering MDI without spacer (demonstrate steps when possible):	Simple step-by-step explanation allows patient to ask questions at any point during procedure.

STEP	RATIONALE
a Remove mouthpiece cover from inhaler after inserting MDI canister into holder.	
b Shake inhaler well for 2 to 5 seconds (five or six shakes).	Ensures mixing of medication in canister.
c Hold inhaler in dominant hand.	
d Instruct patient to position inhaler in one of two ways:	
(1) Place mouthpiece in mouth with opening toward back of throat, closing lips tightly around it (Fig. 39-1).	
(2) Position the device 2 to 4 cm (1 to 2 inches) in front of widely opened mouth (Fig. 39-2), with opening of inhaler toward back of throat. Lips should not touch the inhaler.	Directs aerosol spray toward airway. This is the best way to deliver the medication without a spacer.
e Have patient take a deep breath and exhale completely.	Prepares patient's airway to receive the medication.
f With inhaler positioned, have patient hold it with the thumb at the mouthpiece and the index and middle fingers at the top. This is a three-point or bilateral hand position.	Hand position ensures proper activation of MDI (Lilley et al., 2011).
g Instruct patient to tilt head back slightly, and inhale slowly and deeply	Medication is distributed to airways during inhalation.

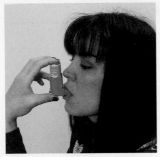

Fig. 39-1 One technique for use of an inhaler. The patient opens lips and places the inhaler in the mouth with the opening toward the back of the throat.

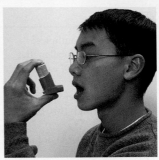

Fig. 39-2 Another technique for use of an inhaler. The patient positions the mouthpiece 2 to 4 cm (1 to 2 inches) from widely opened mouth. This is considered the best way to deliver medication without a spacer.

STEP	RATIONALE
through mouth for 3 to 5 seconds while depressing canister fully.	
h Have patient hold breath for approximately 10 seconds.	Allows tiny drops of aerosol spray to reach deeper branches of airways.
i Remove the MDI from mouth before exhaling and exhale slowly through nose or pursed lips.	Keeps small airways open during exhalation.
12 Explain steps to administer MDI and prepare mouthpiece of spacer device (demonstrate when possible).	
a Remove mouthpiece cover from MDI and mouthpiece of spacer device.	Inhaler fits into end of spacer device.
b Shake inhaler well for 2 to 5 seconds (five or six shakes)	Ensures mixing of medication in canister.

STEP	RATIONALE
c Insert MDI into end of spacer device.	Spacer device traps medication released from MDI; patient then inhales drug from device. These devices improve delivery of correct dose of inhaled medication (Barrons et al., 2011).
d Instruct patient to place spacer device mouthpiece in mouth and close lips. Do not insert beyond raised lip on mouthpiece. Avoid covering small exhalation slots with the lips.	Medication should not escape through mouth.
e Have patient breathe normally through spacer device mouthpiece.	Allows patient to relax before delivering medication.
f Instruct patient to depress medication canister, spraying one puff into spacer device.	Device contains fine spray and allows the patient to inhale more medication.
g Patient breathes in slowly and fully (for 5 seconds).	Ensures particles of medication are distributed to deeper airways.
h Instruct patient to hold full breath for 10 seconds.	Ensures full drug distribution.
13 Instruct patient to wait 20 to 30 seconds between inhalations (if same medication), or 2 to 5 minutes between inhalations (if different medications).	Drugs must be inhaled sequentially. Always administer bronchodilators before corticosteroids so dilators can open airway passages (Lilley et al., 2011).
14 Instruct patient to avoid repeated inhalations before next scheduled dose.	Drugs are prescribed at intervals during day to provide constant drug levels and to minimize side effects. Beta-adrenergic MDIs are used on either an "as needed" basis or on a fixed schedule every 4 to 6 hours.

STEP	RATIONALE
15 Warn patients that they may feel gagging sensation in throat caused by droplets of medication on pharynx or tongue.	This occurs when medication is sprayed and inhaled incorrectly.
16 About 2 minutes after last dose, instruct patient to rinse mouth with warm water and expel water.	Inhaled bronchodilators may cause dry mouth and taste alterations. Corticosteroids may alter normal flora of oral mucosa and lead to development of fungal infection (Lilley et al., 2011).
17 For daily cleaning, instruct patient to remove the medication canister, rinse the inhaler and cap with warm running water, and ensure that inhaler is completely dry before reuse. Do not allow the valve mechanism of the canister to become wet.	Removes residual medication and reduces transmission of microorganisms. Water damages valve mechanism of canister.
18 Complete postprocedure protocol.	

Recording and Reporting

- Record drug administered, dose or strength, route, number of inhalations, and actual time administered on MAR immediately after administration, not before. Include initials or signature. Record patient teaching and validation of understanding in nurses' notes and electronic health record (EHR).
- Record in nurses' notes and EHR the patient's response to MDI (e.g., breath sounds), the evidence of side effects (e.g., dysrhythmia, feelings of anxiety), and the patient's ability to use MDI.
- Report adverse effects/patient response and/or withheld drugs to nurse in charge or health care provider.

UNEXPECTED OUTCOMES	RELATED INTERVENTIONS
1 Patient's respirations are rapid and shallow; breath sounds indicate wheezing.	• Evaluate vital signs and respiratory status. • Notify health care provider.

UNEXPECTED OUTCOMES	RELATED INTERVENTIONS
	• Reassess type of medication and/or delivery method.
2 Patient experiences paroxysms of coughing. Aerosolized particles can irritate posterior pharynx.	• Reassess patient's delivery method. • Notify health care provider.
3 Patient needs bronchodilator more than every 4 hours (may indicate respiratory problem).	• Reassess type of medication and delivery methods needed. • Notify health care provider.
4 Patient experiences cardiac dysrhythmias (light-headedness, syncope), especially if receiving beta-adrenergics.	• Withhold all further doses of medication. • Evaluate cardiac and pulmonary status. • Notify health care provider for reassessment of type of medication and delivery method.
5 Patient is not able to self-administer medication properly.	• Explore alternative delivery routes or devices.
6 Patient is unable to explain technique and risks of drug therapy.	• Further teaching is necessary. • Include family caregivers when possible.

Moist Heat (Compress and Sitz Bath)

A warm compress is a section of sterile or clean gauze moistened with a prescribed heated solution (i.e., normal saline or sterile water) and applied directly to an affected area. Commercially packaged sterile, premoistened compresses are available in some agencies. You heat plain sterile or clean gauze by adding the gauze to a container of warmed solution. Moist heat application also includes the use of warm baths, soaks, and sitz baths. Warm soaks and sitz baths promote circulation, reduce edema and inflammation, promote muscle relaxation, debride wounds, and apply medicated solutions. You give a sitz bath with a special tub or chair basin that allows a patient to sit in water without immersing the legs, feet, and upper trunk.

When preparing a soak or bath, remember that the heated solution is in direct contact with the patient's skin. Be sure to check water temperature frequently to prevent burns. It is desirable to keep the solution temperature constant to enhance the therapeutic effects of the moist heat. Whenever you add heated solution to a soak basin or bath, remove the patient's body part and reimmerse once the solution has mixed.

Delegation Considerations

The skill of applying moist heat can be delegated to nursing assistive personnel (NAP). The nurse must assess the condition of the skin and tissues in the area that is treated, evaluate the patient's response, and explain the purpose of the treatment. The nurse instructs the NAP about:

- Proper temperature of the application.
- Skin changes to immediately report to the nurse (e.g., burning or excessive redness).
- Informing the nurse if the patient complains of dizziness or light-headedness.
- Reporting when treatment is complete so an evaluation of the patient's response can be made.

Equipment

Moist Heat Applications

- Warmed prescribed solution (e.g., normal saline) or commercially prepared compresses or commercial heat pack
- Dry bath towel, bath blanket

- Clean gloves
- Waterproof pad

Clean Compress

- Warmed prescribed solution (e.g., normal saline) or commercially prepared compresses
- Waterproof pad
- Ties or cloth tape
- Aquathermia pad *(optional)*
- Biohazard waste bag
- Clean gloves
- Clean basin
- Clean gauze or towel

Sterile Compress (See Clean Compress)

- Warmed prescribed sterile solution (e.g., normal saline)
- Sterile gloves
- Sterile basin
- Sterile gauze or towel

Soak or Sitz Bath

- Clean basin, tub, or sitz bath (basin may need to be sterile if body part to be soaked has an open wound)
- Prescribed solution warmed to appropriate temperature (tap water is commonly used for sitz baths)
- Prescribed medication (if ordered)

Implementation

STEP	RATIONALE
1 Complete preprocedure protocol.	
2 Assess skin around area to be treated. Perform neurovascular assessments for sensitivity to temperature and pain by measuring light touch, pinprick, and temperature sensation.	Certain conditions alter conduction of sensory impulses that transmit temperature and pain, predisposing patients to injury from heat applications.

STEP	RATIONALE

SAFETY ALERT Patients with diabetes mellitus, stroke or spinal cord injury, peripheral neuropathy, and rheumatoid arthritis are at greater risk for thermal injury (Physiotherapy Canada, 2010).

STEP	RATIONALE
3 Describe the sensation the patient will feel, such as wetness and decreasing warmth. Explain precautions to prevent burning.	Minimizes patient's anxiety and promotes cooperation during procedure.
4 ✏ Perform hand hygiene and apply clean gloves.	Reduces transmission of infection.
5 Apply moist sterile compress:	
a Assist patient in assuming comfortable position in proper body alignment. Expose body part to be covered with compress, and drape patient with bath blanket.	Limited mobility in uncomfortable position causes muscular stress. Prevents cooling.
b Heat prescribed solution to desired temperature by immersing closed bottle of solution in basin of very warm water.	Prevents burns by ensuring proper temperature of solution.
c Remove any existing dressing covering wound. Dispose of gloves and dressings in proper receptacle.	Reduces transmission of microorganisms.
d Inspect condition of wound and surrounding skin. Inflamed wound appears reddened, but surrounding skin is less red in color.	Provides baseline to determine response to moist heat.

SAFETY ALERT If skin surrounding wound is inflamed or reddened or has active drainage, moist heat application may be contraindicated.

STEP	RATIONALE
e Perform hand hygiene.	Reduces risk for transmission of microorganisms.

STEP	RATIONALE
f Prepare compress.	
(1) Open sterile supplies. Pour warmed solution into sterile container.	
(2) Use sterile technique to add sterile gauze into warmed sterile solution to immerse gauze.	Sterile compress is needed when applied to open wound.
(3) If using portable heating source, warm solution. NOTE: *If using a commercially prepared compress, follow manufacturer's instructions for warming.*	

SAFETY ALERT To avoid injury to patient, test temperature of sterile solution by applying a drop to your forearm (without contaminating the solution). It should feel warm to the skin without burning.

g Prepare aquathermia pad *(option)* (see Skill 3) or commercial heat pack (if needed).	Aquathermia pad or heat pack is often needed to maintain temperature of a gauze compress.
h Apply sterile gloves if dressing change is sterile; otherwise, you may use clean gloves.	Allows you to manipulate sterile dressing and touch open wound.
i Grasp one layer of immersed gauze, wring out any excess solution, and apply gauze lightly to open wound, avoiding surrounding skin.	Excess moisture macerates skin and increases risk for burns and infection. Skin is sensitive to sudden change in temperature.
j After a few seconds, lift edge of gauze to assess for redness.	Increased redness indicates burn.
k If patient tolerates compress, pack gauze snugly against wound. Be sure to cover all wound surfaces by warm compress.	Packing of compress prevents rapid cooling from underlying air currents.

STEP	RATIONALE
l Cover moist compress with dry sterile dressing and bath towel. If necessary, secure by pin or tie. Remove and dispose of sterile gloves.	Dry sterile dressing will prevent transfer of microorganisms to wound via capillary action caused by moist compress. Towel insulates compress to prevent heat loss.
m Apply aquathermia, commercial heat pack, or waterproof heating pad over towel (see Skill 3). Keep it in place for desired duration of application.	Provides constant temperature to compress.
n If an aquathermia pad is *not* used, change warm compress using sterile technique every 5 to 10 minutes or as ordered during duration of therapy.	Prevents cooling and maintains therapeutic benefit of compress.
o After prescribed time, apply clean gloves, and remove pad, towel, and compress. Reassess wound and condition of skin, and replace dry sterile dressing as ordered.	Continued exposure to moisture will macerate skin. Prevents entrance of microorganisms into wound site.
6 Sitz bath or soak to intact skin or wound:	
a Apply clean gloves. Remove any existing dressing covering wound. Dispose of gloves and dressings in proper receptacle and perform hand hygiene.	Reduces transmission of microorganisms.
b Inspect condition of wound and surrounding skin. Pay particular attention to suture line.	Provides baseline to determine response to warm soak.

STEP	RATIONALE
c When exudate is present, apply clean gloves and clean intact skin around open area with clean cloth and soap and water or sterile gauze, in which case sterile gloves and sterile normal saline or water are needed. Dispose of gloves and perform hand hygiene.	Cleaning prevents transmission of microorganisms.
d Fill sitz bath or bathtub in bathroom with warmed solution. Check temperature.	Ensures proper temperature and reduces risk for burns.
e Help patient to bathroom to immerse body part in sitz bath, bathtub, or basin. Cover patient with bath blanket or towel as desired.	Prevents falls. Covering patient prevents heat loss through evaporation and maintains constant temperature.
f Assess heart rate. Make sure that patient does not feel light-headed or dizzy and that call light is within reach.	Provides baseline to determine if vascular response to vasodilation occurs during treatment.
g Maintain constant temperature throughout 15- to 20-minute soak.	Ensures proper therapeutic effect.
h After 15 to 20 minutes, remove patient from soak or bath; dry body parts thoroughly. (Wear clean gloves if drainage is present.)	Removing patient from bath before water cools prevents chilling. Enhances patient's comfort.
i Drain solution from basin or tub. Clean and place in proper storage area. Dispose of soiled linen and gloves; perform hand hygiene.	Reduces transmission of microorganisms.
7 Complete postprocedure protocol.	

Recording and Reporting

- Record and report procedure, noting type, location, and duration of application; solution and temperature; condition of body part, wound, and skin before and after treatment; and patient's response to therapy.
- Record preprocedure and postprocedure vital signs (as indicated).
- Record any instructions given and patient's ability to explain and perform procedure.

UNEXPECTED OUTCOMES	RELATED INTERVENTIONS
1 Patient's skin is reddened and sensitive to touch. Extreme warmth caused burning of skin layer.	• Discontinue moist application immediately. • Verify proper temperature, or check device for proper functioning. • Notify health care provider and, if there is a burn, complete an incident report (see agency policy).
2 Patient complains of burning and discomfort.	• Reduce temperature. • Assess for skin breakdown. • Notify health care provider.

Mouth Care:
Unconscious or Debilitated Patients

Unconscious or debilitated patients pose challenges because of their risk for alterations of the oral cavity from the dryness of mucous membranes, the presence of thickened secretions, and the inability to eat or drink. Dryness of the oral mucosa is also caused by mouth breathing and oxygen therapy. Unconscious or debilitated patients are also at risk for aspiration. Although saliva production is decreased, saliva is present and can pool in the back of the oral cavity, which is another contributing factor that places the patient at risk of aspiration. The secretions in the oral cavity change very rapidly to gram-negative pneumonia-producing bacteria if aspiration occurs.

Evaluate the level and frequency of oral care on a daily basis during assessment of the oral cavity. Routine suctioning of the mouth and pharynx is required to manage oral secretions to reduce the risk for aspiration. Chlorhexidine 2% gel or mouth rinse every 12 hours has been shown to effectively prevent ventilator-associated pneumonia (VAP) (Labeau et al., 2011). Research also suggests that toothbrushing provides additional benefit in reducing colonization of dental plaque (Berry et al., 2011).

Delegation Considerations

The skill of providing oral hygiene to an unconscious or debilitated patient can be delegated to nursing assistive personnel (NAP). The nurse must first assess the patient for a gag reflex. The nurse instructs the NAP to:

- Properly position patient for mouth care.
- Be aware of special precautions such as aspiration precautions.
- Use an oral suction catheter for clearing oral secretions.
- Report signs of impaired integrity of oral mucosa to the nurse.
- Report any bleeding of mucosa or gums, excessive coughing, or choking to the nurse.

Equipment

- Small pediatric, soft-bristled toothbrush or toothette sponges for patients for whom brushing is contraindicated
- Antibacterial solution per organization protocol (e.g., chlorhexidine)

- Fluoride toothpaste
- Water-based mouth moisturizer
- Tongue blade
- Penlight
- Oral suction equipment
- Oral airway (uncooperative patient or patient who shows bite reflex)
- Water-soluble lip lubricant
- Water glass with cool water
- Face and bath towel
- Emesis basin
- Clean gloves

Implementation

STEP	RATIONALE
1 Complete preprocedure protocol.	
2 ![hand] Perform hand hygiene, and apply clean gloves.	Reduces transmission of microorganisms in blood or saliva.
3 Test for presence of gag reflex by placing tongue blade on back half of tongue.	Helps in determining aspiration risk.

SAFETY ALERT Patients with impaired gag reflex require oral care but are at risk for aspiration. Keep suction equipment available when caring for patients who are at risk for aspiration.

4 Raise bed to appropriate working height; lower side rail. Unless contraindicated (e.g., head injury, neck trauma), lower side rail and position patient in Sims' or side-lying position. Turn patient's head toward mattress in dependent position with head of bed (HOB) elevated at least 30 degrees.	Use of good body mechanics with bed in high position prevents injury. Allows secretions to drain from mouth instead of collecting in back of pharynx. Prevents aspiration.

STEP	RATIONALE
5 Remove dentures or partial plates if present.	Allows for thorough cleansing of prosthetics later. Provides clearer access to oral cavity.
6 If patient is uncooperative or having difficulty keeping mouth open, insert an oral airway. Insert upside down; then turn the airway sideways and over tongue to keep teeth apart. Insert when patient is relaxed, if possible. Do not use force.	Prevents patient from biting down on nurse's fingers and provides access to oral cavity.

SAFETY ALERT Never place fingers into the mouth of an unconscious or debilitated patient. The normal response is to bite down.

7 Clean mouth using brush moistened in water. Apply toothpaste or use antibacterial solution first to loosen crusts. Clean tooth surfaces using an up-and-down gentle motion. A toothette sponge can be used for patients for whom toothbrushing is contraindicated. Suction any accumulated secretions. Clean chewing and inner tooth surfaces first. Clean outer tooth surfaces. Moisten brush with chlorhexidine solution to rinse. Use brush or toothette to clean roof of mouth, gums, and inside cheeks. Gently brush tongue but avoid stimulating gag reflex (if present). Repeat rinsing several times, and use suction to remove secretions.	Brushing action removes food particles between teeth and along chewing surfaces and removes crusts from mucosa. Repeated rinsing removes all debris and aids in moistening mucosa.

STEP	RATIONALE
8 Use toothbrush or toothette sponge to apply thin layer of water-soluble moisturizer to lips.	Lubricates lips to prevent drying and cracking.
9 Inform patient that procedure is completed. Return patient to comfortable and safe position.	Provides meaningful stimulation to unconscious or less-responsive patient.
10 Complete postprocedure protocol.	

Recording and Reporting

- Record procedure on medical record. Include patient's ability to cooperate and whether suction is necessary for oral care.
- Document and report any pertinent observations (e.g., presence of gag reflex, bleeding gums, dry mucosa, ulcerations, or crusts on tongue).
- Report any unusual findings to nurse in charge or health care provider.

UNEXPECTED OUTCOMES	RELATED INTERVENTIONS
1 Secretions or crusts remain on mucosa, tongue, or gums.	• Provide more frequent oral hygiene.
2 Localized inflammation or bleeding of gums or mucosa is present.	• Provide more frequent oral hygiene with toothette sponges.
	• Apply a water-based mouth moisturizer to provide moisture and maintain integrity of oral mucosa.
	• Chemotherapy and radiation can cause mucositis (inflammation of mucous membranes in mouth) because of sloughing of epithelial tissue. Room temperature saline rinses, bicarbonate and sterile water rinses, and oral care with a soft-bristled

UNEXPECTED OUTCOMES	RELATED INTERVENTIONS
	toothbrush decrease severity and duration of mucositis.
3 Lips are cracked or inflamed.	• Apply moisturizing gel or water-soluble lubricant to lips.
4 Patient aspirates secretions.	• Suction oral airway as secretions accumulate to maintain airway patency.
	• Elevate patient's head of bed to facilitate breathing.
	• If aspiration is suspected, notify the health care provider. Prepare the patient for a chest x-ray examination.

Nail and Foot Care

Feet and nails often require special care to prevent infection, odors, pain, and injury to soft tissues. Often people are unaware of foot or nail problems until discomfort or pain occurs. For proper foot and nail care, instruct patients to protect the feet from injury, to keep the feet clean and dry, and to wear appropriate footwear.

Patients most at risk for developing serious foot problems are those with peripheral neuropathy and peripheral vascular disease. These two disorders, commonly found in patients with diabetes mellitus, cause a reduction in blood flow to the extremities and a loss of sensory, motor, and autonomic nerve function. As a result, the patient is unable to feel heat and cold, pain, pressure, and positioning of the foot or feet. The reduction in blood flow impairs healing and promotes risk for infection.

Delegation Considerations

The skill of nail and foot care of patients *without diabetes* or *circulatory compromise* can be delegated to nursing assistive personnel (NAP). The nurse instructs the NAP about:

- Refraining from trimming patient's nails.
- Implementing special considerations for patient positioning.
- Reporting any breaks in skin, redness, numbness, swelling, or pain.

Equipment

- Wash basin
- Emesis basin
- Washcloth and towel
- Nail clippers (see agency policy)
- Soft nail or cuticle brush
- Plastic applicator stick
- Emery board or nail file
- Body lotion
- Disposable bath mat
- Clean gloves

Implementation

STEP	RATIONALE
1 Complete preprocedure protocol.	

STEP	RATIONALE
2 Apply clean gloves. Inspect all surfaces of fingers, toes, feet, and nails. Pay particular attention to areas of dryness, inflammation, or cracking. Also inspect areas between toes, heels, and soles of feet. Inspect socks for stains.	Integrity of feet and nails determines frequency and level of hygiene required. Heels, soles, and sides of feet are prone to irritation from ill-fitting shoes. Socks may become stained from bleeding or draining ulcer.
3 Assess type of footwear patient wears: Does patient wear socks? Are shoes tight or ill fitting? Are garters or knee-high nylons worn? Is footwear clean?	Some types of shoes and footwear predispose patient to foot and nail problems (e.g., infection, areas of friction, ulcerations).
4 Identify patient's risk for foot or nail problems:	Certain conditions increase likelihood of foot or nail problems.
a Older adult	Poor vision, lack of coordination, or inability to bend over contributes to difficulty in performing foot and nail care. Normal physiological changes of aging also result in brittle nails.
	Discolored, extremely thickened, and deformed nails can indicate infection, fungus, or disease (Malkin and Berridge, 2009).
b Diabetes mellitus	Vascular changes associated with diabetes reduce blood flow to peripheral tissues. Break in skin integrity places patients with diabetes at high risk for skin infection.
c Heart failure, renal disease	Both conditions increase tissue edema, particularly in dependent areas (e.g., feet). Edema reduces blood flow to neighboring tissues.

STEP	RATIONALE
d Cerebrovascular accident (stroke)	Presence of residual foot or leg weakness or paralysis results in altered walking patterns. Altered gait pattern causes increased friction and pressure on feet.
5 Help ambulatory patient sit in chair. Help bedfast patient to supine position with head of bed elevated 45 degrees. Place disposable bath mat on floor under patient's feet or place waterproof pad on mattress.	Sitting in chair facilitates immersing feet in basin. Bath mat protects feet from exposure to soil or debris.
6 Fill wash basin with warm water. Test water temperature. Place basin on floor or pad on mattress. Have patient immerse feet.	Prevents accidental burns to patient's skin.

SAFETY ALERT Patients who have diabetes mellitus, peripheral neuropathy, or peripheral vascular disease (PVD) should not soak their hands and feet because of the increased risk of trauma, inability to sense temperature, and increased risk for infection (American Diabetes Association, 2011; Malkin and Berridge, 2009).

7 Adjust over-bed table to low position and place it over patient's lap.	Easy access prevents accidental spills.
8 Fill emesis basin with warm water and place basin on paper towels on over-bed table. Test water temperature.	Warm water softens nails and thickened epidermal cells. Prevents accidental burns to patient's skin.
9 Instruct patient to place fingers in emesis basin and arms in comfortable position.	Prolonged positioning causes discomfort unless normal anatomical alignment is maintained.
10 Unless patient has diabetes mellitus, peripheral neuropathy, or PVD, allow feet and fingernails to soak 10 minutes.	Goal is to soften debris beneath nails so it can be removed easily.

STEP	RATIONALE
11 Clean gently under fingernails with end of plastic applicator stick while fingers are immersed.	Removes debris under nails that harbors microorganisms.
12 Use soft cuticle brush or nailbrush to clean around cuticles to decrease overgrowth.	Nailbrush helps to prevent inflammation and injury to cuticles.
13 Remove emesis basin, and dry fingers thoroughly.	Thorough drying impedes fungal growth and prevents maceration of tissues.

SAFETY ALERT Check agency policy for appropriate process for cleaning beneath nails. Do not use an orange stick or end of cotton swab; these splinter and can cause injury.

14 Check agency policy on nail care regarding filing and trimming. Trim nails straight across at level of finger or follow curve of finger, ensuring that you do not cut down into nail grooves (Fig. 42-1). Use disposable emery board, and file nail to ensure that there are no sharp corners.	Trimming straight across avoids skin overgrowth at nail edges, which can lead to ingrown nails or infection. Filing nail straight across to eliminate sharp nail edges minimizes risk of injury to adjacent finger (Malkin and Berridge, 2009).

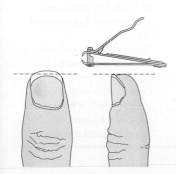

FIG. 42-1 Use nail clipper to clip fingernails straight across.

STEP	RATIONALE

SAFETY ALERT If patient has diabetes or circulatory problems, do not cut nails. Check agency policy.

15	Move over-bed table away from patient. Scrub callused areas with washcloth.	Provides easier access to feet. Friction removes dead skin layers.
16	Dry feet thoroughly, and trim or cut nails following Step 14.	Moisture can cause skin maceration.
17	Apply lotion to feet and hands. Rub in thoroughly. Help patient back to bed and into comfortable position.	Lotion lubricates dry skin by helping to retain moisture.
18	Complete postprocedure protocol.	

Recording and Reporting

- Record procedure and observations in medical record (e.g., breaks in skin, inflammation, ulcerations).
- Report any breaks in skin or ulcerations to nurse in charge or health care provider.

UNEXPECTED OUTCOMES	RELATED INTERVENTIONS
1 Cuticles and surrounding tissues are inflamed and tender to touch.	· Repeat nail care. · Evaluate need for antifungal cream.
2 Localized areas of tenderness occur on feet with calluses or corns at point of friction.	· Change in footwear or corrective foot surgery may be needed for permanent improvement in calluses or corns. · Refer patient to podiatrist.
3 Ulcerations involving toes or feet may remain.	· Institute wound care policies. · Consult with wound care specialist and/or podiatrist. · Increase frequency of assessment and hygiene.

Nasoenteral Tube:
Placement and Irrigation

Tubes used specifically for feeding are composed of either silicone or polyurethane. They are softer and more flexible than nasogastric tubes used for drainage, and patients report that they are more comfortable. These tubes are more difficult to insert. Some tubes are weighted, and research has shown that weighted tubes are superior to nonweighted tubes. Tubes are generally coated with a hydrophilic substance that is activated when exposed to water, making it slippery and easier to insert. A nurse activates the substance immediately before insertion by simply flushing the tube inside and out with water. Wire stylets are included with some tubes, but not all. Stylets are thought to improve insertion success but have also been implicated as increasing the risk for naso-pulmonary intubation. You can pass a feeding tube without the use of a stylet. Nurses often pass feeding tubes through the mouth, especially in critical care when the patient is also intubated for respiratory support.

Placement of a feeding tube requires a physician's order. Patients with facial injuries or craniofacial surgery should not receive a nasogastric (NG) feeding tube. Tubes have been found in the wrong place (e.g., brain) when this is ignored. Tubes should not be used until correct placement is verified by radiological examination.

Delegation Considerations

The skill of feeding tube insertion cannot be delegated to nursing assistive personnel (NAP). However, NAP may help with patient positioning and comfort measures during tube insertion.

Equipment

- Small-bore NG or nasoenteric tube with or without stylet (select the smallest diameter possible to enhance patient comfort)
- 60-mL Luer-Lok or catheter-tip syringe
- Stethoscope and pulse oximeter
- Hypoallergenic tape, semipermeable (transparent) dressing, or tube fixation device
- Tincture of benzoin or other skin barrier protectant
- pH indicator strip (scale 0.0 to 11.0)
- Cup of water and straw or ice chips (for patients able to swallow)
- Emesis basin
- Towel or disposable pad

- Facial tissues
- Clean gloves
- Suction equipment in case of aspiration
- Penlight to check placement in nasopharynx
- Tongue blade

Implementation

STEP	RATIONALE
1 Complete preprocedure protocol.	
Insertion of Nasoenteral Tube	
1 Have patient close each nostril alternately and breathe. Examine each naris for patency and skin breakdown.	Sometimes nares are obstructed or irritated, or septal defect or facial fractures are present.
2 Assess patient's mental status (ability to cooperate with procedure, sedation), presence of cough and gag reflex, ability to swallow, critical illness, and presence of an artificial airway.	These are risk factors for inadvertent tube placement into tracheobronchial tree (Krenitsky, 2011).

SAFETY ALERT Recognize situations in which blind placement of a feeding tube poses an unacceptable risk for placement. Devices designed to detect pulmonary intubation such as CO_2 sensors or electromagnetic tracking devices enhance patient safety. Alternatively, to avoid insertion complications from blind placement in high-risk situations, clinicians trained in the use of visualization or imaging techniques should place tubes (AACN, 2010; Krenitsky, 2011).

STEP	RATIONALE
3 Perform physical assessment of abdomen.	Absent bowel sounds, abdominal pain, tenderness, or distention may indicate medical problem contraindicating feedings.
4 Identify patient using two identifiers (e.g., name and birthday or name and account	Ensures correct patient. Complies with The Joint Commission requirements for patient safety (TJC, 2014).

STEP	RATIONALE
number) according to agency policy. Compare identifiers with information on patient's MAR or medical record.	Some agencies are now using a bar-code system to help with patient identification.
5 Perform hand hygiene.	Reduces transmission of microorganisms.
6 Position patient upright in high-Fowler's position unless contraindicated. If patient is comatose, raise head of bed as tolerated in semi-Fowler's position with head tipped forward, chin to chest. If necessary have an assistant help with positioning of confused or comatose patients. If patient is forced to lie supine, place in reverse Trendelenburg's position.	Reduces risk for pulmonary aspiration in event patient should vomit. Forward head position assists with closure of airway and passage of the tube into the esophagus.
7 Determine length of tube to be inserted, and mark location with tape or indelible ink.	Being aware of proper length to intubate determines approximate depth of insertion.
a Measure distance from tip of nose to earlobe to xiphoid process of sternum (Fig. 43-1).	Length approximates distance from nose to stomach.

SAFETY ALERT Tip of tube must reach stomach to avoid the risk for pulmonary aspiration, which occurs when tubes terminate in the esophagus.

8 Prepare NG for intubation:	
a Inject 10 mL of water from 30- to 60-mL Luer-Lok or catheter-tip syringe into the tube.	Ensures that tube is patent. Avoid using non–Luer-Lok syringes and connectors to reduce risk of tubing misconnection (Simmons et al., 2011).

Fig. 43-1 Determine length of tube to be inserted.

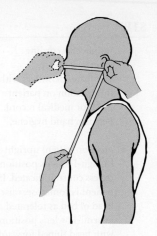

STEP	RATIONALE
b. If using stylet, make certain that it is positioned securely within tube.	Promotes smooth passage of tube into gastrointestinal (GI) tract. Improperly positioned stylet can cause tube to kink or injure patient.
9 Cut hypoallergenic tape 10 cm (4 inches) long, or prepare membrane dressing or other fixation device.	Will be used to secure tubing after insertion.
10 ✋ Apply clean gloves.	Reduces transmission of microorganisms.
11 *Option:* Dip tube with surface lubricant into glass of room temperature water, or apply water-soluble lubricant.	Activates lubricant to facilitate passage of tube into naris and GI tract.
12 Explain the step, and gently insert tube through nostril to back of throat (posterior nasopharynx). This may cause patient to gag. Aim back and down toward ear.	Natural contours facilitate passage of tube into GI tract.

STEP	RATIONALE
13 Have patient flex head toward chest after tube has passed through nasopharynx.	Closes off glottis and reduces risk of tube entering trachea.
14 Encourage patient to swallow by giving small sips of water or ice chips. Advance tube as patient swallows.	Swallowing facilitates passage of tube past oropharynx. Distinct tug may be felt as patient swallows, indicating that tube is following expected path.
15 Emphasize need to mouth breathe and swallow during the procedure.	Helps facilitate passage of tube and alleviates patient's fears during the procedure.
16 When tip of tube reaches carina (approximately 25 to 30 cm [10 to 12 inches] in the adult), stop and listen for air exchange from the distal portion of the tube.	Air may indicate that tube is in the respiratory tract. Remove and start over. Some agency policies require radiograph at 30 to 35 cm (12 to 14 inches) to rule out airway position before proceeding with tube insertion (Krenitsky, 2011).
17 Advance tube each time patient swallows until desired length has been passed.	Reduces discomfort and trauma to patient.

SAFETY ALERT Do not force the tube or push against resistance. If patient starts to cough, experiences a drop in oxygen saturation, or shows other signs of respiratory distress, withdraw the tube into the posterior nasopharynx until normal breathing resumes.

STEP	RATIONALE
18 Check position of tube in back of throat with penlight and tongue blade.	Tube may be coiled, kinked, or inserted into trachea.
19 Temporarily anchor tube to the nose with a small piece of tape.	Movement of the tube stimulates gagging. Assesses general position before anchoring tube more securely.

STEP	RATIONALE
20 Keep tube secure, and check placement of tube by aspirating stomach contents to measure gastric pH.	Proper tube position is essential before initiating feeding.

SAFETY ALERT Insufflation of air into tube while auscultating abdomen is not a reliable means to determine position of feeding tube tip (AACN, 2010; Bourgault and Halm, 2009; Kenny and Goodman, 2010).

STEP	RATIONALE
21 Anchor tube to patient's nose, avoiding pressure on nares. Mark exit site on tube with indelible ink. Select one of the following options for anchoring:	Properly secured tube allows patient more mobility and prevents trauma to nasal mucosa.
a Apply tape:	Prevents pulling of tube. May require frequent changes if tape becomes soiled.
(1) Apply tincture of benzoin or other skin adhesive on tip of patient's nose, and allow it to become "tacky."	Helps tape adhere better. Protects skin.
(2) Remove gloves, and split one end of the adhesive tape lengthwise 5 cm (2 inches).	
(3) Place intact end of tape over bridge of patient's nose. Wrap each of the 5-cm strips in opposite directions around tube as it exits nose (Fig. 43-2).	Secures tube firmly.

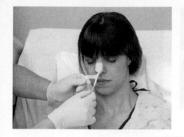

Fig. 43-2 Wrap tape to anchor nasoenteral tube.

STEP	RATIONALE
b Apply membrane dressing or tube fixation device:	Permits longer securement without need to change dressing.
(1) Membrane dressing:	
(a) Apply tincture of benzoin or other skin protector to patient's cheek and area of tube to be secured.	
(b) Place tube against patient's cheek, and secure tube with membrane dressing, out of patient's line of vision.	Decreases risk for patient's inadvertent extubation.
(2) Tube fixation device:	
(a) Apply wide end of patch to bridge of nose (Fig. 43-3).	

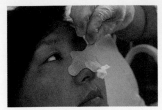

Fig. 43-3 Apply patch to bridge of nose.

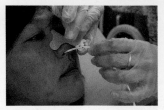

Fig. 43-4 Slip connector around feeding tube.

STEP	RATIONALE
(b) Slip connector around feeding tube as it exits nose (Fig. 43-4).	
22 Fasten end of NG tube to patient's gown using a clip or piece of tape. Do not use safety pins to pin the tube to the patient's gown.	Reduces traction on the naris if tube moves. Safety pins can become unfastened and cause injury to the patient.
23 Assist patient to a comfortable position. Remove gloves and perform hand hygiene.	

SAFETY ALERT Leave stylet in place until correct position is verified by x-ray. Never try to reinsert a partially or fully removed stylet while feeding tube is in place. This can cause perforation of the tube and injure the patient.

24 Obtain x-ray film of chest/abdomen.	X-ray film examination is most accurate method to determine feeding tube placement (Bankhead et al., 2009).
25 Apply clean gloves and administer oral hygiene. Clean tubing at nostril with washcloth dampened in mild soap and water.	Promotes patient comfort and integrity of oral mucous membranes.

STEP	RATIONALE
26 Remove gloves, dispose of equipment, and perform hand hygiene.	Reduces transmission of microorganisms.
Irrigating Feeding Tube	
1 Perform hand hygiene, prepare equipment at patient's bedside, and apply gloves.	Reduces transmission of microorganisms. Ensures an organized approach to irrigation.
2 Verify tube placement if fluid can be aspirated for pH testing.	With tip of tube correctly placed in stomach, irrigation will not increase risk for aspiration.
3 Draw up 30 mL of water in a syringe (Fig. 43-5). Do not use irrigation fluids from multidose bottles that are used on other patients. Patient should have his or her own bottle of solution.	This amount of solution will flush length of tube. Water is most effective agent for preventing tube clogging. Alternative flushing solutions such as cola and fruit juices increase clogging of tubes because of acidity of these fluids (Bankhead et al., 2009; Dandeles and Lodolce, 2011).
4 Change irrigation bottle every 24 hours.	Ensures sterile solution.
5 Kink feeding tube while disconnecting it from administration tubing or while removing plug at end of tube (Fig. 43-6).	Prevents leakage of gastric secretions.
6 Insert tip of syringe into end of feeding tube. Release kink, and slowly instill irrigating solution.	Infusion of fluid clears tubing.
7 If unable to instill fluid, reposition patient on left side, and try again.	Tip of tube may be against stomach wall. Changing patient's position may move tip away from stomach wall.

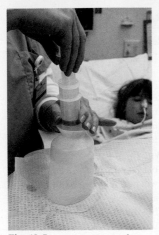

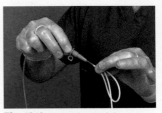

Fig. 43-5 Draw up 30 mL of solution into syringe.

Fig. 43-6 Kink tubing while unplugging feeding tube.

STEP	RATIONALE
8 When water has been instilled, remove syringe. Reinstitute tube feeding, or administer medication as ordered. Flush each medication completely through tube.	Tubing is clear and patent. Ensures that full dose reaches stomach and medications do not mix with formula.
9 Remove and discard gloves; dispose of supplies. Perform hand hygiene.	Reduces transmission of microorganisms.

Recording and Reporting

- Record and report type and size of tube placed, location of distal tip of tube, patient's tolerance of procedure, and confirmation of tube position by x-ray film examination.
- Report any type of unexpected outcome and the interventions performed.
- Record time of irrigation and amount and type of fluid instilled.
- Report if tubing has become clogged.

UNEXPECTED OUTCOMES	RELATED INTERVENTIONS
1 Aspiration of stomach contents into respiratory tract (delayed response or small-volume aspiration), evidenced by auscultation of crackles or wheezes, dyspnea, or fever.	• Report change in patient condition to health care provider; if there has not been a recent chest x-ray film, suggest ordering one. • Position patient on side. • Suction nasotracheally and orotracheally. • Prepare for possible initiation of antibiotics.
2 Displacement of feeding tube to another site (e.g., from duodenum to stomach) possibly occurs when patient coughs or vomits.	• Aspirate GI contents and measure pH. • Remove displaced tube, and insert and verify placement of new tube. • If there is a question of aspiration, obtain chest x-ray film.
3 Tube cannot be irrigated and remains obstructed.	• Repeat irrigation; if unsuccessful, notify health care provider. Tube may need to be removed and a new tube placed.
4 Fluid and electrolyte imbalances occur. Insufficient irrigation can cause water deficiency; excessive irrigations can cause fluid volume excess.	• Notify health care provider of abnormal electrolyte levels or imbalanced intake and output.

Nasogastric Tube for Gastric Decompression:
Insertion and Removal

There are times following major surgery or with conditions affecting the gastrointestinal (GI) tract when normal peristalsis is temporarily altered. Because peristalsis is slowed or absent, a patient cannot eat or drink fluids without causing abdominal distention. The temporary insertion of a nasogastric (NG) tube into the stomach serves to decompress the stomach, keeping it empty until normal peristalsis returns.

The Levin and Salem sump tubes are the most common for stomach decompression. The Levin tube is a single-lumen tube with holes near the tip. You connect the tube to a drainage bag or an intermittent suction device to drain stomach secretions. The Salem sump tube is preferable for stomach decompression. The tube has two lumens: one for removal of gastric contents and one to provide an air vent. A blue "pigtail" is the air vent that connects with the second lumen. When the main lumen of the sump tube is connected to suction, the air vent permits free, continuous drainage of secretions. *Never clamp off the air vent, connect to suction, or use for irrigation.*

Delegation Considerations

The skill of inserting and maintaining an NG tube cannot be delegated to nursing assistive personnel (NAP). The nurse directs the NAP to:

- Measure and record the drainage from an NG tube.
- Provide oral and nasal hygiene measures.
- Perform selected comfort measures, such as positioning or offering ice chips if allowed.
- Anchor the tube to the patient's gown during routine care to prevent accidental displacement.

Equipment

- 14 or 16 French NG tube (smaller-lumen catheters are not used for decompression in adults because they must be able to remove thick secretions)
- Water-soluble lubricant
- pH test strips (measure gastric aspirate acidity); use paper with a range of at least 1.0 to 11.0 or higher
- Tongue blade
- Flashlight

- Emesis basin
- Asepto bulb or catheter-tipped syringe
- 1-inch (2.5-cm) wide hypoallergenic tape or commercial fixation device
- Safety pin and rubber band
- Clamp, drainage bag, or suction machine or pressure gauge if wall suction is to be used
- Towel
- Glass of water with straw
- Facial tissues
- Normal saline
- Tincture of benzoin *(optional)*
- Suction equipment
- Stethoscope
- Clean gloves

Implementation

STEP	RATIONALE
1 Complete preprocedure protocol.	
2 Compare patient identifiers with information on patient MAR.	

SAFETY ALERT If patient is confused, disoriented, or unable to follow commands, obtain assistance from another staff member to insert the tube.

3 Verify health care provider order for type of NG tube to be placed and whether tube is to be attached to suction or drainage bag.	Requires an order from health care provider. Adequate decompression depends on NG suction.
4 ✂ Perform hand hygiene, and apply clean gloves.	Reduces transmission of microorganisms.
5 Stand on patient's right side if right-handed, left side if left-handed. Lower side rail.	Allows easiest manipulation of tubing.
6 Curve 10 to 15 cm (4 to 6 inches) of end of tube tightly around index finger and release.	Aids insertion and decreases stiffness of tube.

STEP	RATIONALE
7 Lubricate 7.5 to 10 cm (3 to 4 inches) of end of tube with water-soluble lubricant.	Minimizes friction against nasal mucosa and aids insertion of tube. Water-soluble lubricant is less toxic than oil-soluble lubricant if aspirated.
8 Alert patient when procedure will begin.	Decreases patient anxiety and increases patient cooperation.
9 Initially, instruct patient to extend neck back against pillow; insert tube gently and slowly through naris with curved end pointing downward.	Facilitates initial passage of tube through naris and maintains clear airway for open naris.
10 Continue to pass tube along floor of nasal passage, aiming down toward patient's ear. If resistance occurs, apply gentle downward pressure to advance tube (do not force past resistance).	Minimizes discomfort of tube rubbing against upper nasal turbinates. Resistance is caused by posterior nasopharynx. Downward pressure helps tube curl around corner of nasopharynx.
11 If there is continued resistance, try to rotate tube and see if it advances. If still resistant, withdraw it, allow patient to rest, lubricate tube again, and then insert tube into other naris.	Forcing against resistance causes trauma to mucosa. Allowing patient to rest helps relieve anxiety.

SAFETY ALERT If unable to insert tube in either naris, stop procedure and notify health care provider.

12 Continue insertion of tube until just past nasopharynx by gently rotating it toward opposite naris.	
a Once past nasopharynx, stop tube advancement, allow patient to relax, and provide tissues.	Relieves patient's anxiety; tearing is natural response to mucosal irritation, and excessive salivation may occur because of oral stimulation.

STEP	RATIONALE
b Explain to patient that next step requires that patient swallow. Give patient glass of water unless contraindicated.	Sipping water aids passage of NG tube into esophagus.
13 With tube just above oropharynx, instruct patient to flex head forward, take a small sip of water, and swallow. Advance tube 2.5 to 5 cm (1 to 2 inches) with each swallow of water. If patient is not allowed fluids, instruct to dry-swallow or suck air through straw. Advance tube with each swallow.	Flexed position closes off upper airway to trachea and opens esophagus. Swallowing closes epiglottis over trachea and helps move tube into esophagus. Swallowing water reduces gagging or choking. Remove water from stomach by suction after insertion.
14 If patient begins to cough, gag, or choke, withdraw slightly and stop tube advancement. Instruct patient to breathe easily and take sips of water.	Cough reflex is initiated when tube accidentally enters larynx. Withdrawal of the tube reduces risk for laryngeal entry. Small sips of water frequently reduce gagging. Give water cautiously to reduce the risk for aspiration.

SAFETY ALERT If vomiting occurs, assist patient in clearing airway. Perform oral suctioning as needed.

15 If patient continues to cough during insertion, pull tube back slightly.	Tube may enter larynx and obstruct airway.
16 If patient continues to gag and cough or complains that tube feels as though it is coiling behind throat, check back of oropharynx using flashlight and tongue blade. Withdraw the tube until tip is back in oropharynx, if coiled. Reinsert with patient swallowing.	Tube may coil around itself in the back of the throat and stimulate gag reflex.

STEP	RATIONALE
17 After patient relaxes, continue to advance tube with swallowing until you reach tape or mark on tube that signifies that tube is in the desired distance. Temporarily anchor tube to patient's cheek with piece of tape until tube placement is verified.	Tip of tube needs to be within stomach to decompress properly. Anchoring of tube prevents accidental displacement while tube placement is verified.
18 Verify tube placement. Check agency policy for preferred methods for checking tube placement:	
a Ask patient to talk.	Patient is unable to talk if NG tube has passed through vocal cords.
b Inspect posterior pharynx for presence of coiled tube.	Tube is pliable and may coil up behind the pharynx instead of advancing into esophagus.
c Place towel under end of NG tube and attach Asepto or catheter-tipped syringe to end of tube. Aspirate gently back on syringe to obtain gastric contents, observing color.	Gastric contents are usually grassy green, clear, and odorless. Postpyloric tube placement appears golden yellow, yellow-brown, or greenish brown with pH of greater than 6.0 (Hockenberry and Wilson, 2011; Lewis et al., 2011).
d Use gastric (Gastroccult) pH paper to measure aspirate for pH with color-coded pH paper. Be sure that paper range of pH is at least from 1.0 to 11.0 or greater.	Gastric aspirates have decidedly acidic pH values typically less than 5.0 (Durai, Venkatraman, and Ng, 2009; Hockenberry and Wilson, 2011). Respiratory secretions usually have pH values greater than 6.0.
e Obtain x-ray film examination of chest and abdomen as ordered.	Radiography is gold standard to verify initial placement of tube (Farrington et al., 2009; Hockenberry and Wilson, 2011; Lewis et al., 2011).

STEP	RATIONALE
f If tube is not in stomach, advance another 2.5 to 5 cm (1 to 2 inches), and repeat Steps a through e to check tube position.	Tube must be in stomach to provide decompression.
19 Anchor tube (see Skill 43, Step 21).	
20 Removal of NG tube:	
a Verify order to remove NG tube.	An order is required for procedure.
b Auscultate abdomen for presence of bowel sounds.	Verifies return of peristalsis.
c Explain procedure to patient, and reassure that removal is less distressing than insertion.	Minimizes anxiety and increases cooperation. Tube passes out smoothly.
d ⚡ Perform hand hygiene, and apply clean gloves.	Reduces transmission of microorganisms.
e Turn off suction and disconnect NG tube from drainage bag or suction. With irrigating syringe, insert 20 mL of air into lumen of NG tube. Remove tape or fixation device from bridge of nose, and unpin tube from gown.	Have tube free of connections before removal. Clears gastric fluids from tube to prevent aspiration of contents or soiling of clothing and bedding.
f Stand on patient's right side if right-handed, left side if left-handed.	Allows easiest manipulation of tube.
g Hand patient facial tissue; place clean towel across chest. Instruct patient to take and hold breath.	Some patients wish to blow nose after tube removed. Towel keeps gown from soil. Temporary airway obstruction occurs during tube removal.

STEP	RATIONALE
h Clamp or kink tubing securely and then pull tube out steadily and smoothly into towel held in other hand while patient holds breath.	Clamping prevents tube contents from draining into oropharynx. Reduces trauma to mucosa and minimizes patient's discomfort. Towel covers tube, which is an unpleasant sight. Holding breath helps to prevent aspiration.
i Inspect intactness of tube.	
j Measure amount of drainage, and note character of content. Dispose of tube and drainage equipment into proper container.	Provides accurate measure of fluid output. Reduces transfer of microorganisms.
k Clean nares, and provide mouth care.	Promotes comfort.
l Position patient comfortably, and explain procedure for drinking fluids, if not contraindicated. Instruct patient to notify you if nausea occurs.	Sometimes patients are not allowed anything by mouth (NPO) for up to 24 hours. When fluids are allowed, orders usually begin with small amount of ice chips each hour and increase as patient is able to tolerate more.

21 Complete postprocedure protocol.

Recording and Reporting

- Record length, size, and type of gastric tube inserted and in which naris it was inserted. In addition, record patient's tolerance of procedure, confirmation of tube placement, character of gastric contents, pH value, results of radiography, whether the tube is clamped or connected to drainage bag or to suction, and amount of suction supplied.
- Record difference between amount of normal saline instilled and amount of gastric aspirate removed on intake and output (I&O) sheet. Record the amount and character of contents draining from NG tube every shift.

UNEXPECTED OUTCOMES	RELATED INTERVENTIONS
1 Patient's abdomen is distended and painful.	• Assess patency of tube. NG tube may not be in stomach. • Irrigate tube. • Verify that suction is on as ordered. • Notify health care provider if distention is unrelieved.
2 Patient complains of sore throat from dry, irritated mucous membranes.	• Perform oral hygiene more frequently. • Ask health care provider whether patient can suck on ice chips, throat lozenges, or local anesthetic medication.
3 Patient develops irritation or erosion of skin around naris.	• Provide frequent skin care to area. • Tape tube on naris to avoid pressure. • Consider switching tube to other naris.
4 Patient develops signs and symptoms of pulmonary aspiration: fever, shortness of breath, or pulmonary congestion.	• Perform complete respiratory assessment. • Notify health care provider. • Obtain chest x-ray film examination as ordered.

Negative-Pressure Wound Therapy

Negative-pressure wound therapy (NPWT) is the application of a vacuum (negative pressure) to a wound through suction to draw edges of a wound together while providing a moist environment to promote healing and collect wound fluid (Figs. 45-1 and 45-2) (AHRQ, 2009; Campbell, Smith, and Smith, 2008; Netsch, 2011). The therapy is commonly used for dehisced wounds, diabetic foot ulcers, pressure ulcers, vascular ulcers (includes venous and arterial ulcers), burn wounds, surgical wounds (especially infected sternal wounds), and trauma-induced wounds (AHRQ, 2009; NPUAP-EPUAP, 2009; Petkar et al., 2011). The WOCN (2010) reports increased rates of healing associated with stage III and IV pressure ulcers when using NPWT.

Added benefits of NPWT include improved patient comfort and a reduction in the frequency of dressing changes. Contraindications to NPWT for chronic wounds are exposed vital organs, inadequately debrided wounds, untreated osteomyelitis or sepsis near a wound, untreated coagulopathy, necrotic tissue with eschar, and malignancy within a wound (AHRQ, 2009; Netsch, 2011).

A health care provider or wound care specialist orders the cycle and amount of negative pressure to a wound. There are different recommendations for the level of negative pressure to use for wound healing. Check your agency policy. The target negative pressures for wound healing tend to range from −50 to −175 mm Hg, but a setting of −125 mm Hg is most common (Netsch, 2011). The schedule for changing NPWT dressings varies based on the type and condition of wound.

Delegation Considerations

The skill of NPWT cannot be delegated to nursing assistive personnel (NAP). The nurse directs the NAP to:

- Use caution in positioning or turning patient to avoid tubing displacement.
- Report any change in integrity of the dressing to the nurse.
- Report any change in patient's temperature or comfort level to the nurse.

Equipment

- Three pairs of gloves, clean and sterile
- Scissors, sterile

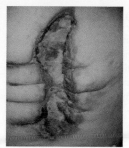

Fig. 45-1 Dehisced wound
before V.A.C. therapy.
(Courtesy KCI USA, Inc.,
San Antonio, TX.)

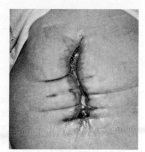

Fig. 45-2 Dehisced wound
after V.A.C. therapy. (Courtesy
KCI USA, Inc., San Antonio,
TX.)

- NPWT unit (requires health care provider's order)
  - NPWT dressing (gauze or foam, see manufacturer's recommendations; transparent dressing; adhesive drape)
  - NPWT suction device
  - Tubing for connection between NPWT unit and NPWT dressing
- Waterproof bag for disposal
- Skin protectant/ostomy adhesive/hydrocolloid dressing/skin barrier
- Protective gown, mask, goggles (used when splashing from wound is a risk)

Implementation

STEP	RATIONALE
1 Complete preprocedure protocol.	
2 Review health care provider's orders for frequency of dressing change, type of negative pressure, type of foam or gauze to use, and cycle (intermittent or continuous).	Health care provider's orders list frequency of dressing changes and special instructions.
3 Ask patient to rate level of pain using pain scale of 0 to 10. Administer prescribed	Comfortable patient will be less likely to move suddenly, causing wound or supply

STEP	RATIONALE
analgesic as needed 30 minutes before dressing change.	contamination. Serves as baseline to measure response to dressing therapy.
4 Cuff top of disposable waterproof bag, and place within reach of work area.	Cuff prevents accidental contamination of top of outer bag.
5 ![icon] Perform hand hygiene, and put on clean disposable gloves. If risk for spray exists, apply protective gown, goggles, and mask.	Reduces transmission of infectious organisms from soiled dressings to nurse's hands.
6 Follow manufacturer's directions for removal and replacement because each NPWT unit varies slightly with approach. Turn off NPWT unit by pushing therapy on/off button.	Deactivates therapy and allows for proper drainage of fluid in drainage tubing.
a Raise tubing above unit and clamp; engage clamp on dressing tubing.	Prevents backflow of any drainage in tubing into wound.
b Allow drainage to flow from tubing into drainage collector.	Prevents drainage from exiting tubing when removed.
c Gently stretch transparent dressing horizontally, and remove slowly from underlying dressing and skin.	Protects periwound skin. Prevents injury to wound tissue.
d Remove old dressing one layer at a time and discard in bag. Keep soiled surfaces away from patient's sight.	Reduces risk of cross contamination.
7 Perform wound assessment. Observe surface area and tissue type, color, odor, and drainage within wound. Measure length, width, and depth of wound.	Measurement of wound is necessary to assess wound healing progression and to justify continuation of NPWT for third-party payers (Netsch, 2011).

STEP	RATIONALE
	Determines condition of wound and need for replacement of dressing.
8 Remove gloves and discard in waterproof bag. Perform hand hygiene.	Reduces transmission of microorganisms.
9 Clean wound.	
a Apply sterile or clean gloves (see agency policy).	
b Clean wound per agency policy. It may be necessary to irrigate with normal saline or other solution ordered by health care provider. Gently blot periwound with gauze to dry thoroughly.	Irrigation removes wound debris and cleans wound bed. Cleaning periwound is essential for an airtight seal.

SAFETY ALERT Health care providers may order wound cultures routinely. However, when drainage looks purulent or has a foul odor or if there is a change in amount or color, obtain wound culture. This may be an indication that NPWT may need to be discontinued (Martindell, 2012).

STEP	RATIONALE
10 Apply skin protectant, barrier film, ostomy wafer, or hydrocolloid dressing to periwound skin. It may be necessary to frame periwound with these products.	Maintains airtight seal needed for NPWT (Netsch, 2011). Protects periwound skin from moisture-associated skin damage (Martindell, 2012).
11 Fill any uneven skin surfaces (e.g., creases, scars, and skinfolds) with skin barrier product (e.g., paste, strip).	Further helps to maintain airtight seal (Netsch, 2011).
12 Remove and discard gloves. Perform hand hygiene.	Prevents transmission of microorganisms.
13 Depending on the type of wound, apply sterile or clean gloves (see agency policy).	Fresh sterile wounds require sterile gloves. Chronic wounds require clean technique, except when sharp

STEP	RATIONALE
	debridement is used at bedside (Wooten and Hawkins, 2005). Do not use same gloves worn to clean wound because cross-contamination may occur.
14 Apply NPWT foam.	
a Prepare NPWT foam (gauze is an option in other types of NPWT devices).	There are several manufacturers; this skill reviews use of foam in KCI VAC.
(1) Check wound measurement and select appropriate foam dressing.	Establishes baseline for wound size. Black polyurethane (PU) foam has larger pores and is most effective in stimulating granulation tissue and wound contraction. White soft foam is denser with smaller pores and is used when the growth of granulation tissue needs to be restricted (Martindell, 2012; Netsch, 2011).
(2) Using sterile scissors, cut foam to exact wound size; make sure to fit size and shape of wound, including tunnels and undermined areas.	Proper size of foam dressing maintains negative pressure to entire wound.

SAFETY ALERT Use of black foam may cause patients to experience more pain because of excessive wound contraction. You may need to switch patient to the polyvinyl alcohol (PVA) soft foam.

(3) *Option:* Instill antimicrobial product (e.g., silver-impregnated gauze) or topical antibiotic into wound.	Limited research suggests that these products may reduce bioburden of wound (Orgill et al., 2009).

STEP	RATIONALE
b Gently place foam in wound, being sure that the foam is in contact with entire wound base, margins, and tunneled areas. Count number of foam dressings and document in patient's chart.	Maintains negative pressure to entire wound. Edges of the foam dressing must be in direct contact with the patient's skin.

SAFETY ALERT For deep wounds, regularly reposition tubing to minimize pressure on wound edges. Reposition patients with restricted mobility or sensation frequently so that they do not lie on the tubing and cause skin damage.

STEP	RATIONALE
c Apply NPWT transparent dressing over foam wound dressing.	
(1) Trim dressing to cover wound so it will extend onto periwound skin approximately 2.5 to 5 cm (1 to 2 inches).	Ensure that the wound is properly covered and that a negative-pressure seal can be achieved (Box 45-1). Dressing should be airtight with no tunnels or gaps to ensure a good seal when suction is activated.
(2) Apply transparent dressing, keeping it wrinkle-free.	Maintains sterility and moist environment.
(3) After wound is completely covered, secure tubing of NPWT unit to transparent film, aligning end of tubing to drainage hole to ensure occlusive seal (Fig. 45-3). Do not apply tension to drape and tubing. Set at ordered suction level.	Excessive tension may compress foam dressing and impede wound healing. It also produces shear force on periwound area (Kinetic Concepts, 2012). Intermittent or continuous negative pressure can be administered at −50 to −175 mm Hg, according to health care provider's orders and patient comfort. Average is −125 mm Hg (Netsch, 2011).

BOX 45-1 Maintaining an Airtight Seal

Once negative-pressure wound therapy (NPWT) is initiated, negative pressure must be maintained, and the wound must stay sealed to avoid wound desiccation. Areas that are difficult to seal include wounds around joints and near the sacrum. Implementation of the following points may help to maintain an airtight seal:

- Choose a wound suitable for therapy.
- Clip hair around wound (check agency policy).
- Cut transparent film to extend 2.5 to 5 cm (1 to 2 inches) beyond wound perimeter.
- Frame the periwound area with skin sealant, skin barrier, hydrocolloid, or transparent film dressing.
- Fill uneven skin surfaces with a skin barrier product.
- Cut or mold transparent dressing to fit wound.
- Avoid wrinkles in transparent film.
- Identify any air leak with a stethoscope and repair with a sealant dressing (e.g., transparent dressing). Only use one or two additional layers for large leaks. Multiple layers reduce moisture vapor transmission and cause maceration of wound.
- Avoid adhesive remover because it leaves a residue that hinders film adherence.

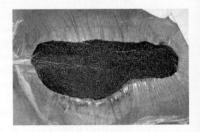

Fig. 45-3 Foam dressing, transparent dressing, and V.A.C. tubing secured over existing wound. (Courtesy KCI USA, Inc., San Antonio, TX.)

STEP	RATIONALE
Examine system to be sure that seal is intact and therapy is working (this step is different for each type of NPWT).	
15 Complete postprocedure protocol.	

Recording and Reporting

- Chart in nurses' notes and electronic health record (EHR) appearance of wound, characteristics of drainage, placement of NPWT (type of dressing, pressure mode and setting), and patient response to dressing change.
- Report brisk, bright-red bleeding; evidence of poor wound healing; evisceration or dehiscence; and possible wound infection to health care provider immediately.

UNEXPECTED OUTCOMES	RELATED INTERVENTIONS
1 Wound appears inflamed and tender, drainage has increased, and an odor is present.	• Notify the health care provider. • Obtain wound culture. • Increase frequency of dressing changes.
2 Patient reports increase in pain.	• Patient may need more analgesia. • Instill normal saline to moisten foam and other filler dressings to allow them to loosen from granulation tissue. • If using black foam, switch to PVA white soft foam. • Decrease pressure setting. • Change from intermittent to continuous cycling. • Change type of NPWT system.
3 Negative-pressure seal has broken.	• Take preventive measures (see Box 45-1).
4 Wound hemorrhages.	• Stop NPWT immediately and notify health care provider
5 Patient or caregiver is unable to perform dressing change.	• Provide additional teaching and support. • Obtain services of home care agency.

Oral Medications

Patients are usually able to ingest or self-administer oral medications with few problems. If oral medications are contraindicated (e.g., inability to swallow, gastric suction), take precautions to protect patients from aspiration. Nurses usually prepare medications in areas designed for medication preparation or at unit-dose carts.

Delegation Considerations

The skill of administering oral medications cannot be delegated to nursing assistive personnel (NAP). The nurse directs the NAP about:

- Potential side effects of medications and to report their occurrence.
- Informing the nurse if the patient's condition changes (e.g., pain, itching, or rash) after medication administration.

Equipment

- Automated, computer-controlled drug dispensing system or medication cart
- Disposable medication cups
- Glass of water, juice, or preferred liquid and drinking straw
- Device for crushing or splitting tablets *(optional)*
- Paper towels
- Medication administration record (MAR) (electronic or printed)
- Clean gloves (if handling an oral medication)

Implementation

STEP	RATIONALE
1 Complete preprocedure protocol.	
2 Assess risk for aspiration using a dysphagia screening tool if available (see Skill 4). Protect patient from aspiration by assessing swallowing ability.	Aspiration occurs when food, fluid, or medication intended for GI administration is inadvertently administered into the respiratory tract. Patients with altered ability to swallow are at higher risk for aspiration (Edmiaston et al., 2010; Kelly et al., 2011).

STEP	RATIONALE
3 Assess patient's medical history, history of allergies, medication history, and diet history. List any drug allergies on each page of the MAR and prominently display on patient's medical record.	These factors influence how certain drugs act. Information reveals previous problems with medication administration.
4 Prepare medications:	
a Perform hand hygiene.	Reduces transmission of microorganisms.
b Plan medication administration to avoid interruptions.	Interruptions contribute to medication administration errors (Hall et al., 2010; Popescu et al., 2011).
c Arrange medication tray and cups in medication preparation area, or move medication cart to position outside patient's room.	Organization of equipment saves time and reduces error.
d Access automated dispensing system (ADS) or unlock medicine drawer or cart.	Medications are safeguarded when locked in cabinet, cart, or ADS.
e Prepare medications for one patient at a time.	Prevents preparation errors.
f Select correct drug from ADS, unit-dose drawer, or stock supply. Compare name of medication label with MAR or computer printout. Be sure to exit ADS after removing drugs.	Reading label first time and comparing it against transcribed order reduces errors. Exiting ADS ensures that no one else can remove medications using your identity. *This is the first check for accuracy.*
g Check or calculate drug dose as necessary. Double-check any calculation. Check expiration date on all medications and return outdated medication to pharmacy.	Double-checking pharmacy calculations reduces risk for error. Agency policy may require you to check calculations of certain medications such as insulin with another nurse. Expired medications may be inactive or harmful to patient.

STEP	RATIONALE
h If preparing a controlled substance, check record for previous medication count and compare current count with supply available. Controlled drugs may be stored in computerized locked cart.	Controlled substance laws require nurses to carefully monitor and count dispensed narcotics.
i **Prepare solid forms of oral medications:**	
(1) To prepare unit-dose tablets or capsules, place packaged tablet or capsule directly into medicine cup without removing wrapper. Administer medications only from containers with labels that are clearly marked.	Wrappers maintain cleanliness and identify drug name and dose, which can facilitate teaching.
(2) When using a blister pack, "pop" medications through foil or paper backing into a medication cup.	Packs provide a 1-month supply, with each "blister" usually containing a single dose.
(3) If it is necessary to give half the dose of medication, pharmacy should split, label, package, and send medication to unit. If you must split medication, use clean, gloved hand to cut with clean pill-cutting device.	In health care agencies, only pharmacy should split tablets to ensure patient safety (ISMP, 2008). Reduces contamination of tablet.
(4) Place all tablets or capsules that patient will receive in one medicine cup, except for those requiring	Keeping medications that require preadministration assessments separate from others serves as a reminder and makes it easier to withhold drugs as necessary.

STEP	RATIONALE
preadministration assessments (e.g., pulse rate or blood pressure). Place in separate additional cup with wrapper intact.	
(5) If patient has difficulty swallowing and liquid medications are not an option, use a pill-crushing device. Clean device before using. Mix ground tablet in small amount (teaspoon) of soft food (custard or applesauce).	Large tablets are often difficult to swallow. Ground tablet mixed with palatable soft food is usually easier to swallow.
j Prepare liquids:	
(1) Thoroughly mix by shaking gently before administration. If drug is in unit-dose container with correct volume, shaking is not needed. If drug is in multidose bottle, remove bottle cap from container and place cap upside down on work surface.	Mixing liquid suspensions just before pouring ensures that correct amount of medication, not just the solvent, is measured for the dose. Prevents contamination of inside of cap.
(2) Hold bottle with label against palm of hand while pouring.	Prevents spilled liquid from dripping and soiling label.
(3) Place medication cup at eye level on countertop and fill to desired level on scale. Scale should be even with fluid level at its surface or base of meniscus, not edges.	Ensures accuracy of measurement.

STEP	RATIONALE
(4) Discard any excess liquid into sink or a place specially designated for wasting of medications. Wipe lip of bottle with paper towel and recap.	Prevents contamination of contents of bottle and prevents bottle cap from sticking.
(5) If giving less than 10 mL of liquid, prepare medication in oral syringe. Do not use hypodermic syringe or syringe with needle or syringe cap.	Allows more accurate measurement of small amounts.

SAFETY ALERT Use only syringes specifically designed for oral use when administering liquid medications. If using hypodermic syringes, the medication may be inadvertently administered parenterally, or the syringe cap or needle, if not removed from the syringe before administration, may become dislodged and accidentally aspirated when the syringe plunger is pressed.

STEP	RATIONALE
(6) Administer liquid medication packaged in single-dose cup directly from the single-dose cup. Do not pour into a medicine cup.	Avoids unnecessary manipulation of dose.
k Before going to patient's room, compare patient's name and name of medication on label of prepared drugs with MAR.	Reading labels a second time reduces errors. *This is the second check for accuracy.*
l Return stock containers or unused unit-dose medications to shelf or drawer, and read label again. Label medication cups and poured medications with patient's name	Ensures that the correct medications are prepared for the correct patient.

STEP	RATIONALE

before leaving medication preparation area. Do not leave drugs unattended.

5 Administer medications:

a Identify patient using two identifiers (e.g., name and birthday or name and account number) according to agency policy. Compare identifiers with information on patient's MAR or medical record.	Ensures correct patient. Complies with The Joint Commission requirements for patient safety (TJC, 2014). Some agencies are now using a bar-code system to help with patient identification.
b At patient's bedside again compare MAR or computer printout with names of medications on medication labels and patient name. Ask patient if he or she has allergies.	*This is the third check for accuracy* and ensures that patient receives correct medication. Confirms patient's allergy history.
c Perform necessary preadministration assessment (e.g., blood pressure, pulse) for specific medications.	Determines whether specific medications should be withheld at that time.
d Discuss purpose of each medication, action, and possible adverse effects. Allow patient to ask any questions about drugs.	Patient has right to be informed, and patient's understanding of purpose of each medication improves adherence to drug therapy.

SAFETY ALERT If patient expresses concern regarding accuracy of a medication, do not give the medication. Explore the patient's concern, and verify the physician's order before administering. Listening to the patient's concerns may prevent a medication error.

e Help patient to sitting or Fowler's position. Use side-lying position if patient is unable to sit. Have patient stay in this position for 30 minutes after administration.	Decreases risk for aspiration during swallowing.

STEP	RATIONALE
f *For tablets:* Patient may wish to hold solid medications in hand or cup before placing in mouth. Offer water or preferred liquid to help patient swallow medications.	Patient can become familiar with medications by seeing each drug. Choice of fluid promotes and can improve fluid intake.
g *For orally disintegrating formulations (tablets or film):* Remove medication from blister packet just before use. Do not push the tablet through the foil. Place medication on top of patient's tongue. Caution patient against swallowing tablet or saliva.	Orally disintegrating formulations begin to dissolve when placed on the tongue. Water is not needed. Careful removal from packaging is necessary because the tablets and strips are thin and fragile.
h *For sublingual medications:* Have patient place medication under tongue and allow it to dissolve completely (Fig. 46-1). Caution patient against swallowing tablet or saliva.	Drug is absorbed through blood vessels of undersurface of tongue. If swallowed, drug is destroyed by gastric juices or so rapidly detoxified by liver that therapeutic blood levels are not attained.
i *For buccal-administered medications:* Have patient place medication in mouth against mucous membranes of cheek and gums until it dissolves (Fig. 46-2).	Buccal medications act locally or systemically because they are swallowed in saliva.

SAFETY ALERT Avoid administering anything by mouth until orally disintegrating, buccal, or sublingual medication is completely dissolved.

j *For powdered medications:* Mix with liquids at bedside, and give to patient to drink.	When prepared in advance, powdered drugs thicken and some even harden, making swallowing difficult.

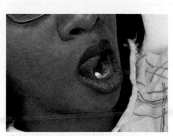

Fig. 46-1 Proper placement of sublingual tablet in sublingual pocket.

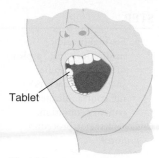

Fig. 46-2 Buccal administration of a tablet.

STEP	RATIONALE
k *For crushed medications mixed with food:* Give each medication separately in teaspoon of food.	Ensures that patient swallows all of the medicine.
l Caution patient against chewing or swallowing lozenges.	Drug acts through slow absorption through oral mucosa, not gastric mucosa.
m Give effervescent powders and tablets immediately after dissolving.	Effervescence improves unpleasant taste of drug and often relieves gastrointestinal problems.
n If patient is unable to hold medications, place medication cup to lips and gently introduce each drug into the mouth, one at a time. A spoon can also be used to place pill in patient's mouth. Do not rush or force medication.	Administering single tablet or capsule eases swallowing and decreases risk for aspiration.

SAFETY ALERT If tablet or capsule falls to the floor, discard it and repeat preparation. Drug is contaminated.

STEP	RATIONALE
o Stay until patient completely swallows each medication completely or takes it by the prescribed route.	Ensures that patient receives ordered dosage. If left unattended, patient may not take dose or may save drugs, causing health risks.

STEP	RATIONALE
p For highly acidic medications (e.g., aspirin), offer patient nonfat snack (e.g., crackers) if not contraindicated by patient's condition.	Reduces gastric irritation. The fat content of foods may delay absorption of the medication.
6 Complete postprocedure protocol.	

Recording and Reporting

- Record drug, dose, route, and time administered on patient's MAR immediately after administration, not before. Include initials or signature. Record patient teaching and validation of understanding in nurses' notes and electronic health record (EHR).
- If drug is withheld, record reason in nurses' notes and EHR, and follow agency policy for noting withheld doses.
- Report adverse effects, patient response, and/or any withheld drugs to nurse in charge or health care provider. Depending on medication, immediate health care provider notification may be required.

UNEXPECTED OUTCOMES	RELATED INTERVENTIONS
1 Patient exhibits adverse effects (e.g., side effect, toxic effect, allergic reaction).	• Withhold further doses. • Assess vital signs. • Notify prescriber and pharmacy. • Symptoms such as urticaria, rash, pruritus, rhinitis, and wheezing may indicate an allergic reaction and need for emergency medications. • Add allergy information to patient's medical record.
2 Patient is unable to explain drug information.	• Further assess the patient's or family caregiver's knowledge of medications and guidelines for drug safety.

UNEXPECTED OUTCOMES	RELATED INTERVENTIONS
3 Patient refuses medication.	• Further instruction or different approach to instruction is necessary. • Assess why patient is refusing medication. • Do not force patient to take medications. • Notify health care provider. • Record refused medication and patient's stated reason.

Oral Medications:
Nasogastric Tube Administration

Nasogastric feeding tubes generally are small-bore tubes that are inserted into the stomach via one of the nares. For long-term enteral feedings, a percutaneous endoscopic gastrostomy (PEG) tube or a jejunostomy tube may be inserted surgically. Do not administer medications into nasogastric tubes that are inserted for decompression.

Preferably, medications administered by enteral tubes should be in liquid form. If a medication is unavailable in liquid form, you will need to prepare an oral medication tablet or capsule by crushing or dissolving it. However, you cannot crush sublingual, sustained-release, chewable, long-acting, or enteric-coated medications. Consult with the hospital pharmacist about whether you can crush or dissolve a medication. Always verify correct placement of a nasogastric tube before administering medications.

Delegation Considerations

The skill of administering medications by enteral feeding tubes cannot be delegated to nursing assistive personnel (NAP). The nurse directs the NAP to:

- Keep the patient's head of the bed elevated a minimum of 30 degrees (preferably 45 degrees) for 1 hour (follow agency policy) after medication administration.
- Report immediately to the nurse signs of aspiration such as coughing, choking, gagging, or drooling of liquid or dissolved pills.

Equipment

- Medication administration record (MAR) (electronic or printed)
- 60-mL syringe, catheter tip for large-bore tubes, Luer-Lok tip for small-bore tubes
- Gastric pH test strip (scale of 0 to 11.0)
- Graduated container
- Medication to be administered
- Pill crusher if medication is in tablet form
- Water
- Tongue blade or straw to stir dissolved medication
- Clean gloves
- Stethoscope (for evaluation)

Implementation

STEP	RATIONALE
1 Complete preprocedure protocol.	
2 Check accuracy and completeness of each MAR with health care provider's medication order. Check patient's name, drug name and dosage, route of administration, and time for administration. Clarify incomplete or unclear orders with health care provider before administration.	The health care provider's order is the most reliable source and only legal record of drugs that patient is to receive. Ensures that patient receives correct medication. Handwritten MARs are a source of medication errors (ISMP, 2010; Jones and Treiber, 2010).
3 Before administration of medications, verify placement of the feeding tube (see Skill 44).	Reduces the risk for aspiration.
4 Perform hand hygiene. Prepare medications for instillation into feeding tube. Check medication label against MAR 2 times. Fill graduated container with 50 to 100 mL of tepid water. Use sterile water for immunocompromised or critically ill patients (Bankhead et al., 2009).	*These are the first and second checks for accuracy.* Preparation process ensures that right patient receives right medication. Tepid water prevents abdominal cramping, which can occur with cold water.

SAFETY ALERT Whenever possible, use liquid medications instead of crushed tablets. If you need to crush tablets, the tubing must be flushed before and after the medication to prevent the drug from adhering to the inside of the tube. In addition, make sure that concentrated medications are thoroughly diluted. Never add crushed medications directly to the feeding tube (Phillips and Endacott, 2011).

a *Tablets:* Crush each tablet into a fine powder. Dissolve each tablet in separate cup of 30 mL of warm water.	Fine powder dissolves more easily, reducing chance of occluding feeding tube.

STEP	RATIONALE
b *Capsules:* Ensure that contents of capsule (granules or gelatin) can be expressed from covering (consult with pharmacist). Open capsule or pierce gel cap with sterile needle and empty contents into 30 mL of warm water (or solution designated by drug company). Gel caps dissolve in warm water, but this may take 15 to 20 minutes.	Ensures that contents of capsules are in solution to prevent occlusion of tube.
5 Identify patient using two identifiers (e.g., name and birthday or name and account number) according to agency policy. Compare identifiers with information on patient's MAR or medical record.	Ensures correct patient. Complies with The Joint Commission requirements for patient safety (TJC, 2014). Some agencies are now using a bar-code system to help with patient identification.
6 At patient's bedside again compare MAR or computer printout with names of medications on medication labels and patient name. Ask patient if he or she has allergies.	*This is the third check for accuracy* and ensures that patient receives correct medication. Confirms patient's allergy history.
7 Discuss purpose of each medication, action, and possible adverse effects. Allow patient to ask any questions about the drugs.	Patient has right to be informed, and patient's understanding of each medication improves adherence to drug therapy.
8 Elevate head of bed to minimum of 30 degrees and preferably 45 degrees (unless contraindicated) or sit patient up in a chair (Bankhead et al., 2009).	Reduces risk for aspiration.

STEP	RATIONALE
9 If continuous enteral tube feeding is infusing, adjust infusion pump to hold tube feeding.	Feeding solution should not infuse while residuals are checked or medications are administered.
10 ![gloves icon] Apply clean gloves. Check placement of feeding tube by observing gastric contents and checking pH of aspirate contents. *Gastric pH for a patient who has fasted for 4 hours is usually 1.0 to 4.0.*	Ensures proper tube placement and reduces risk of introducing fluids into respiratory tract
11 Check for gastric residual volume (GRV). Draw up 10 to 30 mL of air into a 60-mL syringe and connect syringe to feeding tube. Flush tube with air and pull back slowly to aspirate gastric contents. Determine GRV using the scale on either a syringe or a graduate container. Return aspirated contents to stomach unless a single GRV exceeds 500 mL or if two measurements taken 1 hour apart each exceed 250 mL (Bankhead et al., 2009) (check agency policy). When GRV is excessive, hold medication and contact health care provider.	GRV categories have been identified in studies as significant when patients have two or more GRVs of at least 250 mL or one or more GRVs exceeding 500 mL (Bankhead et al., 2009). Large residuals indicate delayed gastric emptying and put patient at increased risk for aspiration (Metheney et al., 2010).
12 Irrigate the tubing.	
a Pinch or clamp enteral tube and remove syringe. Draw up 30 mL of water into syringe. Reinsert tip of syringe into tube, release clamp, and flush tubing. Clamp tube again and remove syringe.	Pinching or clamping tubing prevents leakage or spillage of stomach contents. Flushing ensures that tube is patent.

STEP	RATIONALE
b Some enteral tubes are connected to continuous-feeding tubing with stopcock apparatus such as a Lopez valve that contains a medication port. Attach tip of syringe to medication port on stopcock; turn "off" setting of stopcock away from patient and toward infusion tubing. Flush tube and set stopcock "off" again to medication port. Remove syringe.	
13 Remove bulb or plunger of syringe and reinsert syringe into tip of feeding tube.	Removal of bulb or plunger prepares syringe for delivery of medications.
14 Administer first dose of liquid or dissolved medication by pouring into syringe. Allow to flow by gravity.	

SAFETY ALERT If medication does not flow freely, raise the height of the syringe to increase the rate of flow or try having the patient change position slightly because the end of the feeding tube may be against the gastric mucosa. If these measures do not improve the flow, a gentle push with the bulb of an Asepto syringe or the plunger of the syringe may facilitate the flow of fluid.

a If only giving one dose of medication, flush with 30 mL of water.	Maintains patency of enteral tube and ensures that medication passes through tube to stomach. Allows for accurate identification of medication if dose is spilled. In addition, some medications may be incompatible (Boullata, 2009).
b To administer more than one medication, give each separately, and flush between medications with 15 to 30 mL of water.	

STEP	RATIONALE
c Follow last dose of medication with 30 to 60 mL of water.	Maintains patency of enteral tube and ensures passage of medication into stomach (Boullata, 2009).
15 Clamp the proximal end of the feeding tube if tube feeding is not being administered, and cap end of tube.	Prevents air from entering the stomach between medication doses.
16 When continuous tube feeding is being administered by an infusion pump, follow medication administration Steps 1 to 13. If the medications are not compatible with the feeding solution, then hold the feeding for an additional 30 to 60 minutes.	Allows for adequate absorption of medication and avoids potential drug-food interaction between medication and enteral feeding.
17 Assist patient to comfortable position, but keep the head of the bed elevated for 1 hour after administering the medication.	Prevents aspiration.
18 Complete postprocedure protocol.	

Recording and Reporting

- Record in nurses' notes and electronic health record (EHR) the method used to check placement of enteral tube, GRV, and pH of stomach aspirate. Record actual time that each drug was administered on MAR immediately after administration, not before. Include initials or signature. Record patient teaching and validation of understanding in nurses' notes and EHR.
- Record total amount of water used for medication administration on proper intake and output (I&O) form.
- Report adverse effects, patient response, and/or withheld drugs to nurse in charge or health care provider.

UNEXPECTED OUTCOMES	RELATED INTERVENTIONS
1 Patient exhibits signs of aspiration including respiratory distress, changes in vital signs, or changes in oxygen saturation.	• Stop all medications/fluids through the tube. • Elevate the head of the bed, and stay with the patient. • Assess vital signs and breath sounds while another staff member notifies health care provider.
2 Patient does not receive medication as prescribed because of a blocked nasogastric/enteric tube.	• For newly inserted tube, notify health care provider and obtain x-ray film confirmation of placement. • Requires interventions to unclog tube to ensure drug delivery (Box 47-1).
3 Patient exhibits adverse effects (side effect, toxic effect, allergic reaction).	• Withhold further doses. • Always notify health care provider and pharmacy when the patient exhibits adverse effects. • Symptoms such as urticaria, rash, pruritus, rhinitis, and wheezing indicate an allergic reaction. • Enter patient allergy in medical record.

BOX 47-1   Unclogging a Blocked Feeding Tube

- Prevent tube from becoming blocked by flushing it with at least 15 to 30 mL of tepid water before and after administering each dose of medication, 30 to 60 mL after last dose of medication, before and after checking gastric residual volumes, and every 4 to 12 hours around-the-clock (refer to agency policies) (Bankhead et al., 2009).
- Gently flush tube with large-bore syringe and warm water. Do not use small-bore syringe because this exerts too much pressure and may rupture tube.
- If irrigation with water is not effective, obtain an order for a pancrelipase tablet (e.g., Viokase), and follow manufacturer's guidelines for tube irrigation. In addition, a declogging stylus may be used (see agency policy).
- The tube may have to be removed, and a new one inserted if the medication is urgent.

Ostomy Care (Pouching)

Immediately after a fecal surgical diversion, it is necessary to place a pouch over the newly created stoma to contain effluent when the stoma begins to function. The pouch will keep the patient clean and dry, protect the skin from drainage, and provide a barrier against odor. A cut-to-fit, transparent pouching system is preferred because it will cover the peristomal skin without constricting the stoma and allow for visibility of the stoma.

In the immediate postoperative period, the stoma may be edematous and the abdomen distended. These symptoms will resolve over a 4- to 6-week period after surgery, but, during this time, it will be necessary to revise the pouching system to meet the changing size of the stoma and the changes in body contours (Dietz and Gates, 2010a).

Delegation Considerations

The skill of pouching a new ostomy/ileostomy cannot be delegated to nursing assistive personnel (NAP). In some agencies, care of an established ostomy (4 to 6 weeks or more after surgery) can be delegated to NAP. The nurse directs the NAP about:

- The expected amount, color, and consistency of drainage from the ostomy.
- The expected appearance of the stoma.
- Special equipment needed to complete the procedure.
- Changes in the patient's stoma and surrounding skin integrity that should be reported.

Equipment

- Skin barrier/pouch, clear drainable one-piece or two-piece, cut-to-fit or precut size
- Pouch closure device, such as a clip, if needed
- Ostomy measuring guide
- Adhesive remover (*optional*)
- Clean gloves
- Washcloth
- Towel or disposable waterproof barrier
- Basin with warm tap water
- Scissors
- Waterproof bag for disposal of pouch
- Gown and goggles (*optional*) (for use if there is risk of splashing when emptying pouch)

Implementation

STEP	RATIONALE
1 Complete preprocedure protocol. Perform hand hygiene and apply clean gloves.	Reduces transmission of microorganisms.
2 Observe existing skin barrier and pouch for leakage and length of time in place. Pouch should be changed every 3 to 7 days for colostomy and every 3 to 5 days for ileostomy, not daily (Goldberg et al., 2010). In case of an opaque pouch, remove it to fully observe stoma.	Assesses effectiveness of pouching system and detects potential for problems. To minimize skin irritation, avoid unnecessary changing of entire pouching system. When pouch leaks, skin damage from the effluent causes more skin trauma than early removal of wafer.

SAFETY ALERT Repeated leaking may indicate need for different type of pouch. If the pouch is leaking, change it. Taping or patching it to contain effluent leaves the skin exposed to chemical or enzymatic irritation.

3 Observe amount of effluent in pouch. Empty pouch if it is more than one-third to one-half full by opening clip and draining it into a container for measurement of output. Note consistency of effluent and record output.	Weight of pouch may disrupt seal of adhesive on skin. Monitors fluid balance and bowel function after surgery. Normal colostomy effluent is soft or formed stool, whereas normal ileostomy effluent is liquid.
4 Observe stoma for type, location, color, swelling, presence of sutures, trauma, and healing or irritation of peristomal skin. Remove and dispose of gloves.	Stoma characteristics are one of the factors to consider in selecting an appropriate pouching system. Convexity in the skin barrier is often necessary with a flush or retracted stoma.
5 Position patient semi-reclining or supine during assessment and pouching. (**NOTE:** Some patients with	When patient is semi-reclining, there are fewer skin wrinkles, which allows for ease of application of pouching system.

STEP	RATIONALE
established ostomies prefer to stand.) If possible, provide patient with mirror for observation.	
6 ![hand] Perform hand hygiene, and apply clean gloves.	Reduces transmission of microorganisms.
7 Place towel or disposable waterproof barrier across patient's lower abdomen.	Protects bed linen; maintains patient's dignity.
8 Remove used pouch and skin barrier gently by pushing skin away from barrier. An adhesive remover may be used to facilitate removal of skin barrier.	Reduces skin trauma. Improper removal of pouch and barrier can cause peristomal skin irritation or breakdown.
9 Cleanse peristomal skin gently with warm tap water using a washcloth; do not scrub skin. Pat the skin dry.	Avoid soap. It leaves residue on skin, which may irritate skin. Pouch does not adhere to wet skin.
10 Measure stoma.	Allows for proper fit of pouch that will protect peristomal skin.
11 Trace pattern of stoma measurement on pouch backing or skin barrier (Fig. 48-1).	Prepares for cutting opening in the pouch.
12 Cut opening on backing or skin barrier wafer (Fig. 48-2). Be sure that opening is at least ⅛-inch larger than stoma to avoid pressure on it.	Customizes pouch to provide appropriate fit over stoma.
13 Remove protective backing from adhesive (Fig. 48-3).	Prepares skin barrier for placement.
14 Apply pouch. Press firmly into place around stoma and outside edges. Have patient hold hand over pouch to apply heat to secure seal (Fig. 48-4).	Pouch adhesives are heat activated and will hold more securely at body temperature.

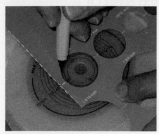

Fig. 48-1 Trace measurement on skin barrier. (Courtesy Coloplast, Minneapolis, MN.)

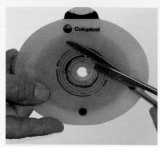

Fig. 48-2 Cut opening in wafer. (Courtesy Coloplast, Minneapolis, MN.)

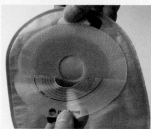

Fig. 48-3 Remove protective backing. (Courtesy Coloplast, Minneapolis, MN.)

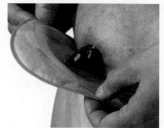

Fig. 48-4 Apply pouch over stoma. (Courtesy Coloplast, Minneapolis, MN.)

STEP	RATIONALE
15 Close end of pouch with clip or integrated closure. Remove drape from patient.	Ensures pouch is secure. Contains effluent.
16 Complete postprocedure protocol.	

Recording and Reporting

- Record type of pouch and skin barrier applied, amount and appearance of effluent in pouch, size and appearance of stoma, and condition of peristomal skin.
- Record patient/family level of participation, teaching that was done, and response to teaching.

- Report any of the following to nurse and/or physician: abnormal appearance of stoma, suture line, peristomal skin, or character of output.

UNEXPECTED OUTCOMES	RELATED INTERVENTIONS
1 Skin around stoma is irritated, blistered, or bleeding, or a rash is noted. May be caused by undermining of pouch seal by fecal contents, allergic reaction, or fungal skin eruption.	• Remove pouch more carefully. • Change pouch more frequently, or use a different type of pouching system. • Consult ostomy care nurse.
2 Necrotic stoma is manifested by purple or black color, dry instead of moist texture, failure to bleed when washed gently, or tissue sloughing.	• Report to nurse/health care provider. • Document appearance.
3 Patient refuses to view stoma or participate in care.	• Obtain referral for ostomy care nurse. • Allow patient to express feelings. • Encourage family support.

Oxygen Therapy:
Nasal Cannula, Oxygen Mask, T Tube, or Tracheostomy Collar

Oxygen therapy is the administration of supplemental oxygen (O_2) to a patient to prevent or treat hypoxia. Selection of the type of oxygen delivery system depends on the level of oxygen support that the patient needs, based on the severity of the hypoxia and the disease process. A *nasal cannula* is a simple, effective, and comfortable device for delivering oxygen to a patient. The two tips of the cannula, about 1.5 cm ($\frac{1}{2}$ inch) long, protrude from the center of a disposable tube and are inserted into the nostrils.

The simple face mask is used for short-term oxygen therapy. It fits loosely and delivers oxygen concentrations from 40% to 60%. A plastic face mask with a reservoir bag and a *Venturi mask* are capable of delivering higher concentrations of oxygen.

Patients with an *artificial airway* require constant humidification to the airway. The two devices that supply humidified gas to an artificial airway are a T tube and a tracheostomy collar. The *T tube*, also called a *Briggs adapter*, is a T-shaped device with a 15-mm ($\frac{3}{5}$-inch) connection that connects an oxygen source to an artificial airway such as an endotracheal (ET) tube or tracheostomy. A *tracheostomy collar* is a curved device with an adjustable strap that fits around the patient's neck.

Delegation Considerations

The skill of applying a nasal cannula or oxygen mask (not adjusting oxygen flow rate) can be delegated to nursing assistive personnel (NAP). The skill of administering oxygen therapy to a patient with an artificial airway cannot be delegated to NAP. The nurse is responsible for assessing the patient's respiratory system, the patient's response to oxygen therapy, and the setup of the oxygen therapy and liter flow, including the adjustment of oxygen flow rate. The nurse directs the NAP by:

- Informing how to safely adjust the device (e.g., loosening the strap on the oxygen cannula or mask).
- Instructing to inform the nurse immediately about any changes in vital signs; changes in level of consciousness (LOC); skin irritation

from the cannula, mask, or straps; patient complaints of pain or breathlessness; any increase in anxiety; and increased secretions associated with the oxygen delivery device.
- Instructing on patient-specific variations for application or adjustment of the T tube or tracheostomy collar (e.g., methods to avoid pressure or pulling on the artificial airway, methods for handling accumulated secretions in devices).

Equipment
- Oxygen delivery device as ordered by health care provider
- Oxygen tubing (consider extension tubing)
- Humidifier, if indicated
- Sterile water for humidifier
- Oxygen source
- Oxygen flowmeter
- Appropriate room signs

For Patients with an Artificial Airway
- T tube or tracheostomy collar
- Large-bore oxygen tubing
- Nebulizer
- Sterile water for nebulizer
- Oxygen or gas source
- Clean gloves
- Goggles (if splash risk exists)
- Flowmeter

Implementation

STEP	RATIONALE
1 Complete preprocedure protocol.	
2 If available, note patient's most recent arterial blood gas (ABG) results or pulse oximetry (SpO_2) value.	Objectively documents the patient's pH, arterial oxygen and arterial carbon dioxide concentrations, or arterial oxygen saturation.
3 Attach oxygen delivery device (e.g., cannula, mask, T tube, tracheostomy collar) to oxygen tubing, and attach end of tubing to humidified	Humidity prevents drying of nasal and oral mucous membranes and airway secretions. Ensures correct O_2 delivery.

STEP	RATIONALE
oxygen source adjusted to prescribed flow rate.	
4 Apply oxygen device:	
a Place the two tips of the cannula into patient's nares. If the tips are curved, they should point downward inside the nostrils. Then loop the cannula tubing up and over patient's ears. Adjust the lanyard so the cannula fits snugly but not too tightly.	Directs flow of oxygen into patient's upper respiratory tract. Patient is more likely to keep device in place if it fits comfortably.
b Apply a mask by placing it over patient's mouth and nose. Then bring the straps over patient's head and adjust to form a comfortable but tight seal.	Provides prescribed oxygen rate and reduces pressure on tips of nares.
5 Observe for proper function of oxygen delivery device:	Ensures patency of delivery device and accuracy of prescribed oxygen flow rate.
a *Nasal cannula:* Cannula is positioned properly in nares; oxygen flows through tips.	Provides prescribed oxygen rate and reduces pressure on tips of nares.
b *Reservoir nasal cannula Oxymizer:* Fit as for nasal cannula. Reservoir is positioned under patient's nose or worn as pendant.	Delivers higher flow of oxygen with nasal cannula. Delivers a 2 : 1 ratio (e.g., 6 L/min nasal cannula is approximately equivalent to 3.5 L/min with Oxymizer device).
c *Nonrebreathing mask:* Apply as regular mask. Valves on mask close; thus exhaled air does not enter reservoir bag.	Does not allow exhaled air to be rebreathed. Valves on mask side ports permit exhalation, but close during inhalation to prevent inhalation of room air.

STEP	RATIONALE
d *Venturi mask* (Fig. 49-1): Apply as regular mask. Select appropriate flow rate.	It is used when high-flow device is desired.
e *Face tent:* Apply tent under patient's chin and over the mouth and nose. It will be loose, and a mist is always present.	Excellent source of humidification; however, you cannot control oxygen concentrations, and patient who requires high oxygen cannot use this device.
f *T tube or tracheostomy collar:* If health care provider orders oxygen, adjust flow rate to 10 L/min or as ordered. Adjust nebulizer to proper FiO₂ setting. Attach T tube to ET or tracheostomy tube. Place tracheostomy collar over tracheostomy tube and adjust straps so it fits snugly.	Provides supplemental humidification to avoid drying of the airway. Flow rate ensures humidification; nebulizer regulates FiO_2.
6 Verify setting on flowmeter and oxygen source for proper setup and prescribed flow rate (Fig. 49-2).	Ensures delivery of prescribed oxygen therapy in conjunction with the specific cannula/mask.
7 Check cannula/mask every 8 hours. Keep humidification container filled at all times.	Ensures patency of cannula and oxygen flow. Oxygen is a dry gas; when it is administered via nasal cannula of 4 L/min or more, you must add humidification so patient inhales humidified oxygen (American Thoracic Society, 2012).
8 Post "Oxygen in use" signs on wall behind bed and at entrance to room.	Alerts visitors and care providers that oxygen is in use.
9 Complete postprocedure protocol.	

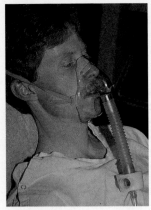

Fig. 49-1 Venturi mask in place.

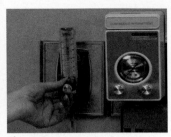

Fig. 49-2 Nurse adjusts flowmeter setting.

Recording and Reporting

- Record respiratory assessment findings; method of oxygen delivery and flow rate; patient's response; any adverse reactions or side effects; change in health care provider's orders.
- Report any unexpected outcome to health care provider or nurse in charge.

UNEXPECTED OUTCOMES	RELATED INTERVENTIONS
1 Patient experiences skin irritation or breakdown (e.g., at ears, bridge of nose, nares, other pressure areas), drying of nasal and oral mucosa, sinus pain, or epistaxis.	• Increase humidification to oxygen delivery system. • Provide appropriate skin care. Do not use petroleum-based gel around oxygen because it is flammable (American Lung Association, 2012).
2 Patient experiences continued hypoxia.	• Notify health care provider. • Obtain health care provider's orders for follow-up SpO_2 monitoring or ABG determinations. • Consider measures to improve airway patency, coughing techniques, and oropharyngeal or orotracheal suctioning.

UNEXPECTED OUTCOMES	RELATED INTERVENTIONS
3 Patient experiences drying of nasal and upper airway mucosa.	• If oxygen flow rate is greater than 4 L/min, use humidification. When oxygen flow is less than 4 L/min, the humidification system of the body is sufficient (British Thoracic Society Guidelines, 2008). • Assess patient's fluid status and increase fluids if appropriate. • Provide frequent oral care. • Obtain health care provider order for use of sterile nasal saline intermittently.

Parenteral Medication Preparation:
Ampules and Vials

Ampules contain single doses of injectable medication in a liquid form. An ampule is made of glass with a constricted, prescored neck that is snapped off to allow access to the medication. A colored ring around the neck indicates where the ampule is prescored. Medication is easily withdrawn from the ampule by aspirating with a filter needle and syringe. Filter needles must be used when preparing medication from a glass ampule to prevent glass particles from being drawn into the syringe (Alexander et al., 2009; Nicholl and Hesby, 2002).

A vial is a single- or multi-dose plastic or glass container with a rubber seal at the top. Vials may contain liquid or dry forms of medications. Some vials have two chambers separated by a rubber stopper. One chamber contains the diluent solution; the other contains the dry medication. Before preparing the medication, push on the upper chamber to dislodge the rubber stopper and allow the powder and the diluent to mix. Unlike an ampule, a vial is a closed system. You must inject air into the vial to permit easy withdrawal of the solution.

Delegation Considerations
The skill of preparing injections from ampules and vials cannot be delegated to nursing assistive personnel (NAP).

Equipment
Medication in an Ampule
- Syringe, needle, and filter needle
- Small sterile gauze pad or unopened alcohol swab

Medication in a Vial
- Syringe and two needles
- Needles:
  - Needleless blunt-tip vial access cannula or needle (with safety sheath) for drawing up medication (if needed)
  - Filter needle if indicated
- Small sterile gauze pad or alcohol swab
- Diluent (e.g., 0.9% sodium chloride or sterile water) (if indicated)

Both

- Medication administration record (MAR) or computer printout
- Sharps with engineered sharps injury protection (SESIP) safety needle for injection
- Medication in vial or ampule
- Puncture-proof container for disposal of syringes, needles, and glass

Implementation

STEP	RATIONALE
1 Complete preprocedure protocol.	
2 Check accuracy and completeness of each MAR or computer printout with prescriber's written medication order. Check patient's name, medication name and dosage, route of administration, and time of administration. Recopy or reprint any portion of MAR that is difficult to read.	The prescriber's order is the most reliable source and legal record of patient's medications. Ensures that patient receives correct medications. Handwritten MARs are a source of medication errors (ISMP, 2010; Jones and Treiber, 2010).
3 Assess the patient's body build, muscle size, and weight if giving subcutaneous or intramuscular (IM) medication.	Determines type and size of syringe and needles for injection.
4 Perform hand hygiene, and prepare supplies.	Reduces transmission of microorganisms.
5 **Prepare medications:**	
a If using a medication cart, move it outside patient's room.	Organization of equipment saves time and reduces error.
b Unlock medication drawer or cart, or log onto computerized medication dispensing system.	Medications are safeguarded when locked in cabinet, cart, or computerized medication dispensing system.

STEP	RATIONALE
c Follow agency's "No-Interruption Zone" policy. Prepare medications for one patient at a time. Keep all pages of MARs or computer printouts for one patient together, or look at only one patient's electronic MAR at a time.	Preventing distractions reduces medication preparation errors (LePorte et al., 2009; Nguyen et al., 2010). No-Interruption Zone has been shown to decrease interruptions during medication preparation (Anthony et al., 2010).
d Select correct drug from stock supply or unit-dose drawer. Compare label of medication with MAR computer printout or computer screen.	Reading label and comparing it with transcribed order reduce errors. *This is the first check for accuracy.*
e Check expiration date on each medication, one at a time.	Medications used past their expiration date are sometimes inactive, less effective, or harmful to patients.
f Calculate drug dose as necessary. Double-check calculation. Ask another nurse to check calculations if needed.	Double-checking reduces error.
g If preparing a controlled substance, check record for previous drug count and compare with supply available.	Controlled substance laws require careful monitoring of dispensed narcotics.
h Do not leave drugs unattended.	Nurse is responsible for safekeeping of drugs.
6 **Preparing ampule:**	
a Tap top of ampule lightly and quickly with finger until fluid moves from its neck (Fig. 50-1).	Dislodges any fluid that collects above neck of ampule. All solution moves into lower chamber.
b Place small gauze pad around neck of ampule.	Protects nurse's fingers from trauma as glass tip is broken off. Do not use opened alcohol swab to wrap around top of ampule because alcohol may leak into ampule.

STEP	RATIONALE
c Snap neck of ampule quickly and firmly away from hands (Fig. 50-2).	Protects your fingers and face from shattering glass.
d Draw up medication quickly, using filter needle long enough to reach bottom of ampule.	System is open to airborne contaminants. Filter needles filter out any fragments of glass (Alexander et al., 2009).
e Hold ampule upside down, or set it on a flat surface. Insert filter needle into center of ampule opening. Do not allow needle tip or shaft to touch rim of ampule.	Broken rim of ampule is considered contaminated. When ampule is inverted, solution dribbles out of ampule if needle tip or shaft touches rim of ampule.
f Aspirate medication into syringe by gently pulling back on plunger (Fig. 50-3).	Withdrawal of plunger creates negative pressure within syringe barrel, which pulls fluid into syringe.
g Keep needle tip under surface of liquid. Tip ampule to bring all fluid within reach of the needle.	Prevents aspiration of air bubbles.

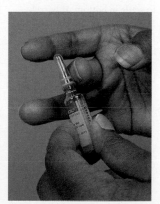

Fig. 50-1 Tapping moves fluid down neck.

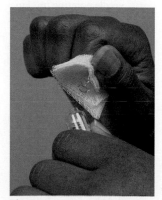

Fig. 50-2 Neck snapped away from hands.

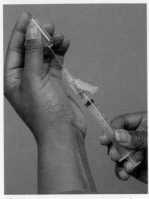

Fig. 50-3 Medication aspirated with ampule inverted.

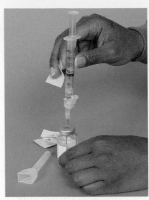

Fig. 50-4 Insert needle's adapter through center of vial's diaphragm.

STEP	RATIONALE
h If you aspirate air bubbles, do not expel air into ampule.	Air pressure forces fluid out of ampule, and medication will be lost.
i To expel excess air bubbles, remove needle from ampule. Hold syringe with needle pointing up. Tap side of syringe to cause bubbles to rise toward needle. Draw back slightly on plunger, and then push plunger upward to eject air. Do not eject fluid.	Withdrawing plunger too far will remove it from barrel. Holding syringe vertically allows fluid to settle in bottom of barrel. Pulling back on plunger allows fluid within needle to enter barrel so fluid is not expelled. You then expel air at top of barrel and within needle.
j If syringe contains excess fluid, use sink for disposal. Hold syringe vertically with needle tip up and slanted slightly toward sink. Slowly eject excess fluid into sink. Recheck fluid level in syringe by holding it vertically.	Safely dispenses excess medication into sink. Position of needle allows you to expel medication without it flowing down needle shaft. Rechecking fluid level ensures proper dose.

STEP	RATIONALE
k Cover needle with its safety sheath or cap. Replace filter needle with regular sharps with engineered sharps injury protection (SESIP) needle.	Minimizes needlesticks. Filter needles cannot be used for injection.
7 **Preparing vial containing a solution:**	
a Remove cap covering top of unused vial to expose sterile rubber seal. If a multi-dose vial has been used, cap is already removed. Firmly and briskly wipe surface of rubber seal with alcohol swab, and allow it to dry.	Vial comes packaged with cap that cannot be replaced after seal is removed. Not all drug manufacturers guarantee that rubber seals of unused vials are sterile. Swabbing with alcohol reduces transmission of microorganisms. Allowing alcohol to dry prevents alcohol from coating needle and mixing with medication.
b Pick up syringe, and remove needle cap or cap covering needleless vial access device. Pull back on plunger to draw amount of air into syringe equivalent to volume of medication to be aspirated from vial.	Injecting air prevents buildup of negative pressure in vial when aspirating medication.

SAFETY ALERT Some medications and agencies require use of a filter needle when preparing medications from vials. Check agency policy or medication reference. If you use a filter needle to aspirate medication, you need to change it to a regular SESIP needle of the appropriate size to administer medication (Alexander et al., 2009).

c With vial on flat surface, insert tip of needle or needleless device through center of rubber seal (Fig. 50-4). Apply pressure to tip of needle during insertion.	Center of seal is thinner and easier to penetrate. Using firm pressure prevents dislodging rubber particles that could enter vial or needle.

STEP	RATIONALE
d Inject air into the vial's air space, holding on to plunger. Hold plunger firmly; plunger is sometimes forced backward by air pressure within vial.	Injection of air creates vacuum needed to get medication to flow into syringe. Injecting into air space of vial prevents formation of bubbles and an inaccurate dose.
e Invert vial while keeping firm hold on syringe and plunger (Fig. 50-5). Hold vial between thumb and middle fingers of nondominant hand. Grasp end of syringe barrel and plunger with thumb and forefinger of dominant hand to counteract pressure in vial.	Inverting vial allows fluid to settle in lower half of container. Position of hands prevents forceful movement of plunger and permits easy manipulation of syringe.
f Keep tip of needle or needleless device below fluid level.	Prevents aspiration of air.

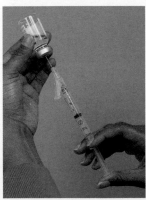

Fig. 50-5 Withdraw fluid with vial inverted.

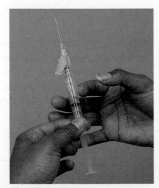

Fig. 50-6 Hold syringe upright; tap barrel to dislodge air bubbles.

STEP	RATIONALE
g Allow air pressure from vial to fill syringe gradually with medication. If necessary, pull back slightly on plunger to obtain correct amount of medication.	Positive pressure within vial forces fluid into syringe.
h When you obtain desired volume, position needle or needleless device into air space of vial; tap side of syringe barrel gently to dislodge any air bubbles. Eject any air remaining at top of syringe into vial.	Forcefully striking barrel while needle is inserted in vial may bend needle. Accumulation of air displaces medication and causes dosage errors.
i Remove needle or needleless access device from vial by pulling back on barrel of syringe.	Pulling plunger rather than barrel causes plunger to separate from barrel, resulting in loss of medication.
j Hold syringe at eye level at 90-degree angle to ensure correct volume and absence of air bubbles. Remove any remaining air by tapping barrel to dislodge any air bubbles (Fig. 50-6). Draw back slightly on plunger; then push it upward to eject air. Do not eject fluid. Recheck volume of medication.	Holding syringe vertically allows fluid to settle in bottom of barrel. Tapping dislodges air to top of barrel. Pulling back on plunger allows fluid within needle to enter barrel so you do not expel fluid. You then expel air at top of barrel and within needle.

SAFETY ALERT When preparing medication from single-dose vial, do not assume that volume listed on label is total volume in vial. Some manufacturers provide small amount of extra liquid, expecting loss during preparation. Be sure to draw up only desired volume.

| k If you need to inject medication into patient's tissue, change needle to appropriate gauge | Inserting needle through a rubber stopper dulls beveled tip. New needle is sharper, and because no fluid is along shaft, |

STEP	RATIONALE
and length according to route of medication administration.	does not track medication through tissues.
l For multi-dose vial, make label that includes date of mixing, concentration of drug per milliliter, and your initials.	Ensures that nurses will prepare future doses correctly. Some drugs must be discarded within a certain time frame after mixing.
8 **Preparing vial containing a powder (reconstituting medications):**	
a Remove cap covering vial of powdered medication and cap covering vial of proper diluent. Firmly swab both rubber seals with alcohol swab, and allow alcohol to dry.	Allowing alcohol to dry prevents alcohol from coating needle and mixing with medication.
b Draw up manufacturer's suggested volume of diluent into syringe following Steps 7b through 7j.	Prepares diluent for injection into vial containing powdered medication.
c Insert tip of needle or needleless device through center of rubber seal of vial of powdered medication. Inject diluent into vial. Remove needle.	Diluent begins to dissolve and reconstitute medication.
d Mix medication thoroughly. Roll in palms. Do not shake.	Ensures proper dispersal of medication throughout solution and prevents formation of air bubbles.
e Reconstituted medication in vial is ready to be drawn into new syringe. Read label carefully to determine dose after reconstitution.	Once you add diluent, concentration of medication (mg/mL) determines dose you give.

STEP	RATIONALE
f Draw up reconstituted medication into syringe. Insert needleless device/needle into vial. Do not add air. Then follow Steps 7c through 7j.	Prepares medication for administration.
9 Compare label of medication with MAR, computer screen, or computer printout.	Ensures that dose is accurate. *This is the second check for accuracy.*
10 Complete postprocedure protocol.	

UNEXPECTED OUTCOMES	RELATED INTERVENTIONS
1 Air bubbles remain in syringe.	Expel air from syringe, and add medication to it until you prepare the correct dose.
2 Incorrect dose of medication is prepared.	Discard prepared dose. Prepare correct new dose.

Parenteral Medications:
Mixing Medications in One Syringe

Some medications need to be mixed from two vials or from a vial and an ampule. Mixing compatible medications avoids the need to give a patient more than one injection. Compatibility charts are in drug reference guides, posted within patient care areas, or available electronically. If you are uncertain about medication compatibilities, consult a pharmacist. When mixing medications, you must correctly aspirate fluid from each type of container. When using multi-dose vials, do not contaminate the contents of the vial with medication from another vial or ampule.

Give special consideration to the proper preparation of insulin, which comes in vials. Insulin is the hormone used to treat diabetes mellitus. Insulin is classified by rate of action, including short duration, intermediate duration, and long duration. Often patients with diabetes mellitus receive a combination of different types of insulin to control their blood glucose levels. Before preparing insulin, gently roll all cloudy insulin preparations (Humulin N) between the palms of your hands to resuspend the insulin (Lehne, 2010).

If more than one type of insulin is required to manage the patient's diabetes, you can mix them into one syringe if they are compatible. Always prepare the short- or rapid-acting insulin first to prevent it from being contaminated with the longer-acting insulin (Lehne, 2010). In some settings insulin is not mixed. Box 51-1 lists recommendations for mixing insulins.

Delegation Considerations

The skill of mixing medications in one syringe cannot be delegated to nursing assistive personnel (NAP). The nurse directs the NAP about:
- Potential side effects of medications and the need to report their occurrence to the nurse.

Equipment

- Single-dose or multi-dose vials and ampules containing medication
- Syringe and two needles
- Needles:
  - Needleless blunt-tip vial access cannula or needle for drawing up medication

BOX 51-1 Recommendations for Mixing Insulins

- Patients whose blood glucose level is well controlled on a mixed-insulin dose should maintain their individual routine when preparing and administering their insulin doses.
- No other medication or diluent should be mixed with any insulin product unless approved by the prescriber.
- Do not mix insulin glargine (Lantus) or insulin detemir (Levemir) with any other types of insulin, and do not administer them intravenously.
- Inject rapid-acting insulins mixed with NPH insulin within 15 minutes before a meal.
- Verify insulin dosages during preparation with another nurse (if required by agency policy).

- Filter needle if indicated
- Sharps with engineered sharps injury protection (SESIP) needle for injection
- Alcohol swab
- Puncture-proof container for disposing of syringes, needles, and glass
- Medication administration record (MAR) or computer printout
- Medication in vial or ampule

Implementation

STEP	RATIONALE
1 Check accuracy and completeness of MAR or computer printout with prescriber's written medication order. Check patient's name, medication name and dosage, route of administration, and time of administration. Recopy or reprint any portion of the MAR that is difficult to read.	Reduces errors and ensures that patient receives correct medication.
2 Review pertinent information related to medication, including action, purpose, side effects, and nursing implications.	Reduces risk of complications.

STEP	RATIONALE
3 Assess patient body build, muscle size, and weight if giving subcutaneous or intramuscular (IM) medication.	Helps ascertain that dosages are correct.
4 Consider compatibility of medications to be mixed and type of injection.	Prevents unwanted medication interactions.
5 Check expiration date of medication printed on vial or ampule.	Expired medications should not be used because potency changes when medications become outdated.
6 Perform hand hygiene.	Reduces risk of infection.
7 Prepare medication for one patient at a time following the six rights of medication. Select an ampule or vial from the unit-dose drawer or automated dispensing system. Compare the label of each medication with the MAR or computer printout. In the case of insulin, ensure that correct type(s) of insulin is prepared. *This is the first check for accuracy.*	Prevents medication error.
8 **Mixing medications from two vials (Fig. 51-1):**	
a Take syringe with needleless device or filter needle and aspirate volume of air equivalent to first medication dose (vial A).	Air must be introduced into vial to create positive pressure needed to withdraw solution.
b Inject air into vial A, making sure that needle or needleless device does not touch solution (Fig. 51-1, *A*).	Prevents cross contamination.

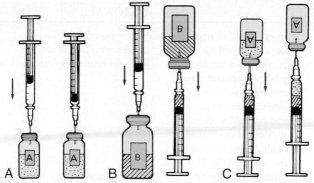

Fig. 51-1 **A,** Injecting air into vial A. **B,** Injecting air into vial B and withdrawing dose. **C,** Withdrawing medication from vial A; medications are now mixed.

STEP	RATIONALE
c Holding plunger, withdraw needle or needleless device and syringe from vial A. Aspirate air equivalent to second medication dose (vial B) into syringe.	If plunger is not held in place, injected air may escape from vial A. Air is injected into vial B to create positive pressure needed to withdraw desired dose.
d Insert needle or needleless device into vial B, inject volume of air into vial B, and withdraw medication from vial B into syringe (Fig. 51-1, *B*).	First portion of dose has been prepared.
e Withdraw needle or needleless device and syringe from vial B. Ensure that proper volume has been obtained.	Ensures that correct dose is prepared.
f Determine on syringe scale what the combined volume of medications should measure.	Prevents accidental withdrawal of too much medication from second vial.

STEP	RATIONALE
g Insert needle or needleless device into vial A, being careful not to push plunger and expel medication within syringe into vial. Invert vial and carefully withdraw the desired amount of medication from vial A into syringe (Fig. 51-1, *C*).	Positive pressure within vial A allows fluid to fill syringe without need to aspirate.
h Withdraw needle or needleless device, and expel any excess air from syringe. Check fluid level in syringe for proper dose. Medications are now mixed.	Air bubbles should not be injected into tissues. Excess fluid causes incorrect dose.

SAFETY ALERT If too much medication is withdrawn from second vial, discard syringe and start over. Do not push medication back into vial.

i Change needle or needleless device for appropriate-size needle if medication is being injected. Keep needle or needleless device capped until administration time.	Needleless vial access device must be changed for needle if medication is to pierce skin. Filter needles cannot be used for injections.
9 Mixing insulin:	
a If patient takes insulin that is cloudy, roll bottle of insulin between hands to resuspend insulin preparation. Wipe off tops of both insulin vials with alcohol swab. Verify insulin dose against MAR.	Rolling between hands prevents mixing with air.
b If mixing rapid- or short-acting insulin with intermediate- or long-acting insulin, take insulin	Air must be introduced into vial to create pressure needed to withdraw solution.

STEP	RATIONALE
syringe and aspirate volume of air equivalent to dose to be withdrawn from intermediate- or long-acting insulin first. If two intermediate- or long-acting insulins are mixed, it makes no difference which vial is prepared first.	

SAFETY ALERT If the long-acting insulin glargine (Lantus) is ordered, note that this is a clear insulin that should not be mixed with other insulin.

---

c Insert needle and inject air into vial of intermediate- or long-acting insulin. Do not let tip of needle touch solution.	Prevents cross contamination.
d Remove syringe from vial of insulin without aspirating medication.	Air will be injected into vial to withdraw desired dose.
e With the same syringe, inject air equal to the dose of rapid- or short-acting insulin into vial and withdraw correct dose into syringe.	Filling syringe with rapid- or short-acting insulin first prevents contamination with intermediate- or long-acting insulin.
f Remove syringe from rapid- or short-acting insulin and expel any air bubbles to ensure accurate dose.	Prevents accidental pulling of plunger, which may cause loss of medication. Ensures that correct dose is prepared.
g Verify short-acting insulin dosage with MAR and show insulin prepared in syringe to another nurse to verify that correct dosage of insulin was prepared. Determine which point on	Accentuates accuracy and prevents medication errors.

STEP	RATIONALE
syringe scale the combined units of insulin should measure by adding the number of units of both insulins (e.g., 4 units Regular + 10 units NPH = 14 units total). Verify combined dosage.	
h Place needle of syringe back into vial of intermediate- or long-acting insulin. Be careful not to push plunger and inject insulin in syringe into vial.	Positive pressure within vial of intermediate- or long-acting insulin allows fluid to fill syringe without need to aspirate.
i Invert vial and carefully withdraw desired amount of insulin into syringe.	
j Withdraw needle and check fluid level in syringe. Keep needle of prepared syringe sheathed or capped until ready to administer medication.	Ensures accurate dose. Inaccurate doses of insulin can cause serious hypoglycemia or hyperglycemia. Keeping needle capped or sheathed keeps needle sterile for insulin administration.
10 Mixing medications from vial and ampule:	
a Prepare medication from vial first (see Skill 50).	Ensures that appropriate amount of medication is prepared.
b Determine on syringe scale what the combined volume of medication should measure.	Ensures accurate dose.

SAFETY ALERT If needleless vial access device was used in preparing medication from vial, change needleless system to filter needle.

| c Next, using the same syringe, prepare second medication from ampule (see Skill 50). | |

STEP	RATIONALE
d Withdraw filter needle from ampule and verify fluid level in syringe. Change filter needle to appropriate SESIP needle. Keep device or needle sheathed or capped until administering medication.	Ensures accurate dose. Keeping needle or needleless device capped maintains sterility for medication administration.
e Check syringe carefully for total combined dose of medications.	Ensures accurate and safe medication administration.
11 Compare MAR, computer screen, or computer printout with prepared medication and labels on vials/ampules. *This is the second check for accuracy.*	Reading label second time reduces error.
12 Complete postprocedure protocol.	

UNEXPECTED OUTCOMES	RELATED INTERVENTIONS
1 Air bubbles remain in syringe.	• Expel air from syringe, and add medication to syringe until you prepare the correct dose.
2 Incorrect dose of medication is prepared.	• Discard prepared dose. • Prepare correct new dose.

Patient-Controlled Analgesia

Patient-controlled analgesia (PCA) is an interactive method of pain management that permits patient control over pain through self-administration of analgesics (D'Arcy, 2008; Wells et al., 2008). A patient depresses the button on a PCA device to deliver a regulated dose of analgesic. It is crucial that candidates for PCA be able to understand how, why, and when to self-administer the medication (APS and AAPM, 2009).

PCA has several advantages. It allows more constant serum levels of an opioid and avoids peaks and troughs of a large bolus. Patients receive better pain relief and fewer side effects from opioids because blood levels are maintained at a level of minimum effective analgesia concentration. Increased patient control and independence are other advantages for patients. Because PCA provides medication on demand, the total amount of opioid use can be reduced.

Delegation Considerations

The skill of administration of PCA cannot be delegated to nursing assistive personnel (NAP). The nurse directs the NAP to:
- Immediately report any new symptom or change in patient status, including unrelieved pain or oversedation, to the nurse.
- Never administer a PCA dose for the patient.

Equipment

- PCA system and tubing
- Identification label and time tape (may come attached and completed by pharmacy)
- Needleless connector
- Alcohol swab
- Adhesive tape
- Clean gloves (when applicable)
- Equipment for vital signs, pulse oximeter, and capnography (CO_2) monitoring equipment

Implementation

STEP	RATIONALE
1 Complete preprocedure protocol.	
2 Check accuracy and completeness of each MAR or computer printout with the health care provider's order for name of medication, dosage, frequency of medication (continuous or demand or both), and lockout settings. Verify that patient is not allergic to medication.	Health care provider's order is required for opioid medication. Ensures that patient receives right medication. *This is the first check for accuracy.*
3 Assess character of patient's pain, including physical, behavioral, and emotional signs and symptoms.	Establishes baseline to determine patient's response to analgesia.
4 When giving an IV, assess existing IV infusion line (peripheral or central) and surrounding tissue for patency and condition of site for infiltration or inflammation (see Skill 54).	IV line must be patent with fluid infusing for medication to reach venous circulation safely and effectively. Never attach PCA to an IV line with blood running or to IV lines with incompatible drugs infusing. If necessary, start another IV site.
5 Assess patient's knowledge and effectiveness of previous pain-management strategies, especially previous PCA use.	Response to pain-control strategies helps to identify learning needs and affects patient's willingness to try therapy.
6 Explain purpose and demonstrate function of PCA to patient and family.	Effective explanations allow patient participation in care and independence in pain control (Pasero and McCaffery, 2011).
7 Perform hand hygiene.	Reduces transmission of microorganisms and possible infection.

STEP	RATIONALE
8 Prepare analgesic while following the "six rights" for administration of medication. NOTE: Pharmacy prepares medication cartridge.	Ensures safe and appropriate medication administration. *This is the second check for accuracy.*
9 Identify patient using two identifiers (e.g., name and birthday or name and account number) according to agency policy. Compare identifiers with information on patient's MAR or medical record.	Ensures correct patient. Complies with The Joint Commission requirements for patient safety (TJC, 2014).
10 At the bedside compare the MAR or computer printout with the name of medication on the drug cartridge. Have a second registered nurse (RN) confirm the health care provider's order and the correct setup of the PCA. The second RN should check the health care provider's order and the device independently and not just look at the existing setup.	Ensures that the correct patient receives the right medication. *This is the third check for accuracy.*
11 Check infuser and patient-control module for accurate labeling or evidence of leaking.	Avoids medication error and injury to patient.
12 Program computerized PCA pump as ordered to deliver prescribed medication dose and lockout interval.	Ensures safe, therapeutic drug administration.
13 Insert drug cartridge into infusion device, and prime tubing.	Locks system and prevents air from infusing into IV tubing.
14 Apply clean gloves.	Prevents transmission of microorganisms.

STEP	RATIONALE
15 Attach needleless adapter to tubing adapter of patient-control module.	Connects device with IV line.
16 Wipe injection port of maintenance IV line with alcohol.	Alcohol is a topical antiseptic that minimizes entry of surface microorganisms during needle insertion.
17 Insert needleless adapter into injection port nearest patient.	Establishes route for medication to enter main IV line.
18 Secure connections with tape, and anchor PCA tubing. Label PCA tubing and remove gloves.	Prevents dislodgment of needleless adapter from port. Label prevents errors caused by connecting tubing from different device to PCA (TJC, 2014).
19 Administer loading dose of analgesia as prescribed.	A one-time dose (bolus) may be given manually by you or programmed into PCA pump.
20 Complete postprocedure protocol.	

Recording and Reporting

- Record drug, concentration, dose (basal and/or demand), time started, lockout time, and amount of IV solution infused and remaining solution. Many agencies have special PCA documentation forms.
- Record regular assessment of patient response to analgesia on PCA medication form, in nurses' notes and electronic health record (EHR), on pain assessment flow sheet, or on other documentation according to agency policy. This includes vital signs, oximetry or capnography results, sedation status, pain rating, status of vascular access site.

UNEXPECTED OUTCOMES	RELATED INTERVENTIONS
1 Patient verbalizes continued or worsening discomfort or displays nonverbal behaviors indicative of pain.	• Perform complete pain assessment. • Assess for possible complications other than pain. • Inspect IV site for possible catheter occlusion or infiltration. • Evaluate number of attempts and deliveries initiated by patient. • Check that maintenance IV fluid is continuously running. • Evaluate pump for operational problems. • Consult with health care provider.
2 Patient is not readily arousable.	• Stop PCA. • Notify health care provider. • Elevate head of bed 30 degrees, unless contraindicated. • Instruct patient to take deep breaths. • Apply oxygen at 2 L/min per nasal cannula (if ordered). • Assess vital signs. • Evaluate amount of opioid delivered within past 4 to 8 hours. • Ask family members if they depressed the button without patient knowledge. • Review MAR for other possible sedating drugs. • Prepare to administer an opioid-reversing agent. • Observe patient frequently (APS and AAPM, 2009).

UNEXPECTED OUTCOMES	RELATED INTERVENTIONS
3 Patient unable to manipulate PCA device to maintain pain control.	• Consult with health care provider regarding alternative medication route or possible basal (continuous) dose. • If agency allows, assess patient support system for significant other who can responsibly manipulate PCA device (Pasero and McCaffery, 2011).

Peripheral Intravenous Care: Dressing Care, Discontinuation

Short peripheral intravenous (IV) catheters require strict adherence to infection-prevention measures to avoid complications associated with these devices. Securely apply catheter dressings and change dressings when wet, soiled, or loosened. Change a transparent dressing during catheter site rotation of a short peripheral device. Change gauze dressings every 48 hours. When using gauze under a transparent dressing (although not recommended), it is considered a gauze dressing and should be changed every 48 hours (INS, 2011).

Discontinue a short peripheral intravenous (IV) catheter when the prescribed length of therapy is completed or a complication occurs (e.g., phlebitis, infiltration, or catheter occlusion). Care must also be taken because the risk of catheter emboli may occur if the catheter breaks during removal.

Delegation Considerations

The skill of changing a short peripheral IV dressing or of discontinuing a short peripheral intravenous line cannot be delegated to nursing assistive personnel (NAP). Delegation to licensed practical nurses (LPNs) varies by state Nurse Practice Act. The nurse instructs the NAP to:

- Report to the nurse if a patient complains of moistness or loosening of an IV dressing.
- Protect the IV dressing during hygiene and activities of daily living (ADLs).
- Report to the nurse any bleeding at the site after the catheter has been removed.
- Report any complaints by the patient of pain or observations of redness at the site.

Equipment

Changing IV Dressing

- Antiseptic swabs (2% chlorhexidine preferred or 70% alcohol, povidone-iodine)
- Adhesive remover (*optional*)
- Skin protectant swab
- Clean gloves

- Strips of sterile, precut tape (or roll of sterile tape), or stabilization device
- Commercially available IV site protection *(optional)*
- Sterile transparent semipermeable dressing

or

- Sterile 2 × 2– or 4 × 4–inch gauze pad

Discontinuing Peripheral Intravenous Access

- Clean gloves
- Sterile 2 × 2– or 4 × 4–inch gauze sponge
- Antiseptic swab
- Tape

Implementation

STEP	RATIONALE
1 Complete preprocedure protocol.	
2 Explain procedure and purpose to patient and family caregiver.	Decreases anxiety, promotes cooperation, and gives patient time frame around which to plan personal activities.
3 ![] Perform hand hygiene. Collect equipment. Apply clean gloves.	Reduces transmission of microorganisms. Infections related to IV therapy are most often caused by catheter hub contamination; thus you need to use careful technique throughout dressing change (INS, 2011).

Changing IV Dressing

1 Remove dressing. *For transparent semipermeable dressing:* Remove by pulling up one corner and pulling side laterally while holding catheter hub with nondominant hand (Fig. 53-1). Repeat on other side. Leave tape or catheter stabilization device that secures IV catheter in place.	Technique minimizes discomfort during removal. Use alcohol swab on transparent dressing next to patient's skin to loosen dressing.

Fig. 53-1 Remove transparent dressing by pulling side laterally.

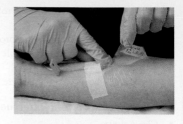

STEP	RATIONALE
For gauze dressing: Stabilize catheter hub while loosening tape and removing old dressing one layer at a time by pulling toward insertion site. Leave intact the tape that secures venous access device (VAD) to skin. Be cautious if IV tubing becomes tangled between two layers of dressing.	
2 Observe insertion site for signs and symptoms of IV-related complications (tenderness, redness, swelling, exudate, or complaints of pain). If complication exists or if ordered by health care provider, discontinue infusion.	Presence of infection or complication indicates need to remove VAD at current site.
3 Prepare new sterile tape strips for use. If IV is infusing properly, gently remove tape or stabilization device securing VAD. Stabilize VAD with one finger. Use adhesive remover to cleanse skin and remove adhesive residue if necessary.	Exposes venipuncture site. Stabilization prevents accidental displacement of VAD. Adhesive residue decreases ability of new tape to adhere securely to skin.

STEP	RATIONALE
4 While stabilizing IV, clean insertion site with chlorhexidine antiseptic swab, using friction vertically and horizontally and moving from insertion site outward with a third swab. Allow antiseptic solution to dry completely.	Allowing antiseptic solutions to air-dry completely effectively reduces microbial counts (INS, 2011). Chlorhexidine 2% takes 30 seconds to dry (INS, 2011).
5 *Optional:* Apply skin protectant solution to area where you will apply tape or dressing. Allow to dry.	Coats the skin with protective solution to maintain skin integrity, prevents irritation from the adhesive, and promotes adhesion of the dressing.
6 While securing catheter, apply sterile dressing over site.	
a Manufactured catheter stabilization device: Apply catheter stabilization device.	Manufactured catheter stabilization device preserves integrity of VAD and minimizes catheter movement at hub (INS, 2011). Must be placed under transparent dressing and is a sterile device.
b Transparent dressing: As directed in Skill 20.	Prevents accidental dislodgment of catheter. Allows continuous inspection of insertion site (Alexander et al., 2010). Occlusive dressing protects site from bacterial contamination. Connection between administration set and hub needs to be uncovered to facilitate changing the tubing if necessary.
c Sterile gauze dressing: See Skill 18.	Use only sterile tape under a sterile dressing to prevent site contamination.

STEP	RATIONALE
	Gauze dressing obscures observation of insertion site and is changed every 48 hours (INS, 2011).
7 Remove and discard gloves.	Prevents transmission of microorganisms.
8 *Option:* Apply site protection device (e.g., I.V. House Ultra Protective Dressing®).	Reduces risk for phlebitis and infiltration from mechanical motion.
9 Anchor IV tubing with additional pieces of tape if necessary. When using transparent dressing, avoid placing tape over dressing.	Prevents accidental displacement of VAD.
10 Label dressing per agency policy. Information on label includes date and time of IV insertion, VAD gauge size and length, and your initials.	Communicates type of device and time interval for dressing change and site rotation (INS, 2011).
11 Discard equipment and perform hand hygiene.	Reduces transmission of microorganisms.

Discontinuing Peripheral IV Access

1 Explain procedure to patient before you remove catheter.

2 Turn IV tubing roller clamp to "off" position or turn electronic infusion device (EID) off and roller clamp to "off" position.

3 ✋ Perform hand hygiene. Apply clean gloves.

4 Carefully remove IV site dressing, and stabilize IV device. Then remove the tape securing the catheter.

5 Place clean sterile gauze above insertion site and withdraw catheter, using a slow, steady motion.

STEP	RATIONALE
6 Apply pressure to site for a minimum of 30 seconds until bleeding has stopped. **NOTE:** Apply pressure for at least 5 to 10 minutes if patient is taking anticoagulants.	
7 Inspect catheter for intactness after removal. Note tip integrity and length.	
8 Apply clean, folded gauze dressing over insertion site and secure with tape.	
9 Complete postprocedure protocol.	

Recording and Reporting

- Record time short peripheral dressing was changed, reason for change, type of dressing material used, patency of system, and description of venipuncture site.
- Report to nurse in charge or oncoming nursing shift that dressing was changed and any significant information about integrity of system.
- Report to health care provider and document any complications.

UNEXPECTED OUTCOMES	RELATED INTERVENTIONS
1 Short peripheral catheter is infiltrated, as evidenced by decreased flow rate or edema, pallor, or decreased temperature around insertion site.	• Stop infusion and remove catheter. • Restart new short peripheral catheter in other extremity or above previous insertion site if continued therapy is necessary.
2 Short peripheral catheter is accidentally removed or dislodged.	• Restart new short peripheral catheter if continued therapy is needed.

Continued

UNEXPECTED OUTCOMES	RELATED INTERVENTIONS
3 Insertion site is red, edematous, painful, or has presence of exudate, indicating infection at venipuncture site.	• Notify health care provider. Culture of catheter tip and/ or exudate may be ordered (confirm before removal of IV). • Remove short peripheral catheter.

Peripheral Intravenous Care: Regulating Intravenous Flow Rate, Changing Tubing and Solution

Appropriate regulation of fluid rates reduces complications associated with intravenous (IV) therapy (INS Policy and Procedures, 2011). Changes in patient position, flexion of the IV site extremity, and occlusion of the IV device influence infusion rates. A patient achieves therapeutic outcomes and fewer complications when the IV system and flow rate are assessed systematically (Alexander et al., 2010).

Electronic infusion devices (EIDs) maintain correct flow rates and catheter patency and prevent an unexpected bolus of IV infusion. Diligence is necessary on your part to assess and monitor patients because use of any EID or controller is not without the risk of malfunction, placing a patient at risk for harm or injury.

Non-EIDs such as a volume-control device deliver small fluid volumes with the aid of gravity. One example of a volume-control device is a calibrated chamber placed between the IV container and the insertion spike and drip chamber of an administration set (Fig. 54-1).

Administration sets used for parenteral nutrition and blood or blood products have specific criteria with which you need to be familiar when administering these advanced therapies (see agency policy). Whenever possible, schedule tubing changes when it is time to hang a new IV container. If the tubing becomes damaged, is leaking, or becomes contaminated, it must be changed, regardless of the tubing change schedule.

Patients receiving intravenous (IV) therapy over time require periodic changes of IV solutions. You change a container when there is an order for a new solution or when it becomes time to add a sequential container to avoid exceeding hang time (Alexander et al., 2010).

Delegation Considerations

The skill of regulating IV flow rate, changing infusion tubing, or changing an IV solution cannot be delegated to nursing assistive personnel (NAP). Delegation to licensed practical nurses (LPNs) varies by state Nurse Practice Act. The nurse instructs the NAP to:

- Inform the nurse when the EID alarm signals.
- Inform the nurse when the fluid container is near completion or empty.

Fig. 54-1 Volume-control device.

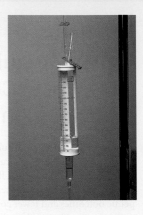

- Report any patient complaints of discomfort related to infusion such as pain, burning, bleeding, or swelling.
- Report to the nurse any leakage from or around the IV tubing.
- Report if tubing has become contaminated (e.g., lying on the floor).
- Report any cloudiness or precipitate in the IV solution.

Equipment

Regulating IV Flow Rate

- Watch with second hand
- Calculator, paper, and pencil
- Tape
- Label
- IV flow-control device: EID *(optional)*, volume-control device *(optional)*

Changing IV Solutions

- IV solution as ordered by health care provider

Changing IV Tubing

- Clean gloves
- Antiseptic wipes (alcohol wipes)
- Label

Continuous IV Infusion

- Microdrip or macrodrip administration set infusion tubing as appropriate

- Add-on device as necessary (e.g., filters, extension set, needleless connector)
- Tubing label

Intermittent Extension Set

- 3- to 5-mL syringe filled with preservative-free normal saline (NS)/0.9% normal saline solution (NSS)
- Short extension tubing (if necessary), injection cap

Implementation

STEP	RATIONALE
1 Complete preprocedure protocol.	
2 Review accuracy and completeness of health care provider's order in patient's medical record for patient name and correct solution: type, volume, additives, rate, and duration of IV therapy. Follow the six rights of medication administration.	Ensures that correct IV fluid is administered.
3 Perform hand hygiene. Inspect IV site for signs and symptoms of IV-related complications such as pain, swelling, or redness.	Observation or reports of any IV-related complications indicate need to reestablish patent IV access.
4 Observe for patency of IV tubing and venous access device (VAD).	IV line and VAD must be free of kinks, knots, and clots for fluid to infuse at proper rate.
5 Know calibration (drop factor) in drops per milliliter (gtt/mL) of infusion set used by agency: *Microdrip:* 60 gtt/mL: Used to deliver rates less than 100 mL/hr	Microdrip tubing universally delivers 60 gtt/mL. Used when small or very precise volumes are to be infused.

STEP	RATIONALE
Microdrip: 10 to 15 gtt/mL (depending on manufacturer): Used to deliver rates greater than 100 mL/hr	There are different commercial parenteral administration sets for macrodrip tubing. Used when large volumes or fast rates are necessary. Know the drip factor for the tubing being used.
6 Determine how long each liter of fluid should run. Calculate milliliters per hour (hourly rate) by dividing volume by hours: mL/hr = Total infusion (mL)/Hours (hr) of infusion 1000 mL/8 hr = 125 mL/hr *Or* If 3 L is ordered for 24 hours: 3000 mL/24 hr = 125 mL/hr	Basis of calculation to ensure infusion of fluid over prescribed hourly rate.
7 Select one of the following formulas to calculate minute flow rate (drops per minute) based on drop factor of infusion set: a mL/hr ÷ 60 min = mL/min Drop factor × mL/min = Drops/min *Or* b (mL/hr × Drop factor) ÷ 60 min = Drops/min Calculate minute flow rate for a bag 1 : 1000 mL with 20 mEq KCl at 125 mL/hr. *Microdrip:* 125 mL/hr × 60 gtt/mL = 7500 gtt/hr 7500 gtt ÷ 60 min = 125 gtt/min	Once you determine hourly rate, these formulas compute correct flow rate. When using microdrip, milliliters per hour (mL/hr) always equals drops per minute (gtt/min).

STEP	RATIONALE

Macrodrip:
125 mL/hr × 15 gtt/mL =
    1875 gtt/hr
1875 gtt ÷ 60 min = 31-
    32 gtt/min
	Multiply volume by drop factor
	and divide product by time (in
	minutes).

8 *For use of EID for infusion:* Follow manufacturer's guidelines for setup of EID.	

a Insert IV tubing
    into chamber of
    control mechanism
    (see manufacturer's
    directions) (Fig. 54-2).
	Most electronic infusion pumps
	use positive pressure to infuse.
	Infusion pumps propel fluid
	through tubing by compressing
	and milking the IV tubing.

b Turn on power button,
    select required drops
    per minute or volume
    per hour, close door to
    control chamber, and
    press start button.	

c Open drip regulator
    completely while EID is
    in use.
	Ensures that pump freely
	regulates infusion rate.

d Monitor infusion rate and
    IV site for complications
    according to agency
    policy. Use watch to verify
    rate of infusion, even
    when using EID.
	Infusion controllers or pumps
	are not perfect and do not
	replace frequent, accurate
	nursing evaluation. EIDs
	continue to infuse IV fluids
	after a complication has begun
	(INS, 2011).

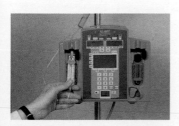

Fig. 54-2 Insert IV tubing into chamber of control mechanism.

STEP	RATIONALE
e Assess patency of system when alarm signals.	Alarm indicates some blockage in the system. Empty solution container, tubing kinks, closed clamp, infiltration, clotted catheter, air in the tubing, and/or low battery will all trigger the EID alarm.
9 *For a volume-control device:*	
a Place volumetric device between IV container and insertion spike of infusion set using aseptic technique.	Delivers small fluid volumes, but needs refilling when volume becomes low. Reduces risk for sudden fluid infusion.
b Place no more than a 2-hour allotment of fluid into device by opening clamp between IV bag and device.	Allows for a continuous infusion of fluid if you do not return in exactly 60 minutes to refill volume. If infusion rate accidentally increases, patient receives only a 2-hour allotment of fluid.
c Assess system at least hourly; add fluid to volume-control device. Regulate flow rate.	Maintains patency of system and patient monitoring.
Hanging New IV Solutions	
1 Prepare new solution for changing. If using plastic bag, hang on IV pole and remove protective cover from IV tubing port. If using glass bottle, remove metal cap and metal and rubber disks.	Permits quick, smooth, and organized change from old to new solution.
2 Close roller clamp on existing solution to stop flow rate. Remove tubing from EID (if used). Then remove old IV fluid container from IV pole. Hold container with tubing port pointing upward.	Prevents solution remaining in drip chamber from emptying while changing solutions. Prevents solution in bag from spilling.

STEP	RATIONALE
3 Quickly remove spike from old solution container and, without touching tip, insert spike into new container.	Reduces risk for solution in drip chamber becoming empty and maintains sterility.
4 Hang new container of solution on IV pole	Gravity helps with delivery of fluid into drip chamber.
5 Check for air in tubing. If air bubbles have formed, remove them by closing roller clamp, stretching tubing downward, and tapping tubing with finger (bubbles rise in fluid to drip chamber).	Reduces risk for air entering tubing. Use of an air-eliminating filter also reduces risk.
6 Regulate flow to ordered rate by using the roller clamp on the tubing or programming EID.	Maintains measures to restore fluid balance and deliver IV fluid as ordered.
7 Place time label on the side of container, and label with the time hung, the time of completion, and appropriate intervals. If using plastic bags, mark only on the label and not the container.	Provides a visual comparison of volume infused compared with prescribed rate of infusion. Ink sometimes leaches into plastic bags (INS, 2011).

Changing Infusion Tubing

Existing Continuous IV Infusion

STEP	RATIONALE
1 Move roller clamp on new IV tubing to "off" position.	Prevents fluid spillage.
2 Slow rate of infusion through old tubing to keep vein open (KVO) rate using EID or roller clamp.	Prevents occlusion of VAD.
3 Compress and fill drip chamber of old tubing.	Ensures fluid chamber remains full until new tubing is changed.
4 Invert container, and remove old tubing. Keep spike sterile and upright. *Optional:* Tape old drip chamber to IV pole without contaminating spike.	Fluid in drip chamber will continue to run and maintain catheter patency.

STEP	RATIONALE
5 Place insertion spike of new tubing into new solution container. Hang solution bag on IV pole, compress and release drip chamber on new tubing, and fill drip chamber one-third to one-half full.	Permits drip chamber to fill and promotes rapid, smooth flow of solution through tubing.
6 Slowly open roller clamp, remove protective cap from adapter (if necessary), and flush new tubing with solution. Stop infusion, and replace cap. Place end of adapter near patient's IV site.	Removes air from tubing and replaces it with IV solution. Equipment is positioned for a quick connection of new tubing.
7 Stop EID or turn roller clamp on old tubing to "off" position.	Prevents fluid spillage.
8 Prepare tubing with extension set or saline lock.	
a If short extension tubing is needed, use sterile technique to connect the new injection cap to new extension set or tubing.	Prepares extension set for connecting with IV.
b Swab injection cap with antiseptic swab. Insert syringe with 3 to 5 mL of saline solution, and inject through the injection cap into extension set.	Maintains patency of catheter. Prevents introduction of microorganisms.
9 Reestablish infusion.	
a Gently disconnect old tubing from extension tubing (or from IV catheter hub), and quickly insert adapter of new tubing or saline lock into extension tubing connection (or IV catheter hub).	Allows smooth transition from old to new tubing, minimizing time system is open.

STEP	RATIONALE
b For continuous infusion, open roller clamp on new tubing, allowing solution to run rapidly for 30 to 60 seconds, and then regulate drip rate using roller clamp or electronic infusion device.	Ensures catheter patency and prevents occlusion.
c Attach a piece of tape or preprinted label with date and time of tubing change onto tubing below the drip chamber.	Provides reference to determine next time for tubing change.
d Form a loop of tubing, and secure it to patient's arm with a strip of tape.	Avoids accidental pulling against site and stabilizes catheter.
10 Remove and discard old IV tubing. If necessary, apply new dressing. Remove and dispose of gloves. Perform hand hygiene.	Reduces transmission of microorganisms.
11 Complete postprocedure protocol.	

Recording and Reporting

- Record rate of infusion in drops per minute or milliliters per hour in nurses' notes and electronic health record (EHR) or on parenteral administration form according to agency policy.
- Document use of any EID or control device and identification number on that device.
- At change of shift or when leaving on break, report rate of infusion and volume left in infusion to nurse in charge or next nurse assigned to care for patient.
- Record solution and tubing change on patient's record. Use parenteral (IV) therapy flow sheet, if available.

UNEXPECTED OUTCOMES	RELATED INTERVENTIONS
1 Sudden infusion of large volume of solution occurs, with patient having symptoms of dyspnea, crackles in lung, and increased urine output, indicating fluid overload.	• Slow infusion rate: KVO rates must have specific rate ordered by licensed independent practitioner (LIP) (INS Policy and Procedures, 2011). • Notify health care provider immediately. • Place patient in high-Fowler's position. • Anticipate new IV orders. • Administer diuretics if ordered.
2 IV fluid container empties with subsequent loss of IV line patency.	• Discontinue present IV and restart new short peripheral catheter in new site.
3 The IV infusion is slower than ordered.	• Check for positional change that affects rate, height of IV container, or kinking/obstruction of tubing. • Check VAD site for complications. • Consult health care provider for new order to provide necessary fluid volume.

Peripheral Intravenous Insertion

Infusion therapy provides access to the venous system to deliver solutions and medications or blood and blood products. Reliable venous access for infusion therapy administration is essential. Your role is to select the appropriate vascular access device (VAD) needed to place a short peripheral intravenous (IV) catheter or to assist clinicians with placement of a midline or central vascular access device (CVAD). In addition, skills are needed to prepare the infusion equipment and become familiar with the various infusion systems used during an infusion. Some solutions and medications can be administered continuously, whereas others are given intermittently. Knowledge about the various types of administration sets, needleless devices, extension sets, flushes, and pumps and skills for their correct and safe use are required. Know and follow INS standards, your agency policy and procedures, and state or government practice guidelines when providing IV therapy.

Delegation Considerations

The skill of initiating IV therapy cannot be delegated to nursing assistive personnel (NAP). Delegation to licensed practical nurses (LPNs) varies by state Nurse Practice Act. The nurse instructs the NAP to:

- Inform the nurse if the patient complains of any IV site–related complications such as pain, redness, swelling, bleeding.
- Inform the nurse if the patient's IV dressing becomes wet.
- Inform the nurse if the solution of fluid in the IV bag is low or the electronic infusion device (EID) alarm is sounding.

Equipment

- Appropriate short peripheral IV catheter for venipuncture (Select the smallest gauge and length possible to administer the prescribed therapy [INS, 2011].)
- IV start kit supplies (available in some agencies): May contain a sterile drape to place under patient's arm, tourniquet, tape, transparent dressing, cleansing agent(s) (2% chlorhexidine preferred or povidone-iodine and 70% alcohol), and 2 × 2–inch gauze pads
- Clean gloves (latex-free for patients with latex allergy)

- Extension set with needleless connection device (also called saline lock, heparin lock, IV plug or adapter)
- Prefilled 5-mL syringe with flush agent (preservative-free normal saline [NS], 0.9% normal saline solution [NSS] [INS, 2011])
- Alcohol pads
- Stabilization device *(optional)* and skin protectant
- Prescribed intravenous solution
- Administration set, either macrodrip or microdrip, depending on prescribed rate; if using EID, appropriate administration set
- 0.2-micron filter for nonlipid (fat emulsions) solutions (may be incorporated into the infusion set)
- Protective equipment: goggles and mask *(optional,* check agency policy)
- IV pole, rolling or ceiling mounted
- EID if available
- Watch with second hand to calculate drip rate
- Special patient gown with snaps at shoulder seams if available (makes removal with IV tubing easier)
- Needle disposal container (also called *sharps container* or *biohazard container)*

Implementation

STEP	RATIONALE
1 Complete preprocedure protocol.	
2 Review accuracy and completeness of health care provider's order for type and amount of IV fluid, medication additives, infusion rate, and length of therapy. Follow six rights of medication administration.	Before administering solutions or medications an order from a licensed independent practitioner (LIP) is needed (Alexander et al., 2010; INS, 2011; INS Policy and Procedures, 2011).
a Check approved online database, drug reference book, or pharmacist about IV fluids' composition, purpose, potential incompatibilities, and side effects.	Ensures safe and correct administration of IV therapy and appropriate selection of vascular access device (VAD).

STEP	RATIONALE
3 Assess for clinical factors/ conditions that will respond to or be affected by administration of IV solutions.	Provides baseline to determine effectiveness of prescribed therapy. A systems approach is recommended to assess for fluid and electrolyte imbalances (Alexander et al., 2010; LeFever Kee et al., 2010).
a Body weight	Changes in body weight reflect fluid loss or gain. One kilogram or 2.2 lbs of body weight is equivalent to gain or loss of 1 L of fluid (Alexander et al., 2010).
b Clinical markers of vascular volume:	
(1) Urine output (decreased, dark yellow)	Kidneys respond to extracellular volume (ECV) deficit by reducing urine production and concentrating urine. Kidney disease can also cause oliguria.
(2) Vital signs: blood pressure, respirations, pulse, temperature	Changes in blood pressure may be associated with fluid volume status (fluid volume deficit [FVD]) seen in postural hypotension. Respirations can be altered in presence of acid-base imbalances. Temperature elevations increase need for fluid requirements (temperatures of 101° F [38.3° C] to 103° F [39.4° C] require at least 500 mL of fluid replacement within a 24-hr period) (Alexander et al., 2010).
(3) Distended neck veins (Normally veins are full when person is supine and flat when person is upright.)	Indicator of fluid volume status: flat or collapsing with inhalation when supine with ECV deficit; full when upright or semi-upright with ECV excess.

STEP	RATIONALE
(4) Auscultation of lungs	Crackles or rhonchi in dependent portions of lung may signal fluid buildup caused by ECV excess.
(5) Capillary refill	Indirect measure of tissue perfusion (sluggish with ECV deficit).
c Clinical markers of interstitial volume	
(1) Skin turgor (Pinch skin over sternum or inside of forearm.)	Failure of skin to return to normal position within 3 seconds indicates ECV deficit. This is called *tenting* (Alexander et al., 2010).
(2) Dependent edema (pitting or nonpitting) 1+ indicates barely detectable edema; 4+ indicates deep pitting edema.	Pitting edema is seen with a weight gain of 10 to 15 lbs (4.5-6.8 kg) of retained fluid (Alexander et al., 2010).
(3) Oral mucous membrane between cheek and gum	More reliable indicator than dry lips or skin. Dry between cheek and gums indicates ECV deficit.
d Thirst	Occurs with hypernatremia and severe ECV deficit. Not a reliable indicator for older adults (Meiner, 2011).
e Behavior and level of consciousness:	
(1) Restlessness and mild confusion	Occurs with FVD or acid-base imbalance.
(2) Decreased level of consciousness (lethargy, confusion, coma)	Occurs with severe ECV deficit.
4 Determine if patient is to undergo any planned surgeries or procedures.	Allows anticipation and placement of appropriate VAD for infusion and avoids placement in an area that

STEP	RATIONALE
	will interfere with medical procedures.
5 Identify patient using two identifiers (e.g., name and birthday or name and account number) according to agency policy. Compare identifiers with information on patient's MAR or medical record.	Ensures correct patient. Complies with The Joint Commission requirements for patient safety (TJC, 2014).
6 *Option:* Prepare short extension tubing with needleless connector or stand-alone saline lock (injection cap) to attach to VAD catheter hub.	Short extension tubing prevents traction on VAD. Many agencies use short extension tubing for continuous infusions and stand-alone saline locks (capped catheters).
a Remove protective cap from needleless connector. Swab injection cap with antiseptic swab. Attach syringe with sterile 0.9% normal saline solution (NS) flush and inject through cap into short extension set, keeping syringe attached.	Removes air from tubing, preventing it from being introduced into vein (Alexander et al., 2010; INS Policy and Procedures, 2011).
b Maintain sterility of end of connector and set aside for attaching to catheter hub after successful venipuncture.	Prevents touch contamination.
7 Prepare IV infusion tubing and solution.	
a Check IV solution using six rights of medication administration. If using bar code, scan code on patient's wristband and then on IV fluid	IV solutions are medications and need to be checked carefully to reduce risk of error. Bar-code system reduces medication errors (Poon et al., 2010). Do not use solutions that are

STEP	RATIONALE
container. Be sure that prescribed additives such as potassium and vitamins have been added. Check solution for color, clarity, and expiration date. Check bag for leaks.	discolored, contain particles, or are expired. Do not use leaking bags because the integrity has been compromised and they present an opportunity for infection (Alexander et al., 2010; INS, 2011; INS Policy and Procedures, 2011).
b Open infusion set, maintaining sterility of both tubing ends. EID pumps sometimes have a special, dedicated administration set.	Prevents touch contamination, which allows microorganisms to enter infusion equipment and bloodstream.
c Place roller clamp about 2 to 5 cm (1 to 2 inches) below drip chamber, and move roller clamp to "off" position.	Close proximity of roller clamp to drip chamber allows more accurate regulation of flow rate. Moving clamp to "off" prevents accidental spillage of IV fluid during priming.
d Remove protective sheath over IV tubing port on plastic IV solution bag (Fig. 55-1) or top of bottle.	Provides access for insertion of infusion tubing into solution using sterile technique.
e Remove protective cap from tubing insertion spike (without touching spike), and insert spike into port of IV bag. Clean rubber stopper on glass-bottled solution with single-use antiseptic, and insert spike into black rubber stopper of IV bottle. Bottles need special vented tubing.	Flat surface on the top of bottled solution may contain contaminants, whereas opening to plastic bag is recessed. Prevents contamination of bottled solution during insertion of spike.

SAFETY ALERT Do not touch spike because it is sterile. If contamination occurs (e.g., spike is accidentally dropped on the floor), discard that IV tubing and obtain new tubing.

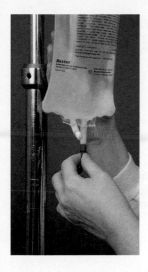

Fig. 55-1 Removing protective sheath from IV bag port.

STEP	RATIONALE
f Compress drip chamber and release, allowing it to fill one-third to one-half full.	Creates suction effect; fluid enters drip chamber to prevent air from entering tubing.
g Prime infusion tubing by filling with IV solution: Remove protective cap on end of tubing (you can prime some tubing without removal), and slowly open roller clamp to allow fluid to travel from drip chamber through tubing to needle adapter. Invert Y connector to displace air. Return roller clamp to "off" position after priming tubing (filled with IV fluid). Replace protective cap on end of infusion tubing.	Priming ensures that tubing is clear of air before connection with VAD. Slow fill of tubing decreases turbulence and chance of bubble formation. Closing clamp prevents accidental loss of fluid.

STEP	RATIONALE
h Be certain tubing is clear of air and air bubbles. To remove small air bubbles, firmly tap IV tubing where air bubbles are located. Check entire length of tubing to ensure that all air bubbles are removed.	Large air bubbles act as emboli.
8 If using optional long extension tubing (not short tubing in Step 6), remove protective cap and attach it to distal end of IV tubing, maintaining sterility. Then prime long extension tubing.	Priming removes air from tubing so it does not enter patient's vascular system.
9 Perform hand hygiene and apply clean gloves. Wear eye protection and mask (see agency policy) if splash or spray of blood is possible.	Reduces transmission of microorganisms. Decreases exposure to human immunodeficiency virus (HIV), hepatitis, and other bloodborne organisms (INS, 2011). Prevents spraying blood from contacting your mucous membranes.
10 Apply tourniquet around arm above antecubital fossa 10 to 15 cm (4 to 6 inches) above proposed insertion site. Do not apply tourniquet too tightly to avoid injury, bruising skin, or occluding artery. Check for presence of radial pulse. (*Option a:* Apply tourniquet on top of a thin layer of clothing such as a gown sleeve to protect fragile or hairy skin.) (*Option b:* Blood pressure cuff may be used in place	Tourniquet should be tight enough to impede venous return but not occlude arterial flow (Alexander et al., 2010; INS Policy and Procedures, 2011). If patient has fragile veins, tourniquet should be applied loosely or not at all to prevent damage to veins and bruising.

STEP	RATIONALE
of tourniquet: Inflate cuff to just below patient's diastolic pressure [less than 50 mg Hg].)	
11 Select vein for VAD insertion. Veins on dorsal and ventral surfaces of arms (e.g., cephalic, basilic, or median) are preferred in adults. Avoid lateral surface of wrist because of potential for nerve damage (INS, 2011).	Ensures adequate vein that is easy to puncture and less likely to rupture. Veins of lower extremities should not be used for routine IV therapy in adults because of risk of tissue damage and thrombophlebitis (INS, 2011).
a Use most distal site in the nondominant arm, if possible.	Patients with VAD placement in their dominant hand have decreased ability to perform self-care.
b Select a well-dilated vein.	Increased volume of blood in vein at venipuncture site makes vein more visible.
Methods to improve venous distention:	
(1) Place extremity in dependent position and stroke from distal to proximal below proposed venipuncture site.	Promotes venous filling.
(2) Apply warmth to extremity for several minutes (e.g., warm washcloth or dry heat).	Heat increases blood supply through vasodilation (INS, 2011).
12 Select a vein large enough for VAD.	
a With your index finger, palpate vein by pressing downward. Note resilient, soft, bouncy feeling while releasing pressure.	Fingertip is more sensitive and better for assessing vein location and condition.

STEP	RATIONALE
b Avoid vein selection in:	
(1) Areas with tenderness, redness, rash, pain, or infection.	It would be difficult to assess for any signs or symptoms of complications if an IV device were inserted in an area already compromised (INS, 2011).
(2) Extremity affected by previous cerebrovascular accident (CVA), paralysis, dialysis shunt, or mastectomy.	Increases risk for complications such as infection, lymphedema, or vessel damage (INS, 2011).
(3) Site distal to previous venipuncture site, sclerosed or hardened veins, infiltrate site, areas of venous valves, or phlebotic vessels.	Such sites cause vessel damage and infiltration around newly placed VAD site.
(4) Fragile dorsal veins in older adults.	Veins have increased risk for infiltration.
c Choose a site that will not interfere with patient's activities of daily living (ADLs), use of assist devices, or planned procedures.	Keeps patient as mobile as possible.
13 Release tourniquet temporarily and carefully.	Restores blood flow and prevents venospasm when preparing for venipuncture.
Option: Clip arm hair with scissors if necessary (explain to patient).	Hair impedes venipuncture or adherence of dressing.
Option: You may apply topical local anesthetic to IV site 30 minutes before insertion. Monitor for allergic reaction.	Local anesthetic reduces discomfort (must have health care provider order for use of local anesthetic).

STEP	RATIONALE
14 Place adapter end of short infusion tubing or extension/injection cap for saline lock nearby on sterile gauze or sterile towel.	Permits smooth, quick connection of infusion to short peripheral catheter once vein is accessed.
15 If area of insertion appears to need cleaning, use soap and water first and dry. Use chlorhexidine antiseptic swab or applicator to clean insertion site, using friction in a horizontal plane with first swab, in a vertical plane with second swab, and in a circular motion moving outward with third swab. Allow to dry completely. Refrain from touching cleaned site unless using sterile technique. Allow drying time between agents if agents are used in combination (alcohol and Betadine).	Mechanical friction in this pattern allows penetration of antiseptic solution to epidermal layer of the skin (Alexander et al., 2010; INS, 2011; INS Policy and Procedures, 2011). Allowing antiseptic solution to air-dry completely effectively reduces microbial counts (INS, 2011). Chlorhexidine 2% dries in 30 seconds (INS, 2011). Touching cleaned area introduces microorganisms from your finger to site. If this happens, prepare site again.
16 Reapply tourniquet 10 to 15 cm (4 to 6 inches) above anticipated insertion site. Check presence of distal pulse.	Diminished arterial flow prevents venous filling. The pressure of the tourniquet causes the vein to engorge.
17 Perform venipuncture. Anchor vein below site by placing thumb over vein and gently stretching skin against direction of insertion 4 to 5 cm ($1\frac{1}{2}$ to 2 inches) distal to the site (Fig. 55-2). Instruct patient to relax hand.	Stabilizes vein for needle insertion and prevents vein from rolling. Skin becomes taut, decreasing drag on insertion of device.

Fig. 55-2 Stabilize vein below insertion site.

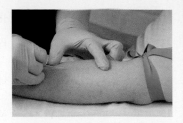

STEP	RATIONALE
a Warn patient of a sharp, quick stick. Insert VAD with bevel up at 10- to 30-degree angle slightly distal to actual site of venipuncture in direction of vein.	Places needle at a 10- to 30-degree angle to the vein. When vein is punctured, risk for puncturing posterior vein wall is reduced. Superficial veins require a smaller angle. Deeper veins require a greater angle.

SAFETY ALERT Use each VAD only once for each insertion attempt.

| 18 | Observe for blood return through flashback chamber of catheter, indicating that bevel of needle has entered vein. Lower catheter until almost flush with skin. Advance catheter approximately 0.6 cm ($\frac{1}{4}$ inch) into vein, and loosen stylet of over-the-needle catheter (ONC). Continue to hold skin taut while stabilizing the needle, and advance catheter off the needle to thread just the catheter into vein until hub rests at venipuncture site. *Do not reinsert stylet once it is loosened.* Advance catheter while safety device automatically retracts the stylet. | Increased venous pressure from tourniquet increases backflow of blood into catheter or tubing. Allows for full penetration of the vein wall, placement of the catheter in the inner lumen of the vein, and advancement of the catheter off the stylet. Reduces risk for introduction of microorganisms along catheter. Advancing the entire stylet into the vein may penetrate the wall of the vein, resulting in a hematoma. Reinsertion of stylet causes catheter shearing in the vein and potential catheter embolization (INS, 2011). |

STEP	RATIONALE

> **SAFETY ALERT** A single nurse should not make any more than two attempts at initiating IV access (INS, 2011). After two attempts the nurse should have another nurse attempt the insertion.

STEP	RATIONALE
19 Stabilize catheter with nondominant hand and release tourniquet or blood pressure cuff with other. Apply gentle but firm pressure with middle finger of nondominant hand 3 cm (1¼ inches) above insertion site. Keep catheter stable with index finger.	Permits venous flow, reduces backflow of blood, and allows connection with administration set with minimal blood loss (INS, 2011).
20 Quickly connect Luer-Lok end of prepared extension set, or saline lock of primary administration set, to end of catheter. Do not touch point of entry of connection. Secure connection.	Prompt connection of infusion set maintains patency of vein and prevents risk of exposure to blood. Maintains sterility.
21 Flush VAD (Fig. 55-3). Slowly flush a primed extension set with remaining saline from attached prefilled syringe, or begin a primary infusion by slowly opening slide clamp or adjusting roller clamp of IV tubing.	Positive-pressure flushing allows fluid to displace removed stylet, creates positive pressure in catheter, and prevents reflux of blood into catheter lumen (INS Policy and Procedures, 2011). Initiates flow of fluid through IV catheter, preventing clotting of device.

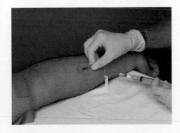

Fig. 55-3 Flush injection cap.

STEP	RATIONALE
Observe for swelling.	Swelling indicates infiltration, and catheter would need to be removed.
Option: Remove syringe. Attach distal end of primary IV tubing to needleless connector on short extension tubing that is attached to catheter.	
22 Secure catheter (procedures differ; follow agency policy).	
a *Manufactured catheter stabilization device:* Wipe selected area with single-use skin protectant and allow it to dry. Apply sterile adhesive strip over catheter hub. Slide device under catheter hub, and center hub over device. Holding catheter in place, peel off half of liner, and press to adhere to skin. Repeat on other side. Holding catheter in place, pull tab out from center of device to create opening, and insert catheter into slit. This frames IV site. Then apply dressing.	Use of a manufactured stabilization device preserves the integrity of access device, minimizes catheter movement at hub, and prevents catheter dislodgment or loss of access (INS, 2011).
b *Transparent dressing:* Secure catheter with nondominant hand while preparing to apply dressing.	Prevents accidental dislodgment of catheter.

STEP	RATIONALE
c *Sterile gauze dressing:* Place narrow piece, 1.27 cm ($\frac{1}{2}$ inch), of sterile tape over catheter hub. Place tape only on catheter, *never* over insertion site. Secure site to allow easy visual inspection. Avoid applying tape or gauze around arm.	Use sterile tape under sterile dressing to prevent site contamination. Regular adhesive tape is potential source of pathogenic bacteria (INS, 2011). Prevents back-and-forth motion of catheter.
23 Apply sterile dressing over site.	
a Transparent dressing (TSM):	
(1) Carefully remove adherent backing. Apply one edge of dressing, and then gently smooth remaining dressing over IV site, leaving connection between IV tubing and catheter hub uncovered. Remove outer covering, and smooth dressing gently over site.	Occlusive dressing protects site from bacterial contamination. Allows for visualization of insertion site and surrounding area for signs and symptoms of IV-related complications (INS, 2011). Connection between administration set and hub needs to be uncovered to facilitate change of tubing if necessary.
(2) Take a 2.5-cm (1-inch) piece of tape and place it over extension tubing or administration set. **Do not apply tape on top of transparent dressing.**	Removal of tape from a transparent dressing can cause accidental removal of catheter. Tape on top of a transparent dressing prevents moisture from being carried away from the skin.

STEP	RATIONALE
b Sterile gauze dressing:	
(1) Place 2 × 2 gauze pad over insertion site and catheter hub. Secure all edges with tape. Do not cover connection between IV tubing and catheter hub.	Optional method of securing device if patient is allergic to transparent dressing. It is not the preferred method to cover and secure IV device because gauze prevents visualization of insertion site (INS, 2011).
(2) Fold a 2 × 2 gauze pad in half, and cover with a 2.5-cm–wide (1 inch) tape extending about 1 inch from each side. Place under the tubing/catheter hub junction.	Tape on top of gauze makes it easier to access hub/tubing junction. Gauze pad elevates hub off skin to prevent pressure area.
24 Loop the short extension tubing or the continuous infusion administration tubing alongside arm, and place second piece of tape directly over tubing and secure.	Securing administration set or extension set reduces risk for dislodging catheter if IV tubing is pulled (i.e., loop comes apart before catheter dislodges).
25 For continuous infusion, insert tubing of IV administration set into electronic infusion device (EID). Check ordered rate of infusion, then turn on EID and program it, and begin infusion at correct rate. If infusing by gravity drip, adjust flow rate to correct drops per minute (see Skill 54)	Manipulation of catheter during dressing application alters flow rate. EID maintains correct rate of flow for IV solution. Flow fluctuates; thus it must be checked at intervals for accuracy.
26 Label dressing per agency policy. Include date and time of IV insertion, VAD gauge size and length, and your initials.	Allows for recognition of type of device and length of time that device has been in place.

STEP	RATIONALE
27 Dispose of used stylet or other sharps in appropriate sharps container. Discard supplies. Remove gloves and perform hand hygiene.	Reduces transmission of microorganisms; prevents accidental needlestick injuries.
28 Complete postprocedure protocol.	

Recording and Reporting

- Record in nurses' notes and electronic health record (EHR) the number of attempts and sites of insertion; precise description of insertion site (e.g., cephalic vein on dorsal surface of right lower arm, 2.5 cm [1 inch] above wrist); flow rate; method of infusion (gravity or EID); size and type, length, and brand of catheter; time infusion started; and patient's response to insertion. Use an infusion therapy flow sheet when available.
- If using an EID, document type and rate of infusion and device identification number.
- Record patient's status, IV fluid, amount infused, and integrity and patency of system according to agency policy.
- Report to oncoming nursing staff: type of fluid, flow rate, status of VAD, amount of fluid remaining in present solution, expected time to hang subsequent IV container, and patient condition.

UNEXPECTED OUTCOMES	RELATED INTERVENTIONS
1 FVD as manifested by decreased urine output, dry mucous membranes, decreased capillary refill, a disparity in central and peripheral pulses, tachycardia, hypotension, shock.	• Notify health care provider. • Requires readjustment of infusion rate.
2 Fluid volume excess (FVE) as manifested by crackles in the lungs, shortness of breath, edema.	• Reduce IV flow rate if symptoms appear. • Notify health care provider.

Continued

UNEXPECTED OUTCOMES	RELATED INTERVENTIONS
3 Electrolyte imbalances indicated by abnormal serum electrolyte levels, changes in mental status, alterations in neuromuscular function, cardiac dysrhythmias, and changes in vital signs.	• Notify health care provider. • Adjust additives in IV or type of IV fluid per order.
4 Infiltration is indicated by slowing of infusion; insertion site is cool to touch, pale, and painful.	• Stop infusion and discontinue IV (see Skill 53). • Elevate affected extremity. • Restart new IV above previous location of infiltrate or opposite extremity if continued therapy is necessary. • Document degree of infiltration and nursing intervention.
5 Phlebitis is indicated by pain and tenderness at IV site with erythema at site or along path of vein. Insertion site is warm to touch, and rate of infusion may be altered (Table 55-1).	• Stop infusion immediately and discontinue IV. • If continued therapy is necessary, restart new IV in area above previous location or using opposite extremity. • Place moist, warm compress over area of phlebitis. • Continue to monitor site for 48 hours after catheter is removed for post-infusion phlebitis (INS, 2011). • Document degree of phlebitis and nursing interventions per agency policy and procedure (see Table 55-1).

TABLE 55-1 Phlebitis Scale

Grade	Clinical Criteria
0	No symptoms
1	Erythema at access site with or without pain
2	Pain at access site with erythema and/or edema
3	Pain at access site with erythema and/or edema Streak formation Palpable venous cord
4	Pain at access site with erythema and/or edema Streak formation Palpable venous cord >2.5 cm (1 inch) in length Purulent drainage

From Infusion Nurses Society: Infusion nursing standards of practice, *J Infus Nurs* 34(1S):S65, 2011.

UNEXPECTED OUTCOMES	RELATED INTERVENTIONS
6 Bleeding occurs at venipuncture site.	• Verify that system is intact and replace dressing if loosened. • Restart new IV if bleeding from site does not stop or if IV is dislodged.
7 IV site infection. Monitor site for signs and symptoms of infection, which may include redness, pain, edema, induration, temperature, and drainage.	• Notify health care provider for appropriate interventions such as culturing of device or site. • If continued therapy is necessary, restart new IV in area above location or using opposite extremity. • Document presence and severity of infection and interventions.

Peripherally Inserted Central Catheter Care

The need for safe and convenient intravenous (IV) therapy has led to the development of vascular access devices (VADs) designed for long-term access to the venous or arterial systems. A central vascular access device (CVAD) has a final tip location in the lower third of the superior vena cava and the junction of the right atrium (INS, 2011). For CVADs placed in the femoral region the final tip placement should be in the inferior vena cava above the level of the diaphragm (INS, 2011). CVADs can have single or multiple lumens. The choice of the number of lumens depends on a patient's condition and prescribed therapy.

Primary complications associated with CVADs are usually related to infections commonly referred to as *central line–associated bloodstream infections (CLABSIs)* caused by contamination of the catheter from the skin of the patient or poor infection-prevention practices during insertion or care and maintenance (Alexander et al., 2010). The Institute for Healthcare Improvement (IHI, 2011) recently introduced a CLABSI bundle. The *IHI Central Line Bundle* is a group of evidence-based interventions for patients with intravascular central catheters that, when implemented together, result in better outcomes than when implemented individually (IHI, 2011).

Delegation Considerations

The skill of caring for a CVAD cannot be delegated to nursing assistive personnel (NAP). Delegation to licensed practical nurses (LPNs) varies by state Nurse Practice Act. The nurse instructs the NAP to:

- Report the following to the nurse immediately: patient's dressing becomes damp or soiled, catheter line appears to be pulled out farther than original insertion position, IV line becomes disconnected, patient has a fever, or patient complains of pain at the site.
- Help with positioning patient during insertion and care.

Equipment

Site Care and Dressing Change

- CVAD dressing change kit, which includes:
  - Sterile gloves
  - Mask
  - Antimicrobial swabs (e.g., 2% chlorhexidine [IHI, 2011] [see agency policy])

- • Transparent antimicrobial dressing (e.g., transparent semipermeable membrane [TSM])
  - • 4 × 4–inch gauze pads
  - • Tape measure
  - • Sterile tape
  - • Label
- Catheter stabilization device (if not sutured) for peripherally inserted central catheter (PICC) or nontunneled catheters
- Needleless injection cap for each lumen
- Noncoring needle for implanted venous port

Blood Sampling

- Clean gloves
- Antimicrobial swabs (e.g., 2% chlorhexidine, alcohol)
- 5-mL Luer-Lok syringes
- 10-mL Luer-Lok syringes
- Vacutainer system or blood transfer device (see agency policy)
- Preservative-free saline flush/0.9% normal saline solution (NSS)
- Blood tubes, including waste tubes, labels
- Needleless injection cap
- Syringe (5 or 10 mL; see agency policy) for discarded blood
- 10-mL syringe with 5- to 10-mL saline flush
- 10-mL syringe with 3-mL heparin flush (100 units/mL)

Implementation

STEP	RATIONALE
1 Complete preprocedure protocol.	
2 Review accuracy and completeness of health care provider's order. Assess treatment schedule: times for administration of IV solutions, medications, and blood sampling. Follow six rights of medication administration.	Identifies patient's need for vascular access, evaluates response to therapy, and determines educational needs.
3 Explain procedure and purpose to patient and family caregiver. Explain to patient that he or she must	Decreases anxiety, promotes cooperation, and prevents sudden movement during sterile procedure.

STEP	RATIONALE
not move during procedure. Offer opportunity at this time to toilet, and offer pain medication (if needed).	
4 Insertion site care and dressing change:	
a Position patient in comfortable position with head slightly elevated or, in the case of a PICC or midline device, have arm extended.	Provides access to patient.
b Prepare dressing materials. *Transparent dressing:* Provide insertion site care every 5 to 7 days and as needed. *Gauze dressing:* Provide insertion site care every 48 hours and as needed.	Transparent semipermeable membrane dressings have the advantage of being able to visualize the IV site. Gauze is preferable to TSM if the patient is diaphoretic or if the site is oozing or bleeding (INS, 2011).
c Perform hand hygiene and apply mask.	Reduces transfer of microorganisms; prevents spread of airborne microorganisms over CVAD insertion site.
d ![gloves icon] Apply clean gloves. Remove old dressing by lifting and removing either TSM or tape and gauze in direction of catheter insertion. Discard in appropriate biohazard container.	Stabilizes catheter as you remove dressing.
e Remove catheter stabilization device if used. Must be removed with alcohol.	

STEP	RATIONALE

Safety Alert If sutures are used for initial catheter stabilization and become loosened or are no longer intact, alternative stabilization measures should be used (INS, 2011). Recent recommendations include use of a stabilization device because of the increased risk for infection when the catheter is sutured (Alexander et al., 2010).

STEP	RATIONALE
f Inspect catheter, insertion site, and surrounding skin. Measure mid-arm circumference above insertion site.	Insertion sites require regular inspection for early detection of signs and symptoms of IV-related complications (infection, pain, redness, swelling, drainage, or bleeding) (INS, 2011).
g Remove and discard clean gloves; perform hand hygiene. Open CVAD dressing kit using sterile technique, and *apply sterile gloves.* Area to be cleaned should be same size as dressing.	Sterile technique is required to apply new dressing.
h Cleanse site:	
(1) 2% chlorhexidine (preferred). Apply using back-and-forth motion vertically and horizontally for at least 30 seconds; allow solution to dry for 30 seconds.	Allowing antiseptic solutions to air-dry completely effectively reduces microbial counts (INS, 2011). Drying allows time for maximum microbicidal activity of agents (INS Policy and Procedures, 2011).
(2) Povidone-iodine may be used in some settings (see agency policy).	
i Apply skin protectant to entire area. Let dry completely so skin is not tacky.	Protects irritated or fragile skin from dressing. It must be used if catheter stabilization device is used.

STEP	RATIONALE
j *Option:* Use chlorhexidine-impregnated dressing for short-term CVADs.	These dressings should be considered for patients older than 2 months of age to prevent catheter-related bloodstream infection (CRBSI) (INS, 2011).
k Apply new catheter stabilization device per manufacturer's instructions if catheter is not sutured in place.	Provides catheter stability to minimize dislodgment or migration.
l Apply sterile, transparent semipermeable dressing or apply gauze dressing over insertion site (see Skill 53).	Transparent dressing allows for clear visualization of catheter site between dressing changes (INS Policy and Procedures, 2011).
m Apply label to dressing with date, time, and your initials.	Provides information about next dressing change.
n Dispose of soiled supplies and used equipment. Remove gloves and perform hand hygiene.	Reduces transmission of microorganisms.
5 **Blood sampling:**	
a ![icon] Perform hand hygiene. Apply clean gloves.	Reduces transmission of microorganisms.
b Turn off all infusions for at least 1 minute before drawing blood. **NOTE:** If you cannot stop infusion, draw blood from peripheral vein.	Prevents interruption of critical fluid therapy.
c When drawing through multilumen catheters, the distal lumen (or one recommended by manufacturer) is preferred.	Distal lumen typically is largest-gauge lumen (Alexander et al., 2010).
d Clean injection cap with antiseptic solution and allow solution to dry	Maximizes bactericidal effectiveness of antiseptic swab.

STEP	RATIONALE
completely. Attach syringe and flush with 3 to 5 mL of preservative-free 0.9% sodium chloride.	Determines catheter patency and clears IV (INS Policy and Procedures, 2011).
e Syringe method: NOTE: Check agency policy for use of Vacutainer with CVADs.	
(1) Remove end of IV tubing or injection cap from catheter hub. Keep end of tubing sterile.	
(2) Disinfect catheter hub with antiseptic solution.	Reduces risk of microorganisms.
(3) Attach an empty 10-mL syringe, unclamp catheter (if necessary), and withdraw blood 1.5 to 2 times fill volume (4 to 5 mL) of catheter for the discard sample.	Discard sample reduces risk of low drug concentrations or diluted specimen (Alexander et al., 2010).
(4) Reclamp catheter (if necessary); remove syringe with blood and discard in appropriate biohazard container.	Open and valved CVADs differ in recommendations for clamping before removal of injection cap and syringe(s) (INS, 2011).
(5) Clean hub with another antiseptic solution.	
(6) Attach second syringe(s) to obtain required volume of blood needed for specimen ordered.	Multiple syringes may be required, depending on specimens required and number of blood tubes needed.

STEP	RATIONALE
(7) Unclamp catheter (if necessary) to withdraw blood.	
(8) Once specimens are obtained, reclamp catheter (if necessary) and remove syringe.	
(9) Clean catheter hub with antiseptic solution.	
(10) Attach prefilled injection cap attached to 10-mL syringe with 10 mL of 0.9% sodium chloride to catheter, unclamp (if necessary), and flush. Reclamp catheter (if necessary).	Flushing with 10 mL of 0.9% sodium chloride after blood draw is minimum volume of solution recommended (INS, 2011). Reduces risk for catheter clotting after procedure.
(11) Remove syringe and discard into appropriate biohazard container.	Reduces transmission of microorganisms.
f Transfer blood using transfer vacuum device.	Reduces risk of blood exposure.
g Flush catheter with syringe containing heparin solution (check agency policy).	Heparin flush volume and concentration vary by agency and type of catheter.
6 Complete postprocedure protocol.	

Recording and Reporting

- Immediately notify health care provider of signs and symptoms of any complications.
- Document catheter site care in nurses' notes and electronic health record (EHR): size of catheter, change of injection caps, appearance of site, condition and type of securement device, date and time of dressing change.
- Document blood draw in nurses' notes. Include date, time, and sample drawn.

UNEXPECTED OUTCOMES	RELATED INTERVENTIONS
1 Patient or family member is unable to explain or perform CVAD care.	• Indicates need for home care referral or additional instruction.
2 Catheter becomes damaged or breaks.	• Clamp the catheter near insertion site, and place sterile gauze over break or hole until repaired. Use permanent repair kit, if available.
	• Remove catheter.
3 Catheter becomes occluded by a thrombus, precipitation, or malposition.	• Reposition patient. Have patient cough and deep breathe. Raise patient's arm overhead. Obtain venogram if ordered.
	• Administer thrombolytics if ordered.
	• Remove catheter (CVAD requires order).
	• Obtain x-ray examination as ordered.
	• If precipitate present, try hydrochloric acid or ethanol solution per orders.
	• Do not use a 1-mL syringe to instill saline because pressure exceeds 200 psi.
4 Infection and/or sepsis develops at exit site, tunnel, or port pocket.	• Obtain blood cultures first, from peripheral and CVAD if ordered.
	• Remove catheter (CVAD requires order).
	• Replace catheter.
5 Catheter becomes dislodged.	• Insert new catheter.
	• Secure with catheter stabilization device.
	• Teach patient not to manipulate catheter.

Continued

UNEXPECTED OUTCOMES	RELATED INTERVENTIONS
6 Catheter migration, pinch-off syndrome, port separation, or catheter fracture.	• Reposition under fluoroscopy as ordered. • Remove catheter as ordered. • Stop all fluid administration.
7 Skin erosion, hematomas, cuff extrusion, scar tissue formation over port.	• Remove CVAD as ordered. • Improve nutrition. • Provide appropriate skin care.
8 Infiltration, extravasation.	• Apply cold/warm compresses according to specific vesicant protocol. • Provide emotional support. • Obtain x-ray examination if ordered. • Use antidotes per protocol. • Discontinue IV fluids.
9 Pneumothorax, hemothorax, air emboli, hydrothorax.	• Administer oxygen as ordered. • Elevate feet. Aspirate air, fluid. • If air emboli are suspected, place patient on left side with head elevated slightly. Remove catheter as ordered. • Assist with insertion of chest tubes as ordered.

Postoperative Exercises

Structured preoperative teaching has a positive influence on a surgical patient's recovery (Lewis et al., 2011). You will provide information and teach skills to help patients understand the surgical experience and participate actively in the recovery process.

Postoperative exercises include diaphragmatic breathing and effective coughing, turning, and leg exercises. The physician may order incentive spirometry for patients especially at risk for atelectasis or pneumonia (e.g., chronic smokers or patients who have experienced prolonged bed rest).

Delegation Considerations

The skill of teaching postoperative exercises cannot be delegated to nursing assistive personnel (NAP). The NAP can reinforce and help patients in performing postoperative exercises. The nurse directs the NAP about:

- Maintaining precautions unique to a particular patient.
- When to report if the patient is unable or unwilling to perform the exercises correctly.

Equipment

- Pillow (*optional;* used to splint the incision when coughing to reduce discomfort)
- Incentive spirometer
- Positive expiratory pressure (PEP) device
- Stethoscope

Implementation

STEP	RATIONALE
1 Complete preprocedure protocol.	
2 Assess patient's risk for postoperative respiratory complications: identify presence of chronic pulmonary condition (e.g., emphysema, chronic bronchitis, asthma); any condition that affects chest wall movement, such as	General anesthesia predisposes patient to respiratory problems because lungs are not fully inflated during surgery, cough reflex is suppressed, and mucus collects within airway passages. After surgery, inadequate lung expansion can lead to atelectasis and pneumonia. Chronic lung

STEP	RATIONALE
obesity, advanced pregnancy, thoracic or abdominal surgery; history of smoking; and presence of reduced hemoglobin level.	conditions create greater risk for developing respiratory complications. Smoking damages ciliary clearance and increases mucus secretion. A reduced hemoglobin level can lead to reduced oxygen delivery.

SAFETY ALERT Assess and report to surgeon and/or anesthesiologist if patient has had a cold or upper respiratory tract infection within past week.

3 Auscultate lungs.	Establishes baseline for postoperative comparison.
4 Assess patient's ability to deep breathe and cough by placing hand on patient's abdomen, having patient take a deep breath, and observing movement of shoulders, chest wall, and abdomen. Measure chest excursion during a deep breath. Ask patient to cough into tissue after taking a deep breath.	Reveals maximum potential for chest expansion and ability to cough forcefully; serves as baseline to measure patient's ability to perform exercises after surgery.
5 Assess patient's risk for postoperative thrombus formation (e.g., older adults, immobilized patients, patients with personal or family history of clots, and women older than 35 who smoke and are taking birth control pills are most at risk). Observe calves for redness, swelling, warmth, or tenderness; assess for swollen calf, or calf swelling more than 3 cm	Following general anesthesia, circulation slows, causing a greater tendency for clot formation. Immobilization results in decreased muscular contraction in lower extremities, which promotes venous stasis. The physical stress of surgery creates a hypercoagulable state in most individuals. Manipulation and positioning during surgery may inadvertently cause trauma to leg veins. Symptoms may

STEP	RATIONALE
(1.2 inches) compared with asymptomatic leg. Compare legs for bilateral equality. Palpate pedal pulses.	indicate phlebitis and thrombus formation.

SAFETY ALERT Homans' sign is not always present when a deep vein thrombosis (DVT) exists (Schick and Windle, 2010). If you suspect a thrombus, notify surgeon and refrain from manipulating extremity any further. Surgery will usually be postponed. Antiembolism stockings or pneumatic compression cuffs may be ordered for patients at risk for thrombus formation.

STEP	RATIONALE
6 Assess patient's ability to move independently while in bed.	Patients confined to bed rest, even for limited periods, will need to turn regularly.
7 Assess patient's willingness and capability to learn exercises.	Capacity to learn depends on readiness, ability, and learning environment.

SAFETY ALERT Highly anxious patients or those in severe pain have difficulty learning and performing postoperative exercises.

STEP	RATIONALE
8 Teach diaphragmatic breathing:	
a Help patient to comfortable sitting or standing position. If patient chooses to sit, raise head of bed to semi-Fowler's or Fowler's position, and help to side of bed or to upright position in chair. If patient is sitting in a chair, knees should be at or higher than hips. Use stool if necessary.	Upright position facilitates diaphragmatic excursion by using gravity to keep abdominal contents away from diaphragm. Prevents tension on abdominal muscles, which allows for greater diaphragmatic excursion. Diaphragmatic breathing allows for complete lung expansion and improved ventilation and increases blood oxygenation. Deep breathing also allows air to pass by partially obstructing mucous plugs, thus increasing force with which to expel plug. Coughing loosens secretions and helps to remove them from pulmonary alveoli and bronchi.

STEP	RATIONALE
b Stand or sit facing patient.	Patient will be able to observe breathing exercises performed by nurse.
c Instruct patient to place palms of hands across from each other along lower borders of anterior rib cage; place tips of third fingers lightly together (Fig. 57-1). Demonstrate for patient.	Position of hands allows patient to feel movement of chest and abdomen as diaphragm descends and lungs expand inside chest wall.
d Have patient take slow, deep breaths, inhaling through nose and pushing abdomen against hands. Explain that patient will feel normal downward movement of diaphragm during inspiration. Demonstrate for patient.	Slow, deep breaths allow for more complete lung expansion and prevent panting or hyperventilation. Inhaling through nose warms, humidifies, and filters air. Explanation and demonstration focus on normal ventilatory movement of chest. Patient learns to understand how diaphragmatic breathing feels.
e Have patient avoid using chest and shoulder muscles while inhaling.	Using auxiliary chest and shoulder muscles during breathing increases unnecessary energy expenditures and does not promote full lung expansion.
f Take slow, deep breath and hold for count of 3; slowly exhale through mouth as if blowing out a candle (pursed lips).	Allows for gradual, controlled expulsion of air.
g Repeat breathing exercise three to five times.	Allows patient to observe slow, rhythmic breathing pattern.
h Have patient practice exercise. Instruct him or her to take 10 slow, deep breaths every hour while awake during postoperative period until	Repetition of exercise reinforces learning. Regular deep breathing will prevent or minimize postoperative respiratory complications. Incentive spirometer gives a

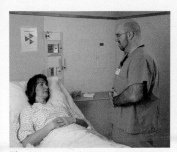

Fig. 57-1 Patient and nurse practice deep breathing.

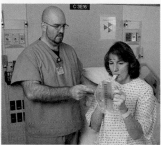

Fig. 57-2 Patient demonstrates incentive spirometry.

STEP	RATIONALE
mobile. Another option is to have patient use incentive spirometry (Fig. 57-2).	visual incentive to breathe as deeply as possible.
9 Teach positive expiratory pressure therapy (PEP) and "huff" coughing:	
a Perform hand hygiene. Set PEP device for setting ordered.	Higher settings require more effort.
b Instruct patient to assume semi-Fowler's or high-Fowler's position, and place nose clip on patient's nose.	Promotes optimum lung expansion and expectoration of mucus.
c Have patient place lips around mouthpiece. Instruct him or her to take a full breath and exhale two or three times longer than inhalation. Repeat pattern for 10 to 20 breaths.	Ensures that patient does all breathing through mouth. Ensures that patient uses device properly.
d Remove device from mouth and have patient take slow, deep breath and hold for 3 seconds.	Promotes lung expansion before coughing.

STEP	RATIONALE
e Instruct patient to exhale in quick, short, forced "huffs."	"Huff" coughing, or forced expiratory technique, promotes bronchial hygiene by increasing expectoration of secretions.
10 Teach controlled coughing:	
a Explain importance of maintaining an upright position.	Position facilitates diaphragm excursion and enhances thorax and abdominal expansion.
b Demonstrate coughing. Take two slow, deep breaths, inhaling through nose and exhaling through (pursed lips) mouth.	Deep breaths expand lungs fully so that air moves behind mucus and facilitates effective coughing.
c Inhale deeply a third time, and hold breath to count of 3. Cough fully for two to three consecutive coughs without inhaling between coughs. (Tell patient to push all air out of lungs.)	Consecutive coughs help remove mucus more effectively and completely than one forceful cough.

SAFETY ALERT Coughing may be contraindicated after brain, spinal, or eye surgery because of an increase in intracranial pressure.

d Caution patient against just clearing throat instead of coughing deeply.	Clearing throat does not remove mucus from deeper airways.
e If a thoracic or abdominal surgical incision was made, teach patient to place either hands or pillow over incisional area and position hands over pillow to splint incision (Fig. 57-3). During breathing and coughing exercises, press gently against incisional area for splinting and support.	Surgical incision cuts through muscles, tissues, and nerve endings. Deep-breathing and coughing exercises place additional stress on suture line and cause discomfort. Splinting incision with hands or pillow provides firm support and reduces incisional pulling and pain.

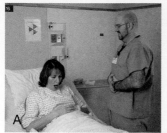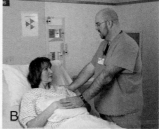

Fig. 57-3 Techniques for splinting incision when coughing or moving.

STEP	RATIONALE
f Patient continues to practice coughing exercises, splinting imaginary incision. Instruct the patient to cough two to three times every hour while awake.	Deep coughing with splinting effectively expectorates mucus with minimal discomfort.
g Instruct patient to examine sputum for consistency, odor, amount, and color changes and to notify nurse if any changes are noted.	Sputum consistency, odor, amount, and color changes indicate the presence of a pulmonary complication such as pneumonia.

SAFETY ALERT For patients with preexisting pulmonary disease, know usual character of mucus to determine if change has occurred.

11 Teach turning (example describes turning to right side):	
a Instruct patient to assume supine position and move toward left side of the bed. He or she can do this by bending knees and pressing heels against mattress to raise and move buttocks.	Positioning begins in this example on left side of bed so that turning to right side will not cause patient to roll off edge of bed. Buttocks lift prevents shearing force from body moving against sheets.

STEP	RATIONALE
b Instruct patient to place right hand or pillow over incisional area to splint it (see Fig. 57-3).	Splinting incision supports and minimizes pulling on suture line during turning.
c Instruct patient to keep right leg straight and flex left knee up.	Straight leg stabilizes the patient's position. Flexed left leg shifts weight for easier turning.
d Have patient grab right side rail with left hand while pulling toward right, and rolling onto right side.	Pulling toward side rail reduces effort needed for turning.
e Instruct patient to turn every 2 hours from side to back to other side while awake. If patient is unable to perform this maneuver, note in chart that staff or primary caregiver must turn patient every 2 hours. You will need to place pillows behind some patients to help maintain side-lying position.	Reduces risk for vascular complications by contraction of leg muscles around veins to improve venous return. Also reduces pulmonary complications by shifting mucus to prevent consolidation.
12 Teach leg exercises:	
a Have patient assume supine position in bed. Demonstrate leg exercises by performing passive range-of-motion exercises and simultaneously explaining exercise.	Provides for normal anatomical position of lower extremities and normal joint motion of each joint of lower extremities.

SAFETY ALERT If patient's surgery involves one or both lower extremities, surgeon must order leg exercises in postoperative period. You can safely exercise leg unaffected by surgery unless patient has preexisting phlebothrombosis (blood clot formation) or thrombophlebitis (inflammation of vein wall).

STEP	RATIONALE
b Rotate each ankle in one direction and then in the other direction. Instruct patient to draw imaginary circles with big toe. Repeat five times.	Ankle circle exercises maintain joint mobility and promote venous return.
c Alternate dorsiflexion and plantar flexion by moving both feet, pointing toes up toward head and then down toward end of mattress. Direct patient to feel calf muscles contract and relax alternately. Repeat five times.	Calf pumping stretches and contracts gastrocnemius muscles, which enhances venous return.
d Perform quadriceps setting by tightening thigh and bringing knee down toward mattress, then relaxing. Repeat five times.	Quadriceps-setting exercises contract muscles of upper legs, maintain knee mobility, and improve venous return to the heart.
e Patient alternately raises each leg from bed surface; patient begins by keeping leg straight and then bends leg at hip and knee. Repeat five times.	Leg raise promotes contraction and relaxation of quadriceps muscles and promotes hip and knee movements by keeping leg straight and bending hip and knee joints.
f Have patient continue to practice exercises at least every 2 hours while awake. Patient is instructed to coordinate turning and leg exercises with diaphragmatic breathing, incentive spirometry, and coughing exercises.	Repetition of exercise sequence reinforces learning. Establishes routine for exercises that develops habit for performance. Sequence of exercises is leg exercises, turning, deep breathing, and coughing. Exercises before coughing enhance ability to move secretions so that they may be expectorated.

STEP	RATIONALE
13 Observe patient performing all exercises independently.	Provides opportunity for practice and return demonstration of exercises. Ensures patient has learned correct technique.
14 Evaluate patient's chest excursion.	Determines extent of lung expansion.
15 Auscultate patient's lungs.	Breath sounds reveal if airways are clear.
16 Gently palpate calves for redness, warmth, and tenderness. Assess pedal pulses.	Absent signs and normal pulses usually indicate that no venous thrombosis is present.
17 Complete postprocedure protocol.	

Recording and Reporting

- Record physical assessment findings in narrative notes or flow sheet.
- Report and record any assessed complications and action taken.
- Record in nurses' notes and electronic health record (EHR) the exercises you have demonstrated to patient and whether or not patient can perform them independently.
- Report to appropriate nurse on next shift any problems that patient has in practicing exercises.

UNEXPECTED OUTCOMES	RELATED INTERVENTIONS
1 Patient is unwilling to perform deep breathing, coughing, turning, or leg exercises because of incisional pain of thorax, abdomen, groin, buttocks, or legs.	• Offer patient pain medication 30 minutes before or have patient use patient-controlled analgesia immediately before performing postoperative exercises.
2 Patient is unable to perform exercises correctly. Anxiety and fatigue alter patient's performance.	• Repeat teaching with more demonstrations. • Patient may benefit from stress-reduction techniques. • Assess for presence of anxiety, pain, and fatigue.

UNEXPECTED OUTCOMES	RELATED INTERVENTIONS
3 Patient develops pulmonary complications such as atelectasis after surgery. Breaths are shallow; cough is ineffective.	• Notify surgeon of findings. • Start oxygen as ordered, and increase frequency of coughing exercises. • Assess breath sounds in all lobes. • Place patient in upright position.
4 Patient develops circulatory complications such as venous stasis or thrombophlebitis after surgery.	• Notify surgeon of findings. • Place patient on bed rest with affected leg elevated as ordered. • Continue to have patient do exercises with unaffected leg.

Pressure Bandages (Applying)

A pressure bandage is a temporary treatment to control excessive, sudden, unanticipated bleeding. Hemorrhage may occur during surgical intervention (e.g., cardiac catheterization, arterial puncture, organ biopsy) or after surgery or be a life-threatening occurrence related to accidental trauma (e.g., stabbing, suicide attempt). Pressure dressings are essential to stopping the flow of blood and promoting clotting at the site until definitive action can be taken to stop the source.

Given the emergent nature of an acute bleeding episode, the aseptic techniques considered essential in most dressing applications are secondary to halting the bleeding. A pressure dressing applied in an emergency is usually temporary; the wound can be cleaned and the dressing changed once the bleeding has been controlled.

Delegation and Collaboration

The skill of applying a pressure dressing in an emergency situation cannot be delegated to nursing assistive personnel (NAP). If application requires more than one person, the NAP can assist. The nurse directs the NAP to:

- Observe the pressure dressing during care activities to make sure that it remains in place and that there is no visible bleeding from the site.
- Observe underneath the patient for bleeding after the dressing has been applied.

Equipment

- Necessary dressings: fine-mesh gauze, abdominal (ABD) pads, hemostatic dressings, roller gauze
- Adhesive tape; hypoallergenic if necessary
- Adhesive remover (optional)
- Clean gloves
- Protective gown, goggles, mask (used when spray from wound is a risk)
- Equipment for vital signs

Implementation

STEP	RATIONALE
Phase I: Immediate action—first nurse	
1 Identify external bleeding site. Look underneath patients with large abdominal dressings. NOTE: Wounds to groin area also can result in large amounts of blood loss, which is not always visible.	Quick identification increases response time to stop bleeding. Maintaining asepsis and privacy is considered only if time and severity of blood loss permit.
2 Apply immediate manual pressure to bleeding site.	Hemostasis is maintained while supplies are prepared.
3 Seek assistance.	Bandage must be secured quickly.
Phase II: Applying pressure bandage—second nurse	
4 Quickly identify source of bleeding.	Determines method of application and which supplies to use.
• *Arterial bleeding* is bright red and flows in waves, related to heart rate; if vessel is very deep, flow is steady.	
• *Venous bleeding* is dark red and flows smoothly.	
• *Capillary bleeding* is oozing of dark red blood; self-sealing controls this bleeding.	
5 Elevate affected body part (e.g., extremity) if possible.	Helps slow rate of hemorrhage.
6 First nurse continues to apply direct pressure as second nurse unwraps roller bandage and places within easy reach. Second nurse quickly cuts three to five lengths of adhesive tape and places them within reach; *do not cleanse wound.*	Pressure dressing controls bleeding temporarily. Preparation allows for quick securement of pressure bandage.

STEP	RATIONALE
7 In simultaneous coordinated actions:	
a Rapidly cover bleeding area with multiple thicknesses of gauze compresses. First nurse slips fingers out as other nurse exerts adequate pressure to continue control of bleeding.	Gauze is absorbent. Layers provide bulk against which local pressure can be applied to the bleeding site.
b Place adhesive strips 7 to 10 cm (3 to 4 inches) beyond width of dressing with even pressure on both sides of fingers as close as possible to central bleeding source. Secure tape on distal end, pull tape across dressing, and keep firm pressure as proximate end of tape is secured.	Tape exerts downward pressure, promoting hemostasis. To ensure blood flow to distal tissues and prevent tourniquet effect, adhesive tape must not be continued around entire extremity.
c Remove fingers temporarily and quickly cover center of area with third strip of tape.	Provides pressure to source of bleeding.
d Continue reinforcing area with tape as each successive strip is overlapped on alternating sides of center strip. Keep applying pressure.	Prevents tape from loosening.
e When pressure bandage is on extremity, apply roller gauze: apply two circular turns tautly on both sides of fingers that are pressing gauze. Compress over bleeding site.	Roller gauze acts as pressure bandage, exerting more even pressure over extremity.

STEP	RATIONALE
Simultaneously remove finger pressure and apply roller gauze over center. Continue with figure-eight turns. Secure end with two circular turns and strip of adhesive.	

SAFETY ALERT Apply pressure bandage in a distal to proximal direction, working toward the heart.

STEP	RATIONALE
8 Observe dressing for control of bleeding.	Effective pressure bandage controls bleeding without blocking distal circulation.
9 Evaluate adequacy of circulation (distal pulse rate, skin characteristics).	Determines level of perfusion to distal body parts.
10 Complete postprocedure protocol.	

Recording and Reporting

- Report immediately to health care provider present status of patient's bleeding control, time bleeding was discovered, estimated blood loss, nursing interventions (including effectiveness of applied pressure bandage), apical and distal pulse rates, blood pressure measurements, mental status, signs of restlessness, and need for health care provider to administer to patient without delay.
- Record interventions taken and patient's response in progress notes and vital signs flow sheet.

UNEXPECTED OUTCOMES	RELATED INTERVENTIONS
1 There is continued bleeding. Fluid and electrolyte imbalance, tissue hypoxia, confusion, hypovolemic shock, and cardiac arrest develop.	• Notify health care provider. • Reinforce or adjust pressure dressing. • Initiate intravenous (IV) therapy per order. • Place patient in Trendelenburg's position. • Provide covers for warmth.

Continued

UNEXPECTED OUTCOMES	RELATED INTERVENTIONS
2 Pressure dressing is too tight and occludes circulation.	• Monitor vital signs every 5 to 15 minutes (apical pulse, distal pulses, and blood pressure). • Inspect areas distal to pressure dressing to ensure that circulation has not been occluded. • Adjust dressing as needed. • Notify health care provider.

Pressure Ulcer Risk Assessment

The goal in preventing the development of pressure ulcers is early identification of an at-risk patient and the implementation of prevention strategies. The overall management goals suggested by the Wound, Ostomy and Continence Nurses Society (WOCN, 2010) include the following:

1. Identify individuals at risk for developing pressure ulcers and initiate an early prevention program.
2. Implement appropriate strategies/plans to:
   a. Attain/maintain intact skin.
   b. Prevent complications.
   c. Promptly identify or manage complications.
   d. Involve patient and caregiver in self-management.
3. Implement cost-effective strategies/plans that prevent and treat pressure ulcers. The WOCN 2010 panel recommends performing a risk assessment on entry to a health care setting and repeating this on a regularly scheduled basis or when there is a significant change in an individual's condition. Use risk assessment tools such as the Braden Scale or the Norton Scale (WOCN, 2010).
4. Inspect the patient's skin and bony prominences at least daily. Remove devices, shoes, socks, antiembolic stockings, and heel and elbow protectors for the skin inspection. Inspect all bony prominences, including back of head, shoulders, rib cage, elbows, hips, ischium, sacrum, coccyx, knees, ankles, and heels (Fig. 59-1). Palpate any reddened or discolored areas with a gloved finger to determine if the erythema (redness of the skin caused by dilation and congestion of the capillaries) blanches (lightens in color).

Delegation Considerations

The skill of pressure ulcer risk assessment cannot be delegated to nursing assistive personnel (NAP). The nurse instructs the NAP to:

- Report any redness or break in the patient's skin.
- Report any abrasion from assistive devices.

Equipment

- Risk assessment tool
- Documentation record

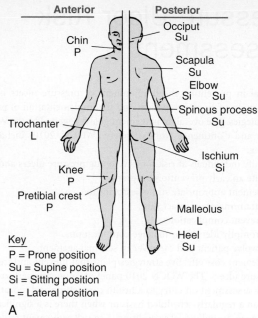

Fig. 59-1 **A,** Bony prominences most frequently underlying pressure sores.

- Pressure-redistribution mattress, bed, and/or chair cushion
- Positioning aids
- Gloves

Implementation

STEP	RATIONALE
1 Complete preprocedure protocol.	
2 Assess patient's risk for pressure ulcer formation:	Determines need to administer preventive care and identifies specific factors placing patient at risk (NPUAP and EPUAP, 2009).
a Paralysis or immobilization caused by restrictive devices	Patient is unable to turn or reposition independently to relieve pressure.

Pressure ulcer sites

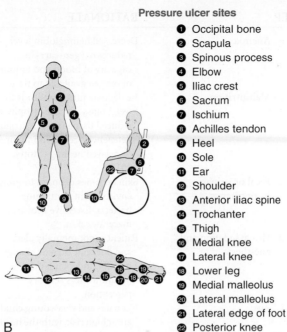

❶ Occipital bone
❷ Scapula
❸ Spinous process
❹ Elbow
❺ Iliac crest
❻ Sacrum
❼ Ischium
❽ Achilles tendon
❾ Heel
❿ Sole
⓫ Ear
⓬ Shoulder
⓭ Anterior iliac spine
⓮ Trochanter
⓯ Thigh
⓰ Medial knee
⓱ Lateral knee
⓲ Lower leg
⓳ Medial malleolus
⓴ Lateral malleolus
㉑ Lateral edge of foot
㉒ Posterior knee

B

Fig. 59-1, cont'd **B,** Pressure ulcer sites. (From Trelease CC: Developing standards for wound care, *Ostomy Wound Manage* 26:50, 1988. Used with permission of HMP Communications.)

STEP	RATIONALE
b Sensory loss (e.g., hemiplegia, spinal cord injury)	Patient is unable to feel discomfort from pressure and does not independently change position.
c Circulatory disorders (e.g., peripheral vascular diseases, vascular changes from diabetes mellitus, neuropathy)	Reduces perfusion of tissue layers of skin.
d Fever	Increases metabolic demands of tissues. Accompanying diaphoresis leaves skin moist.

STEP	RATIONALE
e Anemia	Decreased hemoglobin level reduces oxygen-carrying capacity of blood and amount of oxygen available to tissues.
f Malnutrition	Inadequate nutrition leads to weight loss, muscle atrophy, and reduced tissue mass. Nutrient deficiencies result in impaired or delayed healing (Stotts, 2012).
g Fecal or urinary incontinence	Skin becomes exposed to moist environment containing bacteria. Excessive moisture macerates skin.
h Heavy sedation and anesthesia	Patient is not mentally alert and does not turn or change position independently. Sedation alters sensory perception.
i Age	Neonates and very young children are at high risk, with the head being the most common site of pressure ulcer occurrence (WOCN, 2010). There is a loss of dermal thickness in older adults, impairing the ability to distribute pressure (Pieper, 2012).
j Dehydration	Results in decreased skin elasticity and turgor.
k Edema	Edematous tissues are less tolerant of pressure, friction, and shear.
l Existing pressure ulcers	Limit surfaces available for position changes, placing available tissues at increased risk.
m History of pressure ulcer	Tensile strength of skin from previously healed pressure ulcer is 80% or less; therefore this area cannot tolerate pressure

STEP	RATIONALE
	as well as undamaged skin (Doughty and Sparks-Defriese, 2012).
3 Select an agency-approved risk assessment tool such as the Braden Scale or Norton Scale. Perform risk assessment when patient enters health care setting and repeat on regularly scheduled basis or when there is a significant change in patient's condition (WOCN, 2010).	Valid and reliable risk assessment tools evaluate patient's risk for developing a pressure ulcer. Identifying risk factors that contribute to the potential for skin breakdown allows you to target specific interventions for decreasing risk for skin breakdown.
4 Assess condition of patient's skin over regions of pressure (see Fig. 59-1).	Body weight against bony prominences places underlying skin at risk for breakdown.
a Inspect for skin discoloration (redness in light-tone skin; purplish or bluish in darkly pigmented skin) and tissue consistency (firm or boggy feel), and/or palpate for abnormal sensations (Nix, 2012).	Indicates that tissue was under pressure; hyperemia is a normal physiological response to hypoxemia in tissues.
b Palpate discolored area, release your fingertip, and look for blanching.	If on palpation an area of redness blanches (lightens in color), this indicates normal reactive hyperemia. The tissue is not at risk for skin breakdown. Tissue that does not blanch when palpated indicates abnormal reactive hyperemia, an indication of possible ischemic injury.
c Inspect for pallor and mottling.	Indicates persistent hypoxia in tissues that were under pressure, which is an abnormal physiological response.

STEP	RATIONALE
d Inspect for absence of superficial skin layers.	Represents early pressure ulcer formation, usually a partial-thickness wound that may have resulted from friction and/or shear.
e Inspect for localized heat, edema, or induration, especially in individual with darkly pigmented skin (NPUAP and EPUAP, 2009).	Localized heat, edema, and induration have been identified as warning signs for pressure ulcer development. Because it is not always possible to see signs of redness on darkly pigmented skin (Box 59-1), these additional signs should be considered during the assessment (NPUAP and EPUAP, 2009).
5 Assess patient for additional areas of potential pressure.	Patients at high risk have multiple sites for pressure necrosis (tissue death), in addition to bony prominences.
a Nares: nasogastric (NG) tube, oxygen cannula	
b Tongue and lips: oral airway, endotracheal (ET) tube	
c Ears: oxygen cannula, pillow	
d Drainage tubes or other tubing	Stress against tissue at exit site or if tubing is caught under any part of the body.
e Wound drainage	Wound drainage is caustic to skin and underlying tissues, thereby increasing risk for skin breakdown.
f Indwelling urethral (Foley) catheter	For female patients, the catheter can put pressure on the labia, especially when edematous. For male patients, pressure from a catheter not properly anchored can put pressure on the tip of the penis and urethra.

BOX 59-1 Patient-Centered Care for Skin Assessment of Pressure Ulcers: Patients With Darkly Pigmented Skin

---

Patients with darkly pigmented skin cannot be assessed for pressure ulcer risk by examining only skin color. Teaching points and unique considerations include the following:

1. Assess localized skin color changes. Any of the following may appear:
   - Color remains unchanged when pressure is applied.
   - Color changes that differ from patient's usual skin color occur at site of pressure ulcer.
   - If patient previously had a pressure ulcer, that area of skin may be lighter than original color.
   - Localized area of skin may be purple/blue or violet instead of red.
2. Importance of lighting for skin assessment:
   - Use natural or halogen light.
   - If possible, avoid fluorescent lamps, which can give the skin a bluish tone.
   - Avoid wearing tinted lenses when assessing skin color.
3. Tissue consistency:
   - Edema may occur with induration of more than 15 mm in diameter and may appear taut and shiny.
   - Assess for edema, swelling, and a firm or boggy feel.
4. Skin temperature:
   - Localized heat can be detected by making comparisons with the surrounding skin. An area of coolness may be a sign of tissue devitalization.

STEP	RATIONALE
g Orthopedic and positioning devices	Improperly fitted or applied devices have the potential to cause pressure on adjacent skin and underlying tissue.
6 Observe patient for preferred positions when in bed or chair.	Preferred positions result in weight of body being placed on certain bony prominences. Presence of contractures may result in pressure exerted in unexpected places.

STEP	RATIONALE
7 Observe ability of patient to initiate and help with position changes.	Potential for friction and shear increases when patient is completely dependent on others for position changes.
8 Assess patient and caregiver understanding of risks for the development of pressure ulcers.	Determines baseline knowledge for pressure ulcer risk and identifies areas for patient teaching.
9 Implement prevention guidelines adapted from WOCN Society: *Guideline for Prevention and Management of Pressure Ulcers* (2010).	Reduces patient's risk of developing a pressure ulcer.
10 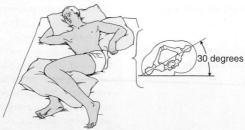 If patient has open, draining wounds, apply clean gloves.	Use of Standard Precautions prevents accidental exposure to body fluids.
11 If immobility, inactivity, or poor sensory perception is a risk factor for patient, consider one of the following interventions:	Immobility and inactivity reduce patient's ability or desire to independently change position. Poor sensory perception decreases patient's ability to feel the sensation of pressure or discomfort.
a Reposition patient at least every 2 hours; use a written schedule (WOCN, 2010).	Reduces the duration and intensity of pressure. Some patients may require more frequent repositioning.
b When patient is in the side-lying position in bed, use the 30-degree lateral position (Fig. 59-2).	Reduces direct contact of the trochanter with the support surface.

30 degrees

Fig. 59-2 Thirty-degree lateral position.

STEP	RATIONALE
c When necessary, use pillow bridging.	Use of pillows prevents direct contact between bony prominences.
d Place patient (when lying in bed) on a pressure-redistribution surface.	Reduces amount of pressure exerted on tissues.
e Place patient (when in a chair) on a pressure-redistribution device and shift the points under pressure at least every hour (WOCN, 2010).	Reduces the amount of pressure on the sacral and ischial areas.
12 If friction and shear are identified as risk factors, consider the following interventions:	Friction and shear damage underlying skin.
a Use two nurses and a pull sheet to reposition patient. Use a slide board to transfer patient from bed to stretcher.	Proper repositioning of patient prevents dragging along the sheets. Slide board provides slippery surface to reduce friction.
b Ensure that heels are free from the surface of the bed by using a pillow under the calves to elevate the heels.	"Floating" the heels from the bed surface eliminates shear and friction.
c Maintain the head of the bed at 30 degrees.	Decreases potential for patient to slide toward foot of bed and incur a shear injury.
13 If patient receives a low score on a moisture subscale, consider one of the following interventions:	Continual exposure of body fluids on the patient's skin increases the risk for skin breakdown and pressure ulcer development.
a Apply clean gloves. Apply a moisture barrier ointment to perineum and surrounding skin after each incontinent episode.	Protects the skin from fecal or urinary incontinence.

STEP	RATIONALE
b If skin is denuded, use a protective barrier paste after each incontinent episode.	Provides a barrier between the skin and the stool/urine, allowing for healing.
c If moisture source is from wound drainage, consider frequent dressing changes and/or skin protection with protective barriers or collection devices.	Removes the frequent exposure of wound drainage from the skin.
14 Educate patient and family caregiver regarding pressure ulcer risk and prevention (WOCN, 2010).	
15 Complete postprocedure protocol.	

Recording and Reporting

- Record any skin changes, patient's risk score, and skin assessment. Describe positions, turning intervals, pressure-redistribution devices, and other prevention measures. Note patient's response to the interventions.
- Report need for additional consultations for the high-risk patient to health care provider.

UNEXPECTED OUTCOMES	RELATED INTERVENTIONS
1 Skin becomes mottled, reddened, purplish, or bluish.	• Refer patient to wound, ostomy, and continence (WOC) nurse; dietitian; clinical nurse specialist (CNS); and/or physical therapist as necessary. Reevaluate position changes and bed surface.
2 Areas under pressure develop persistent discoloration, induration, or temperature changes.	• Refer patient to WOC nurse, dietitian, CNS, and/or physical therapist as necessary. • Modify patient's positioning and turning schedule.

Pressure Ulcer Treatment

The principles of managing patients with pressure ulcers include systematic support of patients, reduction or elimination of the cause of skin breakdown, and management of the wound that provides an environment conducive to healing. Once you find the cause of the pressure ulcer, take steps to control or eliminate it. Next assess the patient's wound-healing abilities.

The principle that guides the selection and use of topical dressings is to provide a wound environment that supports healing (Rolstad, Bryant, and Nix, 2012). The best environment for wound healing is moist and free of necrotic tissue and infection. Choose interventions and dressings designed to support a clean, moist wound bed. Perform a thorough assessment of the wound and the periwound skin before initiating wound therapy.

Choose wound dressings to meet the characteristics of the wound bed (Rolstad et al., 2012). The choice of a wound dressing depends on the type of wound tissue in the base of the wound, the amount of wound drainage, the presence or absence of infection, the location of the wound, the size of the wound, the ease of use and cost-effectiveness of the dressing, and the comfort of the patient.

Delegation Considerations

The skill of treatment of pressure ulcers and dressing changes cannot be delegated to the nursing assistive personnel (NAP). The nurse instructs the NAP to:

- Report any wound drainage that might be on linens or intact skin, indicating the need to change the dressing or use an alternative dressing.
- Report any new areas of redness, blistering, or skin irritation.

Equipment

- Protective equipment: clean gloves, goggles, cover gown (if splash is a risk)
- Sterile gloves *(optional)*
- Plastic bag for dressing disposal
- Measuring device
- Sterile cotton-tipped applicators (check agency policy for use of sterile applicators)

- Topical agent (as ordered)
- Cleansing agent (as ordered)
- Sterile solution container
- Dressing of choice based on wound characteristics
- Hypoallergenic tape (if needed)
- Documentation records

Implementation

STEP	RATIONALE
1 Complete preprocedure protocol.	
2 Assess patient's level of comfort on a pain scale of 0 to 10. If patient is in pain, determine if a prn pain medication has been ordered and administer.	Dressing change should not be a traumatic event for patient; evaluate wound pain before, during, and after wound care management (Hopf et al., 2012).
3 Determine if patient has allergies to topical agents or latex.	Topical agents could contain elements that cause localized skin reactions.
4 Review the order for topical agent(s) and/or dressings.	Ensures administration of proper medication and treatment.

SAFETY ALERT Determine if the order is consistent with established wound care guidelines and outcomes for a patient. If the order is not consistent with guidelines or varies from the identified outcome for a patient, review it with the health care team.

STEP	RATIONALE
5 Perform hand hygiene and apply clean gloves. Position patient to allow dressing removal, and position plastic bag for dressing disposal.	Provides an accessible area for dressing change. Proper disposal of old dressing promotes proper handling of contaminated waste.
6 Assess patient's wounds using wound parameters, and continue ongoing wound assessment per agency policy. NOTE: This may be done during procedure after dressing removal.	Determines effectiveness of wound care and guides the treatment plan of care (WOCN, 2010).

STEP	RATIONALE
a *Wound location:* Describe the body site where the wound is located.	
b *Stage of wound:* Describe the extent of tissue destruction.	Staging is a way of assessing a pressure ulcer based on depth of tissue destruction. Wounds are documented as unstageable if the wound base is not visible (NPUAP and EPUAP, 2009).
c *Wound size:* Length, width, and depth of the wound are measured per agency protocol. Use a disposable measuring guide for length and width. Use a cotton-tipped applicator to assess depth (Fig. 60-1).	Ulcer size changes as healing progresses; therefore the longest and widest areas of the wound change over time. Measuring the width and length by measuring consistent areas provides a consistent measurement (Nix, 2012).
d *Presence of undermining, sinus tracts, or tunnels:* Use a sterile cotton-tipped applicator to measure depth and, if needed, a gloved finger to examine the wound edges.	Wound depth determines amount of tissue loss.

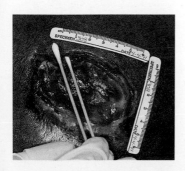

Fig. 60-1 Measuring depth of undermining of skin.

STEP	RATIONALE
e *Condition of wound bed:* Describe the type and percentage of tissue in the wound bed.	The approximate percentage of each type of tissue in the wound provides critical information on the progress of wound healing and the choice of dressing. A wound with a high percentage of black tissue requires debridement, yellow tissue or slough tissue may indicate the presence of an infection or colonization, and granulation tissue indicates that a wound is moving toward healing.
f *Volume of exudate:* Describe the amount, characteristics, odor, and color.	Amount and type of exudate may indicate type and frequency of dressing changes.
g *Condition of periwound skin:* Examine the skin for breaks, dryness, and the presence of a rash, swelling, redness, or warmth. Modify assessment based on patient's skin color.	Impaired skin condition at the edge of an ulcer indicates progressive tissue damage. Maceration on periwound skin shows a need to alter the choice of wound dressing.
h *Wound edges:* Gives information regarding epithelialization, chronicity, and etiology.	
7 Prepare the following necessary equipment and supplies:	
a Normal saline or other wound-cleansing agent in sterile solution container.	Cleans ulcer surface before applying topical agents and a new dressing.
b Prescribed topical agent:	
(1) Enzyme debriding agents (Follow specific manufacturer's	Enzymes debride dead tissue to clean ulcer surface. Enzymes are not applied to healthy tissue.

STEP	RATIONALE
directions for frequency of application.) **OR**	
(2) Topical antibiotics.	Topical antibiotics are used to decrease bioburden of wound and should be considered for use if no healing is noted after 2 to 4 weeks of optimal care (WOCN, 2010).
c Select an appropriate dressing based on pressure ulcer characteristics, principles of wound management, and patient care setting. Dressings options include:	The dressing should maintain a moist environment for the wound while keeping the surrounding skin dry (AHCPR, 1994).
(1) Gauze. Apply as a moist dressing, as a dry cover dressing when using enzymes or topical antibiotics, or as a means to deliver solution to a wound.	Gauze delivers moisture to a wound and is absorptive.

SAFETY ALERT Make sure that the absorbency of the dressing is adequate for the amount of wound drainage. Check that wound does not dry out and that surrounding skin does not become macerated.

(2) Transparent film dressing. Apply over superficial ulcers with minimal or no exudate and skin subjected to friction.	Maintains a moist environment and offers intact skin protection.

STEP	RATIONALE

SAFETY ALERT Use transparent dressings for autolytic debridement of noninfected pressure ulcers.

STEP	RATIONALE
(3) Hydrocolloid dressing.	Maintains moist environment to facilitate wound healing while protecting the wound base.
(4) Hydrogel. Available in a sheet or in tube.	Maintains moist environment to facilitate wound healing.
(5) Calcium alginate.	Highly absorbent of wound exudate in heavily draining wounds.
(6) Foam dressings.	Protective and prevent wound dehydration; also absorb moderate to large amounts of drainage.
(7) Silver-impregnated dressings/gels.	Control bacterial burden in wound.
(8) Wound fillers.	Fill shallow wounds, hydrate, and absorb.
d Obtain hypoallergenic tape or adhesive dressing sheet.	Used to secure nonadherent dressing. Prevents skin irritation and tearing.
8 ⚡ Assemble needed supplies at bedside. Close room door or bedside curtains. Perform hand hygiene, and apply clean gloves. Open sterile packages and topical solution containers. Wear goggles, mask, and moisture-proof cover gown if potential for contamination from spray exists when cleansing the wound.	Maintains patient privacy. Reduces transmission of microorganisms.
9 Remove bed linen, and arrange patient's gown to expose ulcer and surrounding skin. Keep remaining body parts draped.	Prevents unnecessary exposure of body parts.

STEP	RATIONALE
10 Remove old dressing and discard in appropriate receptacle.	With each dressing change, note progress of wound healing.
11 Perform hand hygiene, and change gloves.	Maintains aseptic technique during cleansing, measuring, and application of dressings. Refer to institutional policy regarding use of clean or sterile gloves.
12 Clean wound thoroughly with normal saline or prescribed wound-cleansing agent from least contaminated to most contaminated area.	Cleansing wound removes wound exudates and/or dressing residue and reduces surface bacteria.
13 Apply topical agents to wound using cotton-tipped applicators or gauze as ordered:	
a Enzymes	Follow manufacturer's directions for method and frequency of application. Be aware of which solutions inactivate enzymes, and avoid their use in wound cleansing.
(1) Apply a small amount of enzyme debridement ointment directly to necrotic areas in pressure ulcer. Do not apply enzyme to surrounding skin.	Proper distribution of ointment ensures effective action.
(2) Position moist gauze dressing directly over ulcer, and tape in place. Follow specific manufacturer's recommendation for type of dressing	Protects wound and prevents removal of ointment during turning or repositioning.

STEP	RATIONALE
material to use to cover a pressure ulcer when using enzymes.	
b **Antibacterials**	Reduce bacterial growth.
Examples include bacitracin, metronidazole, and silver sulfadiazine.	
14 Apply prescribed wound dressing:	
a **Hydrogel**	
(1) Cover surface of ulcer with a thick layer of amorphous hydrogel, or cut a sheet to fit wound base.	Provides a moist environment to facilitate wound healing.
(2) Apply secondary dressing such as dry gauze; tape in place.	Holds hydrogel against wound surface because amorphous hydrogel (in tube or sheet form) does not adhere to the wound base and requires a secondary dressing to hold it in place.
(3) If using impregnated gauze, pack loosely into wound; cover with secondary gauze dressing and tape.	A loosely packed dressing delivers the gel to the wound base and allows any wound debris to be trapped in the gauze.
b **Calcium alginate**	Use in heavily draining wounds.
(1) Lightly pack wound with alginate using sterile cotton-tipped applicator or gloved finger.	The dressing swells and increases in size; tight packing can compromise blood flow to the tissues.
(2) Apply a secondary dressing, and tape in place.	Holds alginate against wound surface.
c **Transparent film dressing; hydrocolloid; and foam dressings (see Skill 19)**	

STEP	RATIONALE
15 Reposition patient comfortably off pressure ulcer.	Prevents pressure to ulcer.
16 Observe skin surrounding ulcer for inflammation, edema, and tenderness.	Determines progress of wound healing.
17 Inspect dressings and exposed ulcers, observing for drainage, foul odor, and tissue necrosis. Monitor patient for signs and symptoms of infection: fever and elevated white blood cell (WBC) count.	Ulcers can become infected.
18 Compare subsequent ulcer measurements, using one of the scales designed to measure wound healing, such as the PUSH Tool or the BWAT Assessment.	Provides a standard method of data collection that demonstrates wound progress or deterioration.
19 Complete postprocedure protocol.	

Recording and Reporting

- Record type of wound tissue present in ulcer, ulcer measurements, periwound skin condition, character of drainage or exudate, type of topical agent used, dressing applied, and patient's response.
- Report any deterioration in ulcer appearance to nurse in charge or health care provider.

UNEXPECTED OUTCOMES	RELATED INTERVENTIONS
1 Skin surrounding ulcer becomes macerated.	• Reduce exposure of surrounding skin to topical agents and moisture. • Select a dressing that has increased moisture-absorbing capacity.
2 Ulcer becomes deeper with increased drainage and/or	• Review current wound care management.

Continued

UNEXPECTED OUTCOMES	RELATED INTERVENTIONS
development of necrotic tissue.	• Consult with multidisciplinary team regarding changes in wound care regimen.
	• Obtain wound cultures.
3 Pressure ulcer extends beyond original margins.	• Monitor for systemic signs and symptoms of poor wound healing, such as abnormal laboratory results (WBC count, hemoglobin/hematocrit levels, serum albumin and serum prealbumin levels, amount of total proteins), weight loss, and fluid imbalances.
	• Assess and revise current turning schedule.
	• Consider further pressure-redistribution devices.

Pulse Oximetry

Pulse oximetry is the noninvasive measurement of arterial blood oxygen saturation, the percent to which hemoglobin is filled with oxygen. A pulse oximeter is a probe with a light-emitting diode (LED) connected by cable to an oximeter. The more hemoglobin saturated by oxygen, the higher the oxygen saturation. Normally oxygen saturation (SpO_2) is greater than 95%. The measurement of oxygen saturation is simple and painless, and has few of the risks associated with more invasive measurements of oxygen saturation such as arterial blood gas sampling. A vascular, pulsatile area is needed to detect the change in the transmitted light when making measurements with a digit or earlobe probe.

Delegation Considerations

The skill of oxygen saturation measurement can be delegated to nursing assistive personnel (NAP). The nurse instructs the NAP by:

- Communicating specific factors related to the patient that can falsely lower oxygen saturation.
- Informing NAP about appropriate sensor site and probe.
- Advising NAP of frequency of oxygen saturation measurements for specific patient.
- Advising NAP to notify nurse immediately of any SpO_2 reading lower than 95% or a predetermined value for a specific patient.
- Requesting NAP refrain from using pulse oximetry to obtain heart rate because oximeter will not detect an irregular pulse rate.

Equipment

- Oximeter
- Oximeter probe appropriate for patient and recommended by oximeter manufacturer
- Acetone or nail polish remover if needed
- Pen and vital sign flow sheet or electronic health record (EHR)

Implementation

STEP	RATIONALE
1 Complete preprocedure protocol.	
2 Assess for signs and symptoms of alterations in oxygen saturation	Physical signs and symptoms indicate abnormal oxygen saturation.

STEP	RATIONALE
(e.g., altered respiratory rate, depth, or rhythm; adventitious breath sounds; cyanotic nails, lips, mucous membranes, or skin; restlessness; difficulty breathing).	
3 Assess for factors that influence measurement of SpO_2 (e.g., oxygen therapy, respiratory therapy such as postural drainage and percussion, hemoglobin level, hypotension, temperature, nail polish [Cicek et al., 2011], and medications such as bronchodilators).	Allows nurse to assess oxygen saturation variations accurately. Peripheral vasoconstriction related to hypothermia can interfere with SpO_2 determination.
4 Determine most appropriate patient-specific site (e.g., finger, earlobe, bridge of nose, forehead) for sensor probe placement by measuring capillary refill time. If capillary refill time is less than 2 seconds, select alternative site.	Changes in SpO_2 level are reflected in the circulation of finger capillary beds within 30 seconds and in the capillary beds of earlobes within 5 to 10 seconds.
a Site must have adequate local circulation and be free of moisture.	Finger and earlobe sensors require pulsating vascular bed to identify hemoglobin molecules that absorb emitted light. Forehead sensor detects saturation in low perfusion conditions. Moisture impedes ability of sensor to detect SpO_2 levels.
b A finger free of nail polish or acrylic is preferred (Cicek et al., 2011).	Research on the influence of nail polish is contradictory. Brown and blue nail polish can falsely

STEP	RATIONALE
	lower SpO$_2$ values, but findings are not clinically significant (Rodden et al., 2007).
c If patient has tremors or is likely to move, use earlobe or forehead.	Detection of motion by the sensor probe creates false waves, or motion artifact, which is the most common cause of inaccurate readings (Giuliano and Liu, 2006).
d If patient's finger is too large for the clip-on probe, as may be the case with obesity or edema, the clip-on probe may not fit properly (Mininni et al., 2009); obtain a disposable (tape-on) probe.	
5 Bring equipment to the bedside and perform hand hygiene.	
6 Attach sensor to monitoring site. If using finger, remove fingernail polish from digit with acetone or polish remover. Instruct patient that clip-on probe will feel like a clothespin on the finger but will not hurt.	Select sensor site based on peripheral circulation and extremity temperature. Peripheral vasoconstriction alters SpO$_2$ reading. Pressure of sensor's spring tension on a finger or earlobe is sometimes uncomfortable.

SAFETY ALERT Do not attach probe to finger, ear, or bridge of nose if area is edematous or skin integrity is compromised. Do not use earlobe and bridge of nose sensors for infants and toddlers because of skin fragility. Do not attach sensors to fingers that are hypothermic. Select ear or bridge of nose if adult patient has a history of peripheral vascular disease. Do not use disposable adhesive sensors if patient has a latex allergy. Do not place sensors on same extremity as electronic blood pressure cuff because blood flow to finger will be temporarily interrupted when cuff inflates and cause inaccurate reading that can trigger alarms (Skirton et al., 2011).

STEP	RATIONALE
7 Once sensor is in place, turn on oximeter by activating power. Observe pulse waveform/intensity display and audible beep. Correlate oximeter pulse rate with patient's radial pulse rate.	Pulse waveform/intensity display enables detection of valid pulse or presence of interfering signal. Pitch of audible beep is proportional to SpO_2 value. Double-checking pulse rate ensures oximeter accuracy.
8 Leave sensor in place 10 to 30 seconds or until oximeter readout reaches constant value and pulse display reaches full strength during each cardiac cycle. Inform patient that oximeter alarm will sound if sensor falls off or patient moves it. Read SpO_2 value on digital display.	Reading usually takes 10 to 30 seconds, depending on site selected.
9 If you plan to monitor oxygen saturation continuously, verify SpO_2 alarm limits preset by the manufacturer at a low of 85% and a high of 100%. Determine limits for SpO_2 value and pulse rate as indicated by patient's condition. Verify that alarms are activated. Assess skin integrity under sensor probe every 2 hours; relocate sensor at least every 4 hours and more frequently if skin integrity is altered or tissue perfusion compromised.	Alarms must be set at appropriate limits and volumes to avoid frightening patients and visitors. Spring tension of sensor or sensitivity to disposable sensor adhesive causes skin irritation and leads to disruption of skin integrity.
10 If you plan on intermittent or spot-checking of SpO_2 values, remove probe, and turn oximeter power off. Cleanse sensor and store sensor in appropriate location.	Batteries will die if oximeter is left on. Sensors are expensive and vulnerable to damage.

STEP	RATIONALE
11 Discuss findings with patient. Perform hand hygiene.	
12 Compare SpO$_2$ reading with patient's previous baseline and acceptable SpO$_2$ values.	Allows nurse to assess for change in patient's condition and presence of respiratory alteration.
13 Complete postprocedure protocol.	

Recording and Reporting

- Record SpO$_2$ value on vital sign flow sheet, EHR, or nurses' notes; indicate type and amount of oxygen therapy used by patient during assessment.
- Record any signs and symptoms of alterations in oxygen saturation in narrative form in nurses' notes and EHR.
- Report abnormal findings to nurse in charge or health care provider.

UNEXPECTED OUTCOMES	RELATED INTERVENTIONS
1 SpO$_2$ is less than 90%.	• Verify that oximeter probe is intact and that outside light is not influencing probe. Reposition probe if needed.
	• Assess for signs and symptoms of decreased oxygenation, including anxiety, restlessness, tachycardia, and cyanosis.
	• Verify that supplemental oxygen is delivered as ordered and is functioning properly.
	• Minimize factors that decrease SpO$_2$ value, such as lung secretions, increased activity, and hyperthermia.
	• Implement measures to reduce energy consumption.

Continued

UNEXPECTED OUTCOMES	RELATED INTERVENTIONS
2 Pulse waveform/intensity display is dampened or irregular.	• Assist patient to a position that maximizes ventilatory effort; for example, place an obese patient in a high-Fowler's position. • Locate different peripheral vascular bed, and reposition pulse oximeter probe. • Use another sensor if available. • Protect sensor from room light by covering sensor site with opaque covering or washcloth.

Rectal Suppository Insertion

Rectal medications exert either local effects on gastrointestinal (GI) mucosa (e.g., promoting defecation) or systemic effects (e.g., relieving nausea or providing analgesia). The rectal route is not as reliable as the oral and parenteral routes in terms of drug absorption and distribution. However, the medications are relatively safe because they rarely cause local irritation or side effects. Rectal medications are contraindicated in patients with recent surgery on the rectum, bowel, or prostate gland; rectal bleeding or prolapse; and very low platelet counts (Lilley et al., 2011).

Rectal suppositories are thinner and more bullet-shaped than vaginal suppositories. The rounded end prevents anal trauma during insertion. When you administer a rectal suppository, placing it past the internal anal sphincter and against the rectal mucosa is important. Improper placement can result in expulsion of the suppository before the medication dissolves and is absorbed into the mucosa. If a patient prefers to self-administer a suppository, give specific instructions so the medication is deposited correctly. Do not cut the suppository into sections to divide the dosage; the active drug may not be distributed evenly within the suppository, and the result may be an inaccurate dose (Lilley et al., 2011).

Delegation Considerations

The skill of rectal medication administration cannot be delegated to nursing assistive personnel (NAP). The nurse directs the NAP about:

- Reporting expected fecal discharge or bowel movement to the nurse.
- Potential side effects of medications and to report their occurrence to the nurse.
- Informing the nurse of any rectal discharge, pain, or bleeding.

Equipment

- Rectal suppository
- Water-soluble lubricating jelly
- Clean gloves
- Tissue
- Drape
- Medication administration record (MAR) (electronic or printed)

Implementation

STEP	RATIONALE
1 Complete preprocedure protocol.	
2 Check accuracy and completeness of each medication administration record (MAR) with health care provider's medication order. Check patient's name, drug name and dosage, route, and time for administration. Clarify incomplete or unclear orders with health care provider before administration.	The health care provider's order is the most reliable source and only legal record of drugs that the patient is to receive. Ensures that patient receives correct medication. Handwritten MARs are a source of medication errors (ISMP, 2010; Jones and Treiber, 2010).
3 Review patient's medical history for history of rectal surgery or bleeding, cardiac problems, history of allergies, and medication history.	Certain conditions and medications contraindicate use of suppository.
4 Assess patient's ability to hold suppository and to position self to insert medication.	Mobility restriction indicates need for nurse to help with drug administration.
5 Review patient's knowledge of purpose of drug therapy and interest in self-administering suppository.	Indicates need for health teaching. Level of motivation influences teaching approach.
6 Prepare suppository for administration. Check label of medication against MAR 2 times. Check expiration date on container.	*These are the first and second checks for accuracy.* Process ensures that right patient receives right medication.
7 Identify patient using two identifiers (e.g., name and birthday or name and account number) according	Ensures correct patient. Complies with The Joint Commission requirements for patient safety (TJC, 2014).

STEP	RATIONALE
to agency policy. Compare identifiers with information on patient's MAR or medical record.	Some agencies are now using a bar-code system to help with patient identification.
8 At patient's bedside, again compare MAR or computer printout with names of medications on medication labels and patient name. Ask patient if he or she has allergies.	*This is the third check for accuracy* and ensures that patient receives correct medication. Confirms patient's allergy history.
9 Perform hand hygiene, arrange supplies at bedside, and apply clean gloves. Close room curtain or door.	Reduces transfer of microorganisms. Maintains privacy and minimizes embarrassment.
10 Help patient assume a left side-lying Sims' position with upper leg flexed upward.	Position exposes anus and relaxes external anal sphincter. Left side-lying Sims' position lessens likelihood of the suppository or feces being expelled.
11 If patient has mobility impairment, help into lateral position. Obtain assistance to turn patient, and use pillows under patient's upper arm and leg.	
12 Keep patient draped with only anal area exposed.	Maintains privacy and facilitates relaxation.
13 Examine condition of anus externally. *Option:* Palpate rectal walls as needed (e.g., if impaction is suspected). Dispose of gloves by turning them inside out and placing them in proper receptacle if they become soiled.	Determines presence of active rectal bleeding. Palpation determines whether rectum is filled with feces, which interferes with suppository placement. Reduces transmission of infection.
14 Apply new pair of clean gloves (if previous gloves were soiled and discarded).	Minimizes contact with fecal material to reduce transmission of microorganisms.

STEP	RATIONALE
15 Remove suppository from foil wrapper, and lubricate rounded end with water-soluble lubricant. Lubricate gloved index finger of dominant hand. If patient has hemorrhoids, use liberal amount of lubricant, and touch area gently.	Lubrication reduces friction as suppository enters rectal canal (Fig. 62-1).
16 Ask patient to take slow, deep breaths through mouth and to relax anal sphincter.	Forcing suppository through constricted sphincter causes pain.
17 Retract patient's buttocks with nondominant hand. With gloved index finger of dominant hand, insert suppository gently through anus, past internal sphincter, and against rectal wall, 10 cm (4 inches) in adults (Fig. 62-2) or 5 cm (2 inches) in infants and children. You should feel rectal sphincter close around your finger.	Suppository needs to be against rectal mucosa for eventual absorption and therapeutic action.

SAFETY ALERT Do not insert suppository into a mass of fecal material; this reduce effectiveness of medication.

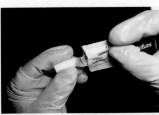

Fig. 62-1 Lubricate tip of suppository.

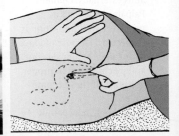

Fig. 62-2 Insert rectal suppository past sphincter and against rectal wall.

STEP	RATIONALE
18 *Option:* A suppository may be given through a colostomy (not ileostomy) if ordered. Patient should lie supine. Use small amount of water-soluble lubricant for insertion.	
19 Withdraw finger, and wipe patient's anal area.	Provides comfort.
20 Ask patient to remain flat or on side for 5 minutes.	Prevents expulsion of suppository.
21 Discard gloves by turning them inside out, and dispose of them and used supplies in appropriate receptacle. Perform hand hygiene.	Reduces transfer of microorganisms.
22 If suppository contains laxative or fecal softener, place call light within reach so patient can obtain assistance to reach bedpan or toilet.	Ability to call for assistance provides patient with sense of control over elimination.
23 If the suppository was given for constipation, remind the patient *not* to flush the commode after the bowel movement.	Allows staff to evaluate results of the suppository.
24 Perform postprocedure protocol.	
25 Return within 5 minutes to determine if suppository was expelled.	Determines if drug is properly distributed. Reinsertion may be necessary.
26 Evaluate patient for relief of symptoms for which medication was prescribed (within time expected action of drug occurs).	Determines medication's effectiveness.

Recording and Reporting

- Record the drug, dosage, route, and actual time and date of administration on MAR immediately after administration, not before. Include initials or signature. Record patient teaching and validation of understanding and self-administration of suppository in nurses' notes.
- Report adverse effects, patient response, and/or withheld drugs to nurse in charge or health care provider.

UNEXPECTED OUTCOMES	RELATED INTERVENTIONS
1 Patient's symptoms are unrelieved.	• Explore alternative therapy.
2 Patient experiences decreased heart rate during rectal suppository insertion.	• Unintended vagal stimulation may occur, resulting in bradycardia in some patients.
	• Monitor heart rate of patient. Rectal route may not be suitable for certain cardiac conditions.
3 Patient reports rectal pain during insertion.	• Suppository may need more lubrication.
	• Rectal route may not be suitable; assess and notify prescriber.
4 Patient is unable to explain purpose of drug therapy.	• Reinstruction is necessary, or patient is unwilling or unable to learn.

Respiration Assessment

You assess ventilation by observing the rate, depth, and rhythm of respiratory movements. Accurate assessment of respiration depends on recognizing normal thoracic and abdominal movements. Normal breathing is both active and passive. On inspiration, the diaphragm contracts, and the abdominal organs move down to increase the size of the chest cavity. At the same time the ribs and sternum lift outward to promote lung expansion. On expiration, the diaphragm relaxes upward, and the ribs and sternum return to their relaxed position. Expiration is an active process only during exercise, with voluntary hyperventilation, and in the presence of certain disease states.

Delegation Considerations

The skill of counting respirations can be delegated to nursing assistive personnel (NAP) unless the patient is considered unstable (i.e., complains of dyspnea). The nurse instructs the NAP by:

- Communicating the frequency of measurement and factors related to patient history or risk for increased or decreased respiratory rate or irregular respirations.
- Reviewing any unusual respiratory values or significant changes to report to the nurse.

Equipment

- Wristwatch with second hand or digital display
- Pen and vital sign flow sheet or electronic health record (EHR)

Implementation

STEP	RATIONALE
1 Complete preprocedure protocol.	
2 Assess for signs and symptoms of respiratory alterations such as the following: • Bluish or cyanotic appearance of nail beds, lips, mucous membranes, and skin	Physical signs and symptoms indicate alterations in respiratory status related to ventilation.

STEP	RATIONALE
• Restlessness, irritability, confusion, reduced level of consciousness • Pain during inspiration • Labored or difficult breathing • Orthopnea • Use of accessory muscles • Adventitious breath sounds • Inability to breathe spontaneously • Thick, frothy, blood-tinged, or copious sputum production	
3 Assess for factors that influence character of respirations:	Allows you to anticipate factors that influence respirations.
a Exercise	Respirations increase in rate and depth to meet the need for additional oxygen and rid the body of carbon dioxide.
b Anxiety	Anxiety causes increase in respiration rate and depth because of sympathetic nervous system stimulation.
c Acute pain	Pain alters rate and rhythm of respirations; breathing becomes shallow. Patient inhibits or splints chest wall movement when pain is in area of chest or abdomen.
d Smoking	Chronic smoking changes pulmonary airways, resulting in an increased respiratory rate at rest when not smoking.
e Medications	Narcotic analgesics, general anesthetics, and sedative hypnotics depress rate and depth; amphetamines and

STEP	RATIONALE
	cocaine increase rate and depth; bronchodilators cause dilation of airways, which ultimately slows respiratory rate.
f Body position	Standing or sitting erect promotes full ventilator movement and lung expansion; stooped or slumped posture impairs ventilator movement; lying flat prevents full chest expansion.
g Neurological injury	Damage to the brainstem impairs the respiratory center and inhibits rate and rhythm.
h Hemoglobin function	Decreased hemoglobin levels lower amount of oxygen carried in blood, which results in increased respiratory rate to increase oxygen delivery.
4 Assess pertinent laboratory values:	
a *Arterial blood gases (ABGs):* normal ranges are (values vary slightly among agencies): (1) pH, 7.35 to 7.45 (2) $PaCO_2$, 35 to 45 mm Hg (3) HCO_3, 22 to 28 mEq/L (4) PaO_2, 80 to 100 mm Hg (5) SaO_2, 95% to 100%	ABG values measure arterial blood pH, partial pressures of oxygen and carbon dioxide, and arterial oxygen saturation, which reflect patient's oxygenation status.
b *Pulse oximetry (SpO_2):* normal SpO_2 ≥95% to 100%; 90% is a red flag; anything less indicates hypoxemia (Valdez-Lowe et al., 2009).	SpO_2 less than 85% is often accompanied by changes in respiratory rate, depth, and rhythm.

STEP	RATIONALE
c *Complete blood count (CBC):* normal CBC for adults (values vary within agencies): • Hemoglobin: 14 to 18 g/100 mL, males; 12 to 16 g/100 mL, females • Hematocrit: 42% to 52%, males; 37% to 47%, females • Red blood cell count: 4.7 to 6.1 million/mm^3, males; 4.2 to 5.4 million/mm^3, females	CBC measures red blood cell count; volume of red blood cells; and concentration of hemoglobin, which reflects patient's capacity to carry oxygen.
5 If patient has been active, wait 5 to 10 minutes before assessing respirations.	Exercise increases respiratory rate and depth. Assessing respirations while patient is at rest allows for objective comparison of values.
6 Assess respirations after pulse measurement in adult.	Inconspicuous assessment of respirations immediately after pulse assessment prevents patient from consciously or unintentionally altering rate and depth of breathing.

Safety Alert Assess patients with difficulty breathing (dyspnea), such as those with heart failure, with abdominal ascites, or in late stages of pregnancy, in the position of greatest comfort. Repositioning may increase the work of breathing, which will increase respiratory rate.

7 Place patient's arm in relaxed position across abdomen or lower chest, or place nurse's hand directly over patient's upper abdomen.	A similar position used during pulse assessment allows respiratory rate assessment to be inconspicuous. Patient's or nurse's hand rises and falls during respiratory cycle.
8 Observe complete respiratory cycle (one inspiration and one expiration).	Rate is accurately determined only after nurse has viewed complete respiratory cycle.

STEP	RATIONALE
9 If rhythm is regular, count number of respirations in 30 seconds and multiply by 2. If rhythm is irregular, less than 12, or greater than 20, count for 1 full minute.	Respiratory rate is equivalent to number of respirations per minute. Suspected irregularities require assessment for at least 1 minute.
10 Note depth of respirations, by observing degree of chest wall movement while counting rate. In addition, assess depth by palpating chest wall excursion or auscultating the posterior thorax after you have counted rate. Describe depth as shallow, normal, or deep.	Character of ventilatory movement reveals specific disease states restricting the volume of air from moving into and out of the lungs.
11 Note rhythm of ventilatory cycle. Normal breathing is regular and uninterrupted. Do not confuse sighing with abnormal rhythm.	Character of ventilations shows specific types of alterations. Periodically, people unconsciously take single deep breaths or sighs to expand small airways prone to collapse.
12 If assessing respirations for the first time, establish rate, rhythm, and depth as baseline if within acceptable range.	Used to compare future respiratory assessment.
13 Compare respirations with patient's previous baseline and usual rate, rhythm, and depth.	Allows nurse to assess for changes in patient's condition and for presence of respiratory alterations.
14 Complete postprocedure protocol.	

Recording and Reporting

- Record respiratory rate on vital sign flow sheet, nurses' notes, or electronic health record (EHR).
- Record abnormal depth and rhythm in appropriate area in nurses' notes and EHR.
- Document measurement of respiratory rate after administration of specific therapies in nurses' notes and EHR.

- Record type and amount of oxygen therapy, if used, in nurses' notes and EHR.
- Report abnormal findings to nurse in charge or health care provider.

UNEXPECTED OUTCOMES	RELATED INTERVENTIONS
1 Patient's respiratory rate is less than 12 breaths/min (bradypnea) or greater than 20 breaths/min (tachypnea). Breathing pattern is sometimes irregular. Depth of respirations increased or decreased. Patient complains of feeling short of breath.	• Assess for related factors, including obstructed airway, abnormal breath sounds, productive cough, restlessness, anxiety, and confusion. • Assist patient to supported sitting position (semi- or high-Fowler's) unless contraindicated. • Provide oxygen as ordered. • Assess for environmental factors that influence patient's respiratory rate such as secondhand smoke, poor ventilation, or gas fumes. • Notify health care provider or nurse in charge if alteration continues.
2 Patient demonstrates Kussmaul's, Cheyne-Stokes, or Biot's respirations.	• Notify health care provider for additional evaluation and possible medical intervention.

Restraint Application

A physical restraint is any manual method, physical or mechanical device, material, or equipment that immobilizes or reduces the ability of a patient to move his or her extremities, body, or head freely (CMS, 2008). Physical or chemical restraints should be the last resort and used only when reasonable alternatives fail. The use of physical restraints is no longer a safe strategy, yet many nurses still believe that restraints are needed to control behavioral symptoms and prevent falls in older adults with dementia (Evans and Cotter, 2008).

The CMS (2008) requires that a restraint be used only under the following circumstances: (1) to ensure the immediate physical safety of the patient, a staff member, or others; (2) when less restrictive interventions have been ineffective; (3) in accordance with a written modification to the patient's plan of care; (4) when it is the least restrictive intervention that will be effective to protect the patient, staff member, or others from harm; (5) in accordance with safe and appropriate restraint techniques as determined by hospital policies; and (6) restraint use should be discontinued at the earliest possible time.

The use of restraints is associated with serious complications, including pressure ulcers, hypostatic pneumonia, constipation, incontinence, and death. Most patient deaths in the past have resulted from strangulation from a vest or jacket restraint. Numerous agencies no longer use vest restraints. For these reasons this text does not describe their use.

Delegation Considerations

The skills of assessing a patient's behavior and level of orientation, the need for restraints, the appropriate restraint type, and the ongoing assessments required while a restraint is in place cannot be delegated to nursing assistive personnel (NAP). Applying and routinely checking a restraint can be delegated to NAP. The Joint Commission (2009) requires first aid training for anyone who monitors patients in restraints. The nurse directs the NAP by:

- Reviewing correct placement of the restraint and how to routinely check the patient's circulation, skin condition, and breathing.
- Reviewing when and how to change a patient's position and provide range-of-motion (ROM) exercises, toileting, and skin care.
- Instructing NAP to notify the nurse immediately if there is a change in level of patient agitation, skin integrity, circulation of extremities, or patient's breathing.

Equipment

- Proper restraint (e.g., belt, wrist, mitten)
- Padding (if needed)

Implementation

STEP	RATIONALE
1 Complete preprocedure protocol.	
2 Assess patient's behavior (e.g., confusion, disorientation, agitation, restlessness, combativeness, repeated removal of tubing or other therapeutic devices, and inability to follow directions).	If patient's behavior continues despite treatment or restraint alternatives, use of restraint is indicated.
3 Follow agency policies regarding restraints. Check health care provider's order for purpose, type, location, and time or duration of restraint. Determine if signed consent for use of restraint is necessary.	In acute care settings a licensed health care provider who is responsible for care of patient must order least restrictive type of restraint. Each original restraint order is limited to 4 hours for adults 18 years of age and older, 2 hours for children ages 9 through 17, and 1 hour for children younger than age 9 (TJC, 2009). Original orders may be renewed up to a maximum of 24 hours (CMS, 2008).
4 Review manufacturer's instructions for correct restraint application and determine most appropriate size restraint.	You need to be familiar with all devices used for patient care and protection. Incorrect application of restraint device can result in patient injury or death.
5 Inspect areas where restraint is to be placed. Note if there is any nearby tubing or devices. Assess condition of	Provides baseline to monitor patient's response to restraint. Provides baseline data to monitor patient's skin integrity.

STEP	RATIONALE
skin, sensation, adequacy of circulation, and ROM.	
6 Identify patient using two identifiers (e.g., name and birthday or name and account number) according to agency policy. Compare identifiers with information on patient's medication administration record (MAR) or medical record.	Ensures correct patient. Complies with The Joint Commission requirements for patient safety (TJC, 2014).
7 Provide privacy. Explain to patient and family purpose of restraint. Be sure patient is comfortable and in correct anatomical position.	May promote cooperation. Positioning prevents contractures and neurovascular impairment.
8 Pad skin and bony prominences (as necessary) that will be covered by restraint.	Reduces friction and pressure from restraint to skin and underlying tissue.
9 Apply proper size restraint: *Follow manufacturer's directions.*	
a *Belt restraint:* Have patient in a sitting position. Apply belt over clothes, gown, or pajamas. Make sure to place restraint at waist, not the chest or abdomen. Remove wrinkles or creases in clothing. Bring ties through slots in belt. Help patient lie down if in bed. Avoid applying the belt too tightly (Fig. 64-1).	Restrains center of gravity and prevents patient from rolling off stretcher, from sitting up while on stretcher, or from falling out of bed. Tight application or misplacement can interfere with ventilation. This type of restraint may be contraindicated in patient who had abdominal surgery.

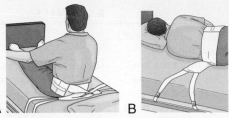

Fig. 64-1 Roll belt restraint tied to the bed frame and to an area that does not cause the restraint to tighten when the bed frame is raised or lowered. (*A* and *B* from Sorrentino SA: *Mosby's textbook for nursing assistants,* ed 7, St Louis, 2008, Mosby.)

STEP	RATIONALE
b *Extremity (ankle or wrist) restraint:* Commercially available limb restraints are composed of sheepskin with foam padding. Wrap limb restraint around wrist or ankle with soft part toward skin and secured snugly (not tightly) in place by Velcro straps. Insert two fingers under secured restraint (Fig. 64-2).	Restraint immobilizes one or all extremities to protect patient from fall or accidental removal of therapeutic device (e.g., intravenous [IV] tube, Foley catheter). Tight application will interfere with circulation and cause neurovascular injury.

SAFETY ALERT Patient with extremity restraints is at risk for aspiration if placed in supine position. Place patient in lateral position rather than supine.

c *Mitten restraint:* Thumbless mitten device restrains patient's hands. Place hand in mitten, being sure Velcro strap(s) is (are) around the wrist and not the forearm (Fig. 64-3).	Prevents patients from dislodging invasive equipment, removing dressings, or scratching yet allows greater movement than a wrist restraint.

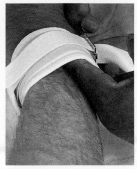

Fig. 64-2 Securing an extremity restraint. (Provided courtesy Posey Co., Arcadia, CA.)

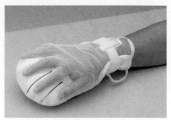

Fig. 64-3 Mitten restraint. (Provided courtesy Posey Co., Arcadia, CA.)

STEP	RATIONALE
d *Elbow restraint (freedom splint):* Restraint consists of rigidly padded fabric that wraps around arm and is closed with Velcro. Upper end has a clamp that hooks to patient's gown sleeve. Insert patient's arm so elbow joint rests against padded area, keeping joint rigid.	Commonly used with infants and children to prevent elbow flexion (e.g., when IV line is placed in antecubital fossa). May also be used for adults.
10 Attach restraint straps to portion of bed frame that moves when raising or lowering head of bed. Be sure that straps are secure. **Do not attach to side rails.** Restraints can be attached to frame of chair or wheelchair as long as ties are out of patient's reach.	Patient will be injured if restraint is secured to side rail and side rail is lowered.

STEP	RATIONALE
11 Secure restraints with a quick-release tie (Fig. 64-4), buckle, or adjustable seat belt–like locking device. *Do not tie in a knot.*	Allows for quick release in an emergency.
12 Double check and insert two fingers under secured restraint.	Checking for constriction prevents neurovascular injury.
13 Remove restraints at least every 2 hours (TJC, 2014) or according to agency policy, and assess patient each time. If patient is violent or noncompliant, remove one restraint at a time and/ or have staff assist while removing restraints.	Removal provides opportunity to change patient's position, offer nutrients, perform full ROM, toilet, and exercise patient.

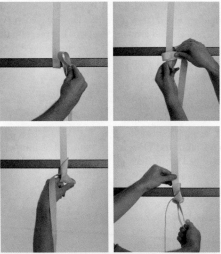

Fig. 64-4 The Posey quick-release tie. (Provided courtesy Posey Co., Arcadia, CA.)

STEP	RATIONALE
14 Secure call light or intercom system within reach.	Allows patient, family, or caregiver to obtain assistance quickly.
15 Leave bed or chair with wheels locked. Keep bed in lowest position.	Locked wheels prevent bed or chair from moving if patient tries to get out. Placing bed in lowest position reduces chance of injury if patient falls out of bed.
16 Complete postprocedure protocol.	

Recording and Reporting

- Record patient's behavior before and after restraints were applied, level of orientation, and patient's or family member's statement of understanding of purpose of restraint and consent (when required).
- Record restraint alternatives tried and patient's response in nurses' notes and electronic health record (EHR).
- Record reason for restraint, the type and location, the time applied, the time removed, and the routine observations made every 15 minutes (e.g., skin color, pulses, sensation, vital signs, behavior) in the nurses' notes and EHR and flow sheets.

UNEXPECTED OUTCOMES	RELATED INTERVENTIONS
1 Patient experiences impaired skin integrity.	• Reassess need for continued use of restraint and determine if you can use alternative measures. If restraint is necessary to protect patient or others from injury, ensure that you applied restraint correctly and provide adequate padding.
	• Check skin under restraint for abrasions, and remove restraints more frequently.
	• Institute appropriate skin/wound care.

Continued

UNEXPECTED OUTCOMES	RELATED INTERVENTIONS
	• Change wet or soiled restraints to prevent skin breakdown.
2 Patient has altered neurovascular status of an extremity (e.g., cyanosis, pallor, and coldness of skin) or complaints of tingling, pain, or numbness.	• Remove restraint immediately, and notify health care provider.
3 Patient exhibits increased confusion, disorientation, and agitation.	• Evaluate cause for altered behavior, and attempt to eliminate cause. • Provide appropriate sensory stimulation, reorient as needed, attempt restraint alternatives, and involve family.
4 Patient releases restraint and suffers a fall or other traumatic injury.	• Attend to patient's immediate physical needs, inform health care provider of fall or injury, and reassess type of restraint and its correct application.

Restraint-Free Environment

Patients at risk for falls or wandering present special safety challenges when trying to create a restraint-free environment. Wandering is the meandering, aimless, or repetitive locomotion that exposes a patient to harm and is often in conflict with boundaries, limits, or obstacles (NANDA International, 2012). This is a common problem in patients who are confused or disoriented. Interrupting a wandering patient can increase distress. The Department of Veterans Affairs has suggestions for managing wandering, most of which are environmental adaptations. Some of these include hobbies, social interaction, regular exercise, and circular design of a care unit (VA NCPS, 2010). Environmental modifications are effective alternatives to restraints. More frequent observation of patients, involvement of family during visitation, and frequent reorientation are also helpful measures. *There are many alternatives to the use of restraints. Use these alternatives before applying restraints.*

Delegation Considerations

The skills of assessing patient behaviors and orientation to the environment and determining the type of restraint-free interventions to use cannot be delegated to nursing assistive personnel (NAP). However, actions for promoting a safe environment can be delegated to NAP. The nurse instructs the NAP about:

- Using specific diversional or activity measures for making the environment safe.
- Applying appropriate alarm devices.
- Reporting patient behaviors and actions (e.g., confusion, getting out of bed unassisted, combativeness) to the nurse.

Equipment

- Visual or auditory stimuli (e.g., calendar, clock, radio, television, pictures)
- Diversional activities (e.g., puzzles, games, audio books, DVDs)
- Wedge cushion
- Wrap-around belt (Fig. 65-1)
- AmbuAlarm or pressure-sensitive bed or chair alarm
- Bed enclosure system

Fig. 65-1 Wrap-around belt.
(Courtesy Posey Co., Arcadia, CA.)

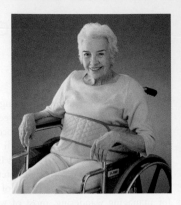

Implementation

STEP	RATIONALE
1 Complete preprocedure protocol.	
2 Assess patient's behavior (e.g., orientation, ability to understand and follow directions, combative behaviors, restlessness, agitation), balance, gait, vision, hearing, bowel/ bladder routine, level of pain, electrolyte and blood count values, and presence of orthostatic hypotension.	Accurate assessment identifies patients with safety risks and the physiological causes for patient behaviors that prompt caregivers to use restraints. Ensures proper selection of nonrestraint interventions.
3 Review over-the-counter (OTC) and prescribed medications for interactions and untoward effects.	Medication interactions or side effects often contribute to falling or altered mental status.
4 Orient patient and family to surroundings and explain all treatments and procedures.	Promotes patient understanding and cooperation.
5 Assign same staff to care for patient as often as possible. Encourage family and friends to stay with patient. In some agencies, volunteers are effective companions.	Increases familiarity with individuals in patient's environment, decreasing anxiety and restlessness. Companions are often helpful, preventing patient from being alone.

STEP	RATIONALE
6 Place patient in a room that is easily accessible to caregivers, close to nurses' station.	Allows for frequent observation to reduce falls in high-risk patients (VA NCPS, 2010).
7 Provide visual and auditory stimuli meaningful to patient (e.g., clock, calendar, radio/MP3 player [with patient's choice of music], television, and family pictures).	Orients patient to day, time, and physical surroundings. You must individualize stimuli for this to be effective.
8 Anticipate patient's basic needs (e.g., toileting, relief of pain, relief of hunger) as quickly as possible.	Provision of basic needs in a timely fashion decreases patient discomfort, anxiety, and restlessness.
9 Provide scheduled ambulation, chair activity, and toileting (e.g., ask patient every hour about toileting needs). Organize treatments so patient has uninterrupted periods throughout the day.	Regular opportunity to void avoids risk of patient trying to reach bathroom alone. Provides for sleep and rest periods. Constant activity overstimulates patients.
10 Position intravenous (IV) catheters, urinary catheters, and tubes/drains out of patient view. Use camouflage by wrapping IV site with bandage or stockinette.	Maintains medical treatment and reduces patient access to tubes/lines.
11 Use stress-reduction techniques, such as backrub, massage, and guided imagery.	Reduced stress allows patient energy to be channeled more appropriately.
12 Use diversional activities such as puzzles, games, music therapy, pet therapy, activity apron, or performance of purposeful activity (e.g., folding towels, drawing, coloring). Be sure that it is an activity in which	Meaningful diversional activities provide distraction, help to reduce boredom, and provide tactile stimulation. Minimize occurrences of wandering.

STEP	RATIONALE
patient has interest. Involve a family member in the activity.	
13 Use pressure-sensitive bed or chair pad with alarms:	Alarms alert staff to patient who is standing or rising without assistance.
a Explain use of device to patient and family.	
b When in the bed, position device so it is under the patient's mid-to-low back rather than under the buttocks.	Alarm activates sooner if placed under back. By the time buttocks are off the sensor, patient may be almost out of bed.
c Test alarm by applying and releasing pressure.	Ensures that alarm is audible through call-light system.
14 Use an AmbuAlarm monitoring device.	
a Explain use of device to patient and family.	Reinforces patient's risk for falling or wandering.
b Measure patient's thigh circumference just above knee to determine appropriate size.	Band that is too loose slips off; one that is too tight irritates skin or interferes with circulation.
c Test battery and alarm by touching snaps to corresponding snaps on leg band.	
d Apply leg band just above knee, and snap battery securely in place.	
e Instruct patient that alarm will sound unless he or she keeps leg in horizontal position.	
f Deactivate alarm to ambulate patient; unsnap device from leg band.	
15 Place patient in bed enclosure system.	Restraint alternative that allows patient freedom of movement within a protected environment.

STEP	RATIONALE
16 Determine need for continuation of invasive treatments and whether you can substitute less invasive treatment.	Eliminates cause and reason for restraint.
17 Complete postprocedure protocol.	

Recording and Reporting

- Record restraint alternatives attempted, patient's behaviors that relate to cognitive status, and interventions to mediate these behaviors in nurses' notes, electronic health record (EHR), and/or care plan.

UNEXPECTED OUTCOMES	RELATED INTERVENTIONS
1 Patient displays behaviors that increase risk for injury to self or others.	• Review episodes for a pattern (e.g., activity, time of day); can indicate alternatives that would eliminate behavior. • Discuss with all caregivers alternative interventions.
2 Patient sustains an injury or is out of control, placing others at risk for injury.	• Notify health care provider, and complete incident or occurrence report according to agency policy. • Identify alternative measures for safety or behavioral control. • Apply physical restraint only after all other interventions are unsuccessful.

Seizure Precautions

The two basic types of seizures are partial (simple and complex) and generalized. In a simple seizure a patient does not lose consciousness. In a partial complex seizure a patient loses consciousness. Generalized seizures affect the whole brain and cause both nonconvulsive and convulsive seizures. Status epilepticus, characterized by prolonged seizures lasting more than 10 minutes or a series of seizures that occur in rapid succession over 30 minutes, is a medical emergency (Eliahu et al., 2008).

Your role as a nurse is to protect patients who have a seizure disorder from harm. The most immediate risks from a generalized seizure are traumatic injury and choking, requiring you to protect the patient physically and assist with airway management as needed. A generalized seizure lasts from 1 to 2 minutes. A cry, loss of consciousness, tonicity (muscle rigidity), clonicity (rhythmic muscle jerking), and incontinence are all characteristics. Following the seizure there is a postictal phase, which lasts for up to an hour.

During a seizure perform interventions to keep the patient's airway open. Insert a bite block or an oral airway only when there is clear access for insertion, possibly after the seizure resolves and there is a need for airway support.

Delegation Considerations

The skill of assessing a patient on seizure precautions cannot be delegated to nursing assistive personnel (NAP). However, the skills for making a patient's environment safe can be delegated. The nurse directs NAP by:

- Explaining the patient's prior seizure history and factors that may trigger a seizure.
- Instructing to inform the registered nurse immediately when seizure activity develops.
- Explaining how to protect the patient in the event of a seizure.
- Emphasizing not to try to restrain the patient or place anything in the patient's mouth during a seizure.

Equipment

- Suction machine
- Oral airway
- Oral Yankauer suction catheter
- Oxygen via nasal cannula or face mask
- Stethoscope, sphygmomanometer, pulse oximeter

- Equipment for vital signs
- Equipment for intravenous access (0.9% saline)
- Emergency medications (e.g., IV diazepam, lorazepam, valproate [Depacon], phenytoin [Dilantin])
- Clean gloves

Implementation

STEP	RATIONALE
1 Complete preprocedure protocol.	
2 Assess patient's seizure history (e.g., new diagnosis, frequent seizures, seizure within last year) and knowledge of precipitating factors. Ask patient to describe frequency of past seizures, presence and type of aura (e.g., metallic taste, perception of breeze blowing on face, or noxious odor), and body parts affected if known. Use family as resource if necessary.	Knowledge about seizure history enables nurse to anticipate onset of seizure activity and take appropriate safety measures.
3 Assess for medical and surgical conditions, including history of head trauma, electrolyte disturbances (e.g., hypoglycemia, hyperkalemia), heart disease, excess fatigue, alcohol or caffeine consumption.	Common conditions that lead to seizures or worsen existing seizure condition.
4 Assess medication history (e.g., antidepressants and antipsychotics). Assess for patient's adherence to anticonvulsants and for therapeutic drug levels if test results are available.	If patient does not take seizure medications as prescribed and stops them suddenly, this often precipitates seizure activity.

STEP	RATIONALE
5 Inspect patient's environment for potential safety hazards (e.g., extra furniture) if seizure occurs.	Protects patient from injury sustained by striking head or body on furniture or equipment.
6 For patients with a history of seizures, keep bed in lowest position with side rails up (see agency policy). Pad rails if patient is at risk for head injury. Have oral suction and oxygen equipment ready for use.	Reduces risk of fall and injury. Equipment ensures prompt intervention directed toward maintaining a patent airway. Padded side rails are used only when patient is at risk for head injury (Clore, 2010; Lewis et al., 2011).
7 Patient with history of seizures should be in room close to nurses' station or room with video monitor.	Improves likelihood of quick response with emergency equipment.
8 Seizure response a Position patient safely. (1) If standing or sitting, guide patient to floor and protect head in your lap or place pillow under head. Turn patient onto side with head tilted slightly forward. Do not lift patient from floor to bed during seizure. (2) If patient is in bed, turn him or her onto side; raise side rails.	Position protects patient from aspiration and traumatic injury, especially head injury.
b Note time seizure began and call for help. Track duration of seizure. Have health care provider notified immediately. Have staff member bring emergency cart to bedside and clear surrounding area of furniture.	Reduces exposure to injury. Description of seizure may help in ultimate identification of type of seizure.

STEP	RATIONALE
c Keep patient in side-lying position, supporting head and keeping it flexed slightly forward.	Position prevents tongue from blocking airway and promotes drainage of secretions, reducing risk of aspiration.
d If possible, provide privacy. Have staff control flow of visitors in area.	Embarrassment is common after a seizure, especially if others witnessed it.
e Do not restrain patient; if patient is flailing limbs, hold them loosely. Loosen restrictive clothing/gown.	Prevents musculoskeletal injury. Promotes free ventilatory movement of chest and abdomen.
f *Never force any object, such as fingers, medicine, or tongue depressor, into patient's mouth* when teeth are clenched.	Prevents injury to mouth and possible aspiration.

SAFETY ALERT Injury can result from forcible insertion of a hard object into the mouth. Soft objects break and become aspirated. Insert a bite block or oral airway in advance if you recognize the possibility of a generalized seizure.

g Maintain patient's airway; suction orally as needed. Check patient's level of consciousness and oxygen saturation. Provide oxygen by nasal cannula or mask if ordered.	Prevents hypoxia during seizure activity.
h Observe sequence and timing of seizure activity. Note type of seizure activity (tonic, clonic, staring, blinking); whether more than one type of seizure occurs; sequence of seizure progression; level of consciousness; character of breathing; presence of incontinence; presence	Continued observation helps to document, diagnose, and treat seizure disorder.

STEP	RATIONALE
of autonomic nervous system signs such as lip smacking, mastication, grimacing, or rolling of eyes.	
i As patient regains consciousness, assess vital signs and reorient and reassure him or her. Explain what happened and answer patient's questions. Stay with patient until fully awake.	Informing patients of type of seizure activity experienced helps them to participate knowledgeably in their care. Some patients remain confused for a period of time after the seizure or become violent.
9 Status epilepticus is a medical emergency.	
a Call health care provider and response team immediately.	Medical emergency requires rapid response.
b Insert oral airway when jaw is relaxed (between seizure activity).	
c Access oxygen and suction equipment; keep airway patent.	
d Prepare for intravenous (IV) insertion (if one is not in place) and administration of IV antiseizure medications.	Provides route for intravenous (IV) medication.
10 After seizure assist patient to side-lying position in bed with padded side rails (if needed) up and bed in lowest position (Fig. 66-1). Place call light or intercom system within reach and provide quiet, nonstimulating environment. Instruct patient not to get out of bed without assistance.	Provides for continued safety. Patients are often confused and lethargic following a seizure (postictal).

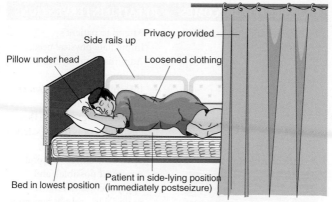

Fig. 66-1 Position of patient following seizure and when on seizure precautions.

STEP	RATIONALE
11 As patient regains consciousness, reorient and reassure. Explain what happened, and provide time for him or her to express feelings and concerns. 12 Complete postprocedure protocol.	Patients may be confused postictal. Patients who understand disease are better prepared to manage their seizure activity and have higher self-esteem.

Recording and Reporting

- Record in nurses' notes and electronic health record (EHR) what you observed before, during, and after seizure. Provide detailed description of the type of seizure activity and sequence of events (e.g., presence of aura [if any], level of consciousness, color, movement of extremities, incontinence, patient's status immediately following seizure, and time frame of events).
- Alert primary health care provider immediately as seizure begins. Status epilepticus is an emergency situation requiring immediate medical therapy.

UNEXPECTED OUTCOMES	RELATED INTERVENTIONS
1 Patient suffers traumatic injury.	• Attend to patient's immediate physical needs. • Administer prescribed treatments. • Inform health care provider. • Reassess patient's environment to ensure that environment is free of safety hazards.
2 Patient aspirates.	• Turn onto side, insert oral airway (if possible), and apply suction to remove material in oral pharynx and maintain patent airway. • Administer oxygen as needed.

Sequential Compression Device and Elastic Stockings

A patient may develop a deep vein thrombosis (DVT) for many reasons. Some common risk factors include injury to a vein from a fracture or surgery, immobility caused by a cast or prolonged sitting, inherited clotting disorders, obesity, smoking, and a family history (Harvard Health Publications, 2009). Three factors (known as *Virchow's triad*)—hypercoagulability of the blood, venous wall damage, and blood flow stasis—contribute to DVT development (Lewis et al., 2011). Prevention, which can include anticoagulant medications, is the best approach for DVTs; however, moving the extremities, wearing compression stockings, and using foot pumps are equally important. Elastic stockings help reduce blood stasis and venous wall injury by promoting venous return and limiting venous dilation, which decreases the risk of endothelial tears. Sequential compression devices (SCDs) pump blood into deep veins, thus removing pooled blood and preventing venous stasis.

Delegation Considerations

The skill of applying elastic stockings and SCDs may be delegated to nursing assistive personnel (NAP). The nurse initially determines the size of elastic stockings and assesses the patient's lower extremities for any signs and symptoms of DVTs or impaired circulation. The nurse directs the NAP to:

- Remove the SCD sleeves before allowing a patient to get out of bed.
- Report to the nurse if a patient's calf appears larger than the other or is red or hot, or if there are signs of allergic reactions to elastic (redness, itching, irritation).

Equipment

- Tape measure
- Powder or cornstarch *(optional)*
- Elastic support stockings
- SCD motor, disposable SCD sleeve(s), tubing assembly

Implementation

STEP	RATIONALE
1 Complete preprocedure protocol.	
2 Explain procedure and reason for applying elastic stockings and SCDs.	Eases patient apprehension and helps ensure compliance with therapy.
3 Position patient in supine position. Elevate head of bed to comfortable level. Use tape measure to measure patient's leg to determine proper elastic stocking or SCD size.	Stockings must be measured according to manufacturer's directions. The choice of length depends on the physician or health care provider's order. However, knee-length stockings are more comfortable for the patient and result in better adherence to therapy. If too large, stockings will not adequately support extremities. If too small, stockings may impede circulation.
4 *Option:* Apply a small amount of powder or cornstarch to legs provided patient does not have sensitivity.	Helps stockings slide on easier. Increases patient comfort.
5 Applying elastic stockings:	
a Turn elastic stocking inside out by placing one hand into sock, holding toe of sock with other hand, and pulling. Pull until reaching the heel (Fig. 67-1).	Allows easier application of stocking.
b Place patient's toes into foot of elastic stocking up to heel, making sure that sock is smooth (Fig. 67-2).	Wrinkles in elastic stocking can cause constrictions and impede circulation to lower region of extremity.
c Slide remaining portion of sock over patient's foot, making sure that the toes are covered. Make sure that foot fits into the toe and heel positions of sock. Sock will now be right side out (Fig. 67-3).	If toes remain uncovered, they will become constricted by elastic, and their circulation can be reduced.

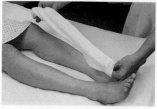

Fig. 67-1 Turn stocking inside out; hold toe and pull through.

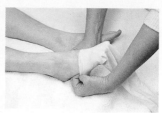

Fig. 67-2 Place toes into foot of stocking.

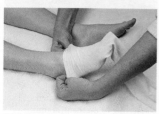

Fig. 67-3 Slide remaining portion of stocking over foot.

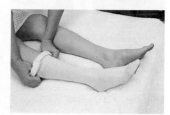

Fig. 67-4 Slide stocking up leg until completely extended.

STEP	RATIONALE
d Slide sock up over patient's calf until sock is completely extended. Be sure stocking is smooth and that no ridges or wrinkles are present (Fig. 67-4).	
e Instruct patient not to roll socks partially down.	Rolling stocking partially down has a constricting effect and impedes venous return.
6 **Applying SCD sleeves:**	
a Remove SCD sleeves from plastic, unfold, and flatten.	
b Arrange the SCD sleeve under the patient's leg according to the leg position indicated on inner lining of sleeve (Fig. 67-5).	Ensures straight and even application.

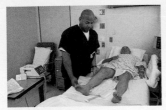

Fig. 67-5 Correct leg position on inner lining.

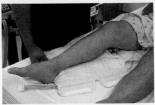

Fig. 67-6 Position back of patient's knee with popliteal opening.

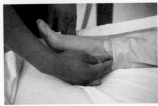

Fig. 67-7 Check fit of SCD sleeve.

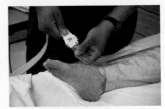

Fig. 67-8 Align arrows when connecting to mechanical unit.

STEP	RATIONALE
c Place patient's leg on SCD sleeve. Back of ankle should line up with the ankle marking on inner lining of sleeve.	
d Position back of knee with the popliteal opening (Fig. 67-6).	Prevents pressure on popliteal artery.
e Wrap SCD sleeve securely around patient's leg. Check fit of SCD sleeves by placing two fingers between patient's leg and sleeve (Fig. 67-7).	Secure fit needed for adequate compression. Ensures proper fit and prevents constriction, which impedes circulation.
f Attach SCD sleeve's connector to plug on mechanical unit. Arrows on connector line up with arrows on plug from mechanical unit (Fig. 67-8).	

STEP	RATIONALE
g Turn mechanical unit on. Green light indicates unit is functioning. Monitor functioning SCD through one full cycle of inflation and deflation.	Power source initiates sequential compression cycle. Ensures proper functioning of unit and determines if SCD sleeves are too loose or constricting.
7 Complete postprocedure protocol.	
8 Remove elastic stockings or SCD sleeves at least once per shift (e.g., long enough to inspect skin for irritation or breakdown).	Compliance in wearing elastic stockings and SCDs poses an issue when patients find them to be uncomfortable or applied incorrectly. Elastic stockings and SCDs are removed long enough to perform an assessment and/or hygiene measures and replaced as soon as possible.

Recording and Reporting

- Record date and time of application of elastic stockings and/or SCD sleeves in MAR. Include condition of skin and circulatory status of lower extremities before application, length and size of elastic stockings and SCD sleeves, time stockings/sleeves are removed, and condition of skin and circulatory status after removal. Initial or sign entry.
- Immediately report to health care provider any signs of thrombophlebitis or impeded circulation in lower extremities.

UNEXPECTED OUTCOMES	RELATED INTERVENTIONS
1 Patient develops decreased circulation in lower extremities.	• Assess lower extremities for coolness, cyanosis, decreased pedal pulses, decreased blanching, and numbness or tingling sensation.
	• Check that elastic stockings are not too small or have wrinkles or folds that impede circulation.

Continued

UNEXPECTED OUTCOMES	RELATED INTERVENTIONS
	• Notify physician immediately; signs and symptoms may indicate obstruction of arterial blood flow.
2 Patient develops deep vein thrombosis.	• Because clinical signs may be vague, an order for more sensitive radiology tests should be obtained from a physician. Doppler compression ultrasonogram (also known as Doppler duplex) or impedance plethysmography may be carried out to rule out the presence of thrombosis.
	• Do not massage lower extremities because of potential for dislodging thrombus.
3 Patient develops pulmonary embolism.	• Signs and symptoms include tachypnea, shortness of breath, anxiety, pleuritic chest pain, cough, hemoptysis, tachycardia, and signs of right ventricular failure (e.g., distended neck veins).
	• Notify health care provider immediately.
	• Monitor vital signs.
	• Administer supplemental oxygen as ordered.
	• Get a new mechanical unit if a reason cannot be found for alarm.

Specialty Beds:
Air-Fluidized, Air-Suspension, and Rotokinetic

The air-suspension bed supports a patient's weight on air-filled cushions. A low-air-loss system minimizes pressure and reduces shear. If a patient has large stage III or IV pressure ulcers on multiple turning surfaces of the skin, a low-air-loss bed or air-fluidized bed may be indicated (WOCN, 2010).

An air-fluidized bed is a powered device designed to distribute a patient's weight evenly over its support surface (Fig. 68-1). Fluidization is created by forcing a gentle flow of temperature-controlled air upward through a mass of fine ceramic microspheres. The microspheres fluidize and assume the appearance of boiling milk and all the properties of a fluid.

The Rotokinetic bed helps maintain skeletal alignment while providing constant rotation. This bed improves skeletal alignment with constant side-to-side rotation up to 90 degrees.

Delegation Considerations

The skill of placing a patient on an air-suspension or air-fluidized bed can be delegated to nursing assistive personnel (NAP), but the skill of placing a patient on a Rotokinetic bed cannot. In all cases, you complete the assessment, determine the need for a support surface, and select the specific surface. Some types of support surfaces require that the manufacturer representative prepare and maintain the support system. The nurse directs the NAP to:

- Notify the nurse of any changes in the patient's skin but warns the NAP to not stop rotation, move, or reposition patient without the assistance of the registered nurse (RN) if the patient is on a Rotokinetic bed.
- Monitor the exact rotation frequency of the bed.
- Continue to regularly turn and reposition the patient and seek assistance for patient position changes as necessary. This is not always necessary for patients who are placed on a lateral rotation air-suspension bed.
- Monitor the normal functioning of the air-suspension bed, such as inflation and deflation cycles, and report to the nurse any changes in these cycles.

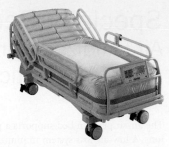

Fig. 68-1 Combination air-fluidized, low-air-loss bed. (©2008 Hill-Rom Services. Reprinted with permission. All rights reserved.)

- Notify the nurse if the patient becomes disoriented or restless or complains of nausea.

Equipment

Air-Fluidized Bed
- Foam positioning wedges, if indicated
- Filter sheet (supplied by rental company)
- Clean gloves *(optional)*

Air-Suspension Bed
- Gore-Tex sheet (supplied by manufacturer)
- Disposable bed pads, if indicated
- Clean gloves *(optional)*

Rotokinetic Bed
- Rotokinetic bed with support packs, bolsters, and safety straps
- Top sheet
- Pillowcases for bolsters

Implementation

STEP	RATIONALE
1 Complete preprocedure protocol.	
2 Determine patient's risk for pressure ulcer formation using a valid assessment tool (e.g., Braden Scale), and assess for risk factors for pressure ulcers, including nutritional deficits, shear stress, friction, alterations in mobility and sensory	Risk assessment tools as suggested by the Agency for Healthcare Research and Quality (AHRQ) and WOCN (e.g., Braden Scale) provide an objective measure of risk consistent between nurse assessors over time (WOCN, 2010).

STEP	RATIONALE
perception, and hemoglobin levels (see Skill 60).	
3 Inspect condition of skin, especially over dependent sites and bony prominences. Note appearance of existing ulcers and determine stage of ulcer.	Provides baseline to determine a change in skin integrity or in an existing pressure ulcer over time.
4 Assess patient's level of comfort using a pain scale of 0 to 10.	Provides baseline to determine the patient's comfort needs. Patients usually require less analgesia while on the bed.
5 Assess risk for complications from air-fluidized beds:	Anticipates need for frequent monitoring once patient is placed on support surface.
a Dehydration	Patients may become dehydrated with use of this bed because of insensible fluid loss.
b Aspiration	Inability to elevate head of bed is limited to placing foam wedges under patient's head and shoulders.
c Difficulty with patient positioning	Repositioning is limited to use of foam wedges.
d Level of orientation	Patients may be at risk for developing delirium from dehydration and floating sensation with air-fluidized bed.
6 For Rotokinetic bed, determine the number of people needed to assist in safe patient transfer from regular bed to Rotokinetic bed.	Reduces risk of injury by ensuring safe patient handling.
7 Review instructions supplied by bed manufacturer.	Promotes safe and correct use of bed.
8 For patients with severe to moderate pain, premedicate approximately 30 minutes before transfer.	Promotes patient's comfort and ability to cooperate during transfer to bed. Decreases patient's energy expenditure.

STEP	RATIONALE
9 ![hand] Perform hand hygiene and apply clean gloves (if linen or surface is soiled or wet).	Reduces transmission of microorganisms.
10 Transfer patient to bed using appropriate transfer techniques. Bed surface is sometimes slippery; thus do not attempt transfers without assistance.	Appropriate patient-handling techniques maintain alignment and reduce risk of injury during procedure. Manufacturer representative adjusts bed to patient's height and weight.
11 Once patient has been transferred, release Instaflate, fluidize, or activate bed by depressing switch; regulate temperature.	Releasing Instaflate or activating bed allows pressure cushions to automatically adjust to preset levels to minimize pressure, friction, and shear.
12 Position patient for comfort, and perform range-of-motion (ROM) exercises as appropriate.	Promotes comfort and reduces contracture formation.
13 To turn patient, position bedpans, or perform other therapies, turn on Instaflate setting. Once you have completed the procedure, release Instaflate. With air-fluidized bed, use foam wedges to position patient as needed.	Instaflate firms bed surface to facilitate turning and handling patient. Patient does not receive pressure relief while bed is in this mode.
14 Use special features of bed as needed:	
a Scales	Facilitates ease of routine weights.
b Portable transport units to maintain inflation when primary power is interrupted	Provides for continuous pressure reduction.
c Specialty cushions for positioning, providing pressure relief, reducing moisture, preventing patient from sliding down	Reduces pressure, friction, and shearing forces.

STEP	RATIONALE
in bed, or relieving weight from orthopedic devices	
d Lateral rotation, which allows approximately 30 degrees of turning	Helps to prevent and reduce risk of pulmonary and urinary complications of reduced mobility (Cullum et al., 2003; WOCN, 2010).
15 Rotokinetic bed (Fig. 68-2):	
a Place Rotokinetic bed in horizontal position and remove all bolsters, straps, and supports. Close posterior hatches.	
b Unplug electrical cord. Lock gatch.	Prevents accidental rotation during transfer.
c Maintaining proper alignment of the patient and using appropriate transfer techniques, transfer patient to Rotokinetic bed.	Reduces risk for further tissue injury during transfer. Will need health care provider available to assist in transfer.
d Secure thoracic panels, bolsters, head and knee packs, and safety straps.	Maintains proper alignment and prevents sliding during rotation.
e Cover patient with top sheet.	Prevents unnecessary exposure.
f Plug in bed.	

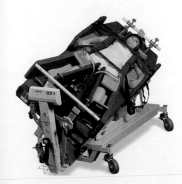

Fig. 68-2 Rotokinetic bed. (RotoRest, courtesy Kinetic Concepts, San Antonio, TX.)

STEP	RATIONALE
g Have manufacturer representative prepare optional angle as ordered by health care provider. Gradually increase rotation.	Health care provider determines rotational angle based on the patient's overall condition and tolerance to constant motion.
h Increase degree of rotation gradually according to patient's tolerance.	Reduces or prevents nausea, dizziness, and orthostatic hypotension.
i Provide space for caregivers and family to move around bed to facilitate communication.	Allows opportunity to meet patient's psychosocial needs.
j Stop bed for assessment and procedures. To stop the bed, permit bed to rotate to the desired position, turn off motor, and push knob into a lock position. If necessary, you can manually reposition the bed.	Allows nurse to easily access patient for any procedure.
k Inform patient that there will be a sensation of light-headedness or falling. However, reassure patient that he or she will not fall because pads prevent this and are checked by two people to ensure proper placement.	Informing patient of what to expect decreases anxiety.
l Inspect condition of skin (occipital region, ears, axillae, elbows, sacrum, groin, and heels) and musculoskeletal alignment every 2 hours or more often if indicated by patient's condition.	Evaluates healing process of any existing pressure ulcers and determines effectiveness of Rotokinetic therapy.

STEP	RATIONALE
m Determine patient's level of orientation once per shift while on bed.	Evaluates if sensory overload has developed from excess kinetic stimulation.
16 Complete postprocedure protocol.	

Recording and Reporting

- Record transfer of patient to bed, amount of assistance needed for transfer, time of transfer, degree of rotation, tolerance of procedure, and condition of skin before placement on bed in nurses' notes, electronic health record (EHR), and/or skin assessment flow sheet. Record patient teaching and validation of understanding in nurses' notes and EHR. Take a photograph to document skin condition and provide a baseline for later assessments for progress in healing.
- Record and report subjective data indicating response to the constant rotation. Record presence/absence of dizziness or nausea or blood pressure changes.
- Use a flow sheet to document routine assessment and care, including the length of time the bed rotation stopped. The bed needs to be rotating at least 20 hours out of every 24 hours and stopped for no more than 30 minutes at a time.
- Report changes in condition of skin, level of orientation, and levels of electrolytes to health care provider.

UNEXPECTED OUTCOMES	RELATED INTERVENTIONS
1 Existing areas of skin breakdown or pressure areas fail to heal or increase in size or depth.	• Evaluate rotation schedule; bed needs to remain in rotation 20 hours a day to prevent skin breakdown. • Modify skin-care regimen.
2 Patient experiences hypotension.	• If severe drop in blood pressure occurs, stop rotation, notify health care provider, remain with patient, and monitor vital signs every 5 minutes.

Continued

UNEXPECTED OUTCOMES	RELATED INTERVENTIONS
	• For less severe blood pressure changes, decrease rotational angle. Gradually increase rotational angle as patient adjusts to rotation.
3 Patient becomes disoriented, confused, and anxious, or complains of nausea.	• Reorient patient to person, place, and time.
	• Provide audio stimulation via radio or recordings.
	• Provide television adapted to Rotokinetic bed (available from manufacturer).
	• Hang mirror on ceiling so patient is able to view surroundings.
	• Provide symptomatic relief of motion sickness.

Sterile Gloving

Sterile gloves help prevent the transmission of pathogens by direct and indirect contact. Nurses apply sterile gloves before performing sterile procedures such as inserting urinary catheters or applying sterile dressings. It is important to select the proper size glove. The gloves should not stretch so tightly over the fingers that they can easily tear, yet they need to be tight enough that objects can be picked up easily. Sterile gloves are available in various sizes (e.g., 6, 6½, 7).

Many patients and health care workers are allergic to latex, the natural rubber used in most gloves (Church and Bjerke, 2009). Box 69-1 lists risk factors for latex allergy. The powder that is used to make latex gloves slip on easily is a carrier of the latex proteins (AORN, 2011; Molinari and Harte, 2009). When you apply or remove gloves, the powder particles become airborne and can remain so for hours. Then the latex can be inhaled or settle on clothing, skin, or mucous membranes. Reactions to latex are mild to severe (Box 69-2). For individuals at high risk or with suspected sensitivity to latex, it is important to choose latex-free or synthetic gloves.

Delegation Considerations

Assisting with skills that include the application and removal of sterile gloves may be delegated to nursing assistive personnel (NAP). However, many procedures that require the use of sterile gloves cannot be delegated to NAP. The nurse instructs the NAP about:

- The reason for using sterile gloves for a specific procedure.

Equipment

- Package of proper-size sterile gloves, latex or synthetic nonlatex (**NOTE:** Hypoallergenic, low-powder, and low-protein latex gloves may still contain enough latex protein to cause an allergic reaction [Molinari and Harte, 2009].)

Implementation

STEP	RATIONALE
1 Consider the type of procedure to be performed, and consult agency policy on use of sterile gloves.	Ensures proper use of sterile gloves when needed.

BOX 69-1 Risk Factors for Latex Allergy

- Spina bifida
- Congenital or urogenital defects
- History of indwelling catheters or repeated catheterizations
- History of using condom catheters
- High latex exposure (e.g., health care workers, housekeepers, food handlers, tire manufacturers, workers in industries that use gloves routinely)
- History of multiple childhood surgeries
- History of food allergies

BOX 69-2 Levels of Latex Reactions

The three types of common latex reactions (in order of severity) are:
1. **Irritant dermatitis:** A nonallergic response characterized by skin redness and itching.
2. **Type IV hypersensitivity:** Cell-mediated allergic reaction to chemicals used in latex processing. Reaction (including redness, itching, and hives) can be delayed up to 48 hours. Localized swelling, red and itchy or runny eyes and nose, and coughing may develop.
3. **Type I allergic reaction:** A true latex allergy that can be life-threatening. Reactions vary based on type of latex protein and degree of individual sensitivity, including local and systemic. Symptoms include hives, generalized edema, itching, rash, wheezing, bronchospasm, difficulty breathing, laryngeal edema, diarrhea, nausea, hypotension, tachycardia, and respiratory or cardiac arrest.

STEP	RATIONALE
2 Consider patient's risk for infection (e.g., preexisting condition and size or extent of area being treated).	Directs you to follow added precautions (e.g., use of additional protective barriers) if necessary.
3 Select correct size and type of gloves and then examine glove package to determine if it is dry and intact with no water stains.	Torn or wet package is considered contaminated. Signs of water stains on package indicate previous contamination by water.

STEP	RATIONALE
4 Inspect condition of hands for cuts, hangnails, open lesions, or abrasions. In some settings you are allowed to cover any open lesions with a sterile, impervious transparent dressing (check agency policy). In some cases the presence of such lesions may prevent you from participating in a procedure.	Cuts, abrasions, and hangnails tend to ooze serum, which possibly contains pathogens. Breaks in skin integrity permit microorganisms to enter and increase the risk of infection for both patient and nurse (AORN, 2011).
5 Assess patient for the following risk factors before applying latex gloves:	Determines level of patient's risk for latex allergy and need to use nonlatex gloves.
a Previous reaction to the following items within hours of exposure: adhesive tape, dental or face mask, golf club grip, ostomy bag, rubber band, balloon, bandage, elastic underwear, intravenous (IV) tubing, rubber gloves, condom	Items known to lead to latex allergy.
b Personal history of asthma, contact dermatitis, eczema, urticaria, rhinitis	
c History of food allergies, especially avocado, banana, peach, chestnut, raw potato, kiwi, tomato, papaya	
d Previous history of adverse reactions during surgery or dental procedure	
e Previous reaction to latex product	

SAFETY ALERT Synthetic nonlatex gloves are necessary for patients at risk or if nurse has sensitivity or allergy to latex.

STEP	RATIONALE
6 Applying gloves:	
a Perform thorough hand hygiene. Place glove package near work area.	Reduces number of bacteria on skin surfaces and transmission of infection. Ensures availability before procedure.
b Remove outer glove package wrapper by carefully separating and peeling apart sides (Fig. 69-1).	Prevents inner glove package from accidentally opening and touching contaminated objects.
c Grasp inner package, and lay it on clean, dry, flat surface at waist level. Open package, keeping gloves on inside surface of wrapper (Fig. 69-2).	Sterile object held below waist is contaminated. Inner surface of glove package is sterile.
d Identify right and left glove. Each glove has cuff approximately 5 cm (2 inches) wide. Glove dominant hand first.	Proper identification of gloves prevents contamination by improper fit. Gloving of dominant hand first improves dexterity.
e With thumb and first two fingers of nondominant hand, grasp edge of cuff of glove for dominant hand by touching only inside surface (Fig. 69-3).	Inner edge of cuff will lie against skin and thus is not sterile.

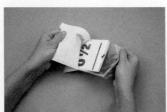

Fig. 69-1 Open outer glove package wrapper.

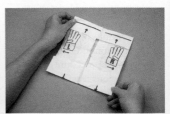

Fig. 69-2 Open inner glove package on work surface.

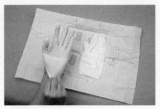

Fig. 69-3 Pick up glove for dominant hand, insert fingers, and pull glove completely over dominant hand (example is for left-handed person).

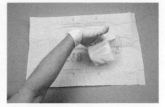

Fig. 69-4 Pick up glove for nondominant hand.

STEP	RATIONALE
f Carefully pull glove over dominant hand, leaving cuff and being sure that cuff does not roll up wrist. Be sure thumb and fingers are in proper spaces.	If glove's outer surface touches hand or wrist, it is contaminated.
g With gloved dominant hand, slip fingers underneath second glove's cuff (Fig. 69-4).	Cuff protects gloved fingers. Sterile touching sterile prevents glove contamination.
h Carefully pull second glove over nondominant hand (Fig. 69-5).	Contact of gloved hand with exposed hand results in contamination.
i After second glove is on, interlock hands together, above waist level. The cuffs usually fall down after application. Be sure to touch only sterile sides.	Ensures smooth fit over fingers.
7 Remove gloves:	
a Grasp outside of one cuff with other gloved hand; avoid touching wrist.	Minimizes contamination of underlying skin.
b Pull glove off, turning it inside out and placing it in gloved hand (Fig. 69-6).	Outside of glove does not touch skin surface.

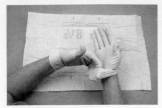

Fig. 69-5 Pull second glove over nondominant hand.

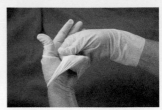

Fig. 69-6 Carefully remove first glove by turning it inside out.

Fig. 69-7 Remove second glove by turning it inside out.

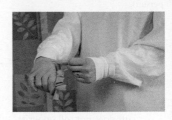

STEP	RATIONALE
c Take fingers of bare hand and tuck inside remaining glove cuff. Peel glove off inside out and over the previously removed glove (Fig. 69-7). Discard both gloves in receptacle.	Fingers do not touch contaminated glove surface.
8 Perform hand hygiene.	

Recording and Reporting

- It is not necessary to record application of gloves. Record specific procedure performed and patient's response and status.
- In the event of a latex allergy reaction, record patient's response in nurses' notes, electronic health record (EHR), and vital sign flow sheet. Note type of response and patient's reaction to emergency treatment.

UNEXPECTED OUTCOMES	RELATED INTERVENTIONS
1 Patient develops localized signs of infection (e.g., urine becomes cloudy or odorous; wound becomes painful, edematous, or reddened with purulent drainage).	• Contact health care provider, and implement appropriate treatments as ordered.
2 Patient develops systemic signs of infection (e.g., fever, malaise, increased white blood cell count).	• Contact health care provider, and implement appropriate treatments as ordered.
3 Patient develops allergic reaction to latex (see Box 69-2).	• Immediately remove source of latex.
	• Bring emergency equipment to bedside. Have epinephrine injection ready for administration, and be prepared to initiate IV fluids and oxygen.

Sterile Technique:
Donning and Removing Cap, Mask, and Protective Eyewear

Although masks and caps are usually worn in surgical procedure areas (e.g., the operating room [OR]), there are certain aseptic procedures performed at a patient's bedside that also might require these barriers. For example, it may be agency policy for a nurse to wear a mask during the changing of a central line dressing or insertion of a peripherally inserted central catheter (PICC). When there is a risk for splattering of blood or body fluid, there is also the need to apply protective eyewear.

Delegation Considerations

The skill of applying and removing cap, mask, and protective eyewear is required of all caregivers when working in sterile areas. However, the procedures performed at a patient's bedside that require cap and mask generally cannot be delegated to nursing assistive personnel (NAP). The nurse determines if protective barriers are necessary for the other staff. The nurse instructs the NAP about:

- The procedure to be performed and how to assist with positioning and obtaining supplies.
- Performing hand hygiene after glove removal.

Equipment

- Surgical mask (different types are available for people with different skin sensitivities)
- Surgical cap (**NOTE:** Use in OR or if agency policy requires. Use to secure hair if there is a possibility of contamination of a sterile field.)
- Hairpins, rubber bands, or both
- Protective eyewear (e.g., goggles or glasses with appropriate side shields)

Implementation

STEP	RATIONALE
1 Review type of sterile procedure to be performed, and consult agency policy for use of mask, cap, and eyewear.	Not all sterile procedures require mask, cap, or protective eyewear. Ensures that patient and nurse are properly protected.
2 If you have symptoms of a cold or respiratory tract infection, either avoid participating in procedure or apply a mask.	A greater number of pathogenic microorganisms reside within the respiratory tract when infection is present.
3 Assess patient's actual or potential risk for infection when choosing barriers for surgical asepsis (e.g., older adult, neonate, or immunocompromised patient).	Some patients are at a greater risk for acquiring an infection; thus use additional barriers.
4 Prepare equipment and inspect packaging for integrity and exposure to sterilization.	Ensures availability of equipment and sterility of supplies before procedure begins.
5 Perform hand hygiene.	Reduces transient microorganisms on skin.
6 Applying cap:	
a If hair is long, comb back behind ears and secure.	Cap must cover all hair entirely.
b Secure hair in place with pins.	Ensures that long hair does not fall down or cause cap to slip and expose hair.
c Apply cap over head as you would apply hairnet. Be sure all hair fits under cap's edges (Fig. 70-1).	Loose hair hanging over sterile field or falling dander will contaminate objects on sterile field.
7 Applying mask:	
a Find top edge of mask, which usually has a thin metal strip along edge.	Pliable metal fits snugly against bridge of nose.
b Hold mask by top two strings or loops, keeping top edge above bridge of nose.	Prevents contact of hands with clean facial portion of mask. Mask will cover all of nose.

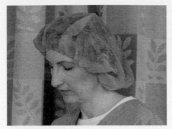

Fig. 70-1 Nurse places cap over head, covering all hair.

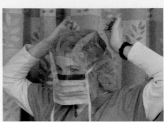

Fig. 70-2 Tie top strings of mask.

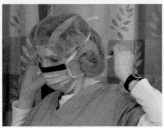

Fig. 70-3 Tie bottom strings of mask.

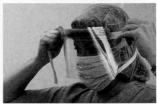

Fig. 70-4 Place face shield over cap.

STEP	RATIONALE
c Tie two top strings at top of back of head, over cap (if worn), with strings above ears (Fig. 70-2).	Position of ties at top of head provides tight fit. Strings over ears may cause irritation.
d Tie two lower ties snugly around neck with mask well under chin (Fig. 70-3).	Prevents escape of microorganisms through sides of mask as you talk and breathe.
e Gently pinch upper metal band around bridge of nose.	Prevents microorganisms from escaping around nose and prevents eyeglasses from steaming up.
8 Applying protective eyewear:	
a Apply protective glasses, goggles, or face shield comfortably over eyes, and check that vision is clear (Fig. 70-4).	Positioning affects clarity of vision.

STEP	RATIONALE
b Be sure that face shield fits snugly around forehead and face.	Ensures that eyes are fully protected.
9 Removing protective barriers:	
a Remove gloves first, if worn (see Skill 69).	Prevents contamination of hair, neck, and facial area.
b Untie bottom strings of mask.	Prevents top part of mask from falling down over the uniform. If mask falls and touches uniform, uniform will be contaminated.
c Untie top strings of mask, and remove mask from face, holding ties securely. Discard mask in proper receptacle (Fig. 70-5).	Avoids contact of nurse's hands with contaminated mask.

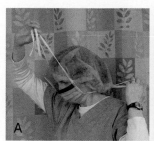
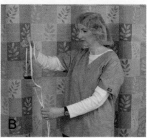
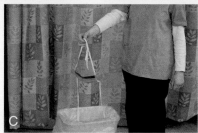

Fig. 70-5 **A,** Untying top mask strings. **B,** Removing mask from face. **C,** Discarding mask.

STEP	RATIONALE
d Remove eyewear. Avoid any touching of soiled lens with hands. If wearing face shield, remove it before removal of mask. **NOTE:** A combination mask and eyewear is available in some agencies.	Prevents transmission of microorganisms.
e Grasp outer surface of cap and lift from hair.	Minimizes contact of hands with hair.
f Discard cap in proper receptacle and perform hand hygiene.	Reduces transmission of infection.

Recording and Reporting

- No recording or reporting is required for this set of skills. Record specific procedure performed in nurses' notes and electronic health record (EHR), and describe patient's status.

Subcutaneous Injections

Subcutaneous injections involve depositing medication into the loose connective tissue underlying the dermis. Because subcutaneous tissue does not contain as many blood vessels as muscles, medications are absorbed more slowly than with intramuscular (IM) injections. Physical exercise or application of hot or cold compresses influences the rate of drug absorption by altering local blood flow to tissues. Any condition that impairs blood flow is a contraindication for subcutaneous injections.

You give subcutaneous medications in small doses of less than 2 mL that are isotonic, nonirritating, nonviscous, and water soluble. The best subcutaneous injection sites include the outer aspect of the upper arms, the abdomen from below the costal margins to the iliac crests, and the anterior aspects of the thighs (Fig. 71-1).

Most patients manage type 1 diabetes mellitus with injections. Anatomical injection site rotation is no longer necessary because newer human insulins carry a lower risk for hypertrophy. Patients choose one anatomical area (e.g., the abdomen) and systematically rotate sites within that region, which maintains consistent insulin absorption from day to day. Absorption rates of insulin vary based on the injection site. Insulin is most quickly absorbed in the abdomen and most slowly in the thighs (Lehne, 2010).

Heparin therapy provides therapeutic anticoagulation to reduce the risk for thrombus formation by suppressing clot formation. Therefore patients receiving heparin are at risk for bleeding, including bleeding gums, hematemesis, hematuria, or melena.

Delegation Considerations

The skill of administering subcutaneous injections cannot be delegated to nursing assistive personnel (NAP). The nurse directs the NAP about:

- Potential medication side effects and to report their occurrence to the nurse.

Equipment

- Proper size syringe with engineered sharps injury protection (SESIP) needle:
  - Subcutaneous syringe (1 to 3 mL) and needle (25 to 27 gauge, $\frac{3}{8}$ to $\frac{5}{8}$ inch)
  - Subcutaneous U-100 insulin: insulin syringe (1 mL) with preattached needle (28 to 31 gauge, $\frac{5}{16}$ to $\frac{1}{2}$ inch)

Fig. 71-1 Common sites for
subcutaneous injections.

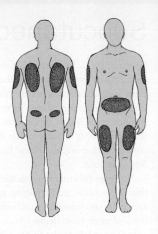

- Subcutaneous U-500 insulin: 1-mL tuberculin (TB) syringe
  with needle (25 to 27 gauge, ½ to ⅝ inch)
- Small gauze pad *(optional)*
- Alcohol swab
- Medication vial or ampule
- Clean gloves
- Medication administration record (MAR) or computer printout
- Puncture-proof container

Implementation

STEP	RATIONALE
1 Complete preprocedure protocol.	
2 Check accuracy and completeness of each MAR or computer printout with prescriber's written medication order. Check patient's name, medication name and dosage, route of administration, and time of administration. Recopy or reprint any portion of MAR that is difficult to read.	The order sheet is the most reliable source and legal record of the patient's medications. Ensures that patient receives the correct medication. Handwritten MARs are a source of medication errors (ISMP, 2010; Jones and Treiber, 2010).

STEP	RATIONALE
3 Perform hand hygiene and prepare medication using aseptic technique. Check label of the medication carefully with the MAR or computer printout two times when preparing medication.	Ensures that medication is sterile. *These are the first and second checks for accuracy* and ensure that correct medication is administered.
4 Identify patient using two patient identifiers (e.g., name and birthday or name and account number) according to agency policy. Compare identifiers with information on patient's MAR or medical record.	Ensures correct patient. Complies with The Joint Commission requirements for patient safety (TJC, 2014).
5 At patient's bedside, again compare MAR or computer printout with names of medications on medication labels and patient name. Ask patient if he or she has allergies.	*This is the third check for accuracy* and ensures that patient receives correct medication. Confirms patient's allergy history.
6 ![icon] Perform hand hygiene and apply clean gloves. Keep sheet or gown draped over body parts not requiring exposure.	Reduces transfer of microorganisms. Respects patient dignity during injection.
7 Select appropriate injection site. Inspect skin surface over sites for bruises, inflammation, or edema. Do not use an area that is bruised or has signs associated with infection.	Injection sites are free of abnormalities that interfere with drug absorption. Sites used repeatedly become hardened from lipohypertrophy (increased growth in fatty tissue).
8 Palpate sites; avoid those with masses or tenderness. Be sure that needle is correct size by grasping skinfold at site with thumb and	You can mistakenly give subcutaneous injections into muscle, especially in the abdomen and thigh sites. Appropriate size of needle

STEP	RATIONALE
forefinger. Measure fold from top to bottom. Make sure needle is one-half length of fold.	ensures that you inject medication into the subcutaneous tissue (Gibney et al., 2010; Hunter, 2008b).
a When administering insulin or heparin subcutaneously, use abdominal injection sites first, followed by thigh injection site.	Risk for bruising is not affected by site (Aschenbrenner and Venable, 2009).
b When administering low-molecular-weight heparin (LMWH) subcutaneously, choose a site on the right or left side of the abdomen, at least 5 cm (2 inches) away from the umbilicus.	Injecting LMWH on the side of the abdomen will help decrease pain and bruising at the injection site (Sanofi-Aventis, 2010).
c Rotate insulin site within an anatomical area (e.g., the abdomen), and systematically rotate sites within that area.	Rotating injection sites within the same anatomical site maintains consistency in day-to-day insulin absorption (Sheeja et al., 2010).

SAFETY ALERT Applying ice to the injection site for 1 minute before the injection may decrease the patient's perception of pain (Hockenberry and Wilson, 2011).

9	Help patient into comfortable position. Have him or her relax arm, leg, or abdomen, depending on site selection.	Relaxation of site minimizes discomfort.
10	Cleanse site with antiseptic swab. Apply swab at center of site and rotate outward in circular direction for about 5 cm (2 inches) (Fig. 71-2).	Mechanical action of swab removes secretions containing microorganisms.
11	Hold swab or gauze between third and fourth fingers of nondominant hand.	Swab or gauze remains readily accessible for use when withdrawing needle after injection.

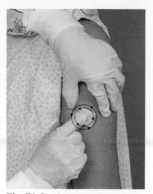

Fig. 71-2 Cleansing site with circular motion.

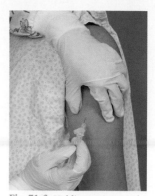

Fig. 71-3 Holding syringe as if grasping a dart.

STEP	RATIONALE
12 Remove needle cap or protective sheath by pulling it straight off.	Preventing needle from touching sides of cap prevents contamination.
13 Hold syringe between thumb and forefinger of dominant hand; hold as dart (Fig. 71-3).	Quick, smooth injection requires proper manipulation of syringe parts.
14 Administer injection:	
a For average-size patient, hold skin across injection site or pinch skin with nondominant hand.	Needle penetrates tight skin more easily than loose skin. Pinching skin elevates subcutaneous tissue and desensitizes area.
b Inject needle quickly and firmly at 45- to 90-degree angle. Release skin, if pinched. *Option:* When using injection pen or giving heparin, continue to pinch skin while injecting medicine.	Quick, firm insertion minimizes discomfort. (Injecting medication into compressed tissue irritates nerve fibers.) Correct angle prevents accidental injection into muscle.
c For obese patient, pinch skin at site and inject needle at 90-degree angle below tissue fold.	Obese patients have fatty layer of tissue above subcutaneous layer.

Fig. 71-4 Subcutaneous injection.

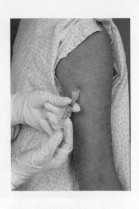

STEP	RATIONALE
d After needle enters site, grasp lower end of syringe barrel with nondominant hand to stabilize it. Move dominant hand to end of plunger, and slowly inject medication over several seconds (Hunter, 2008b) (Fig. 71-4). Avoid moving syringe.	Movement of syringe may displace needle and cause discomfort. Slow injection of medication minimizes discomfort.

SAFETY ALERT Aspiration after injecting a subcutaneous medication is not necessary. Piercing a blood vessel in a subcutaneous injection is very rare (Hunter, 2008b). Aspiration after injecting heparin and insulin is not recommended (Aschenbrenner and Venable, 2009).

e Withdraw needle quickly while placing antiseptic swab or gauze gently over site.	Supporting tissues around injection site minimizes discomfort during needle withdrawal. Dry gauze may minimize patient discomfort associated with alcohol on nonintact skin.
15 Apply gentle pressure to site. *Do not massage site.* (If heparin is given, hold alcohol swab or gauze to site for 30 to 60 seconds.)	Aids absorption. Massage can damage underlying tissue. Time interval prevents bleeding at site.

STEP	RATIONALE
16 Help patient to comfortable position.	Gives patient a sense of well-being.
17 Discard uncapped needle or needle enclosed in safety shield and attached syringe into puncture- and leak-proof receptacle.	Prevents injury to patients and health care personnel. Recapping needles increases risk for a needlestick injury (OSHA, 2012).
18 Complete postprocedure protocol.	

Recording and Reporting

- Immediately after administration, record medication, dose, route, site, time, and date given on MAR. Correctly sign MAR according to institutional policy.
- Record patient teaching, validation of understanding, and patient's response to medication in nurses' notes and electronic health record (EHR).
- Report any undesirable effects from medication to patient's health care provider, and document adverse effects in record.

UNEXPECTED OUTCOMES	RELATED INTERVENTIONS
1 Patient complains of localized pain, numbness, tingling, or burning at injection site.	• Assess injection site; may indicate potential injury to nerve or tissues. • Notify patient's health care provider, and do not reuse site.
2 Patient displays adverse reaction with signs of urticaria, eczema, pruritus, wheezing, and dyspnea.	• Monitor patient's heart rate, respirations, blood pressure, and temperature. • Follow agency policy or guidelines for appropriate response to allergic reactions (e.g., administration of antihistamine such as diphenhydramine [Benadryl] or epinephrine), and notify patient's health care provider immediately.

Continued

UNEXPECTED OUTCOMES	RELATED INTERVENTIONS
	• Add allergy information to patient's record.
3 Hypertrophy of skin develops from repeated subcutaneous injection.	• Do not use site for future injections.
	• Instruct patient not to use site for 6 months.

Suctioning:
Closed (In-Line)

Endotracheal tubes (ETs) and tracheostomy tubes (TTs) are artificial airways inserted to relieve airway obstruction, provide a route for mechanical ventilation, permit easy access for secretion removal, and protect the airway from gross aspiration in patients with impaired cough or gag reflexes. An ET tube is inserted through the nares (nasal ET tube) or the mouth (oral ET tube) past the epiglottis and vocal cords into the trachea. The length of time that an ET tube remains in place is somewhat controversial; however, in most cases a tracheostomy tube (TT) is inserted if a patient still requires an artificial airway after 2 to 4 weeks (AARC, 2010).

A TT can be temporary or permanent, depending on the patient's condition. It is inserted directly into the trachea through a small incision made in the patient's neck. Some agencies use a closed-suction catheter system or in-line suction catheter device to minimize infections, especially in critically ill or immunosuppressed patients (Pedersen et al., 2009). Use of a closed-system catheter (in-line) allows quicker lower airway suctioning without applying sterile gloves or a mask and does not interrupt ventilation and oxygenation in critically ill patients. With a closed-system method, the patient's artificial airway is not disconnected from the mechanical ventilator (Jongerden et al., 2011).

Delegation Considerations

The skill of airway suction with a closed (in-line) suction catheter cannot be delegated to nursing assistive personnel (NAP). In special situations, such as suctioning a permanent tracheostomy, this procedure may be delegated to NAP. The nurse is responsible for cardiopulmonary assessment and evaluation of the patient. The nurse directs the NAP about:

- Any individualized aspects of patient care that pertain to suctioning (e.g., position, duration of suction, pressure settings).
- Expected quality, quantity, and color of secretions and to inform the nurse immediately if there are changes.
- Patient's anticipated response to suction and to immediately report to the nurse changes in vital signs, complaints of pain, shortness of breath, confusion, or increased restlessness.

Equipment

- Closed-system or in-line suction catheter
- Suction machine
- Connecting tubing (6 feet)
- Two clean gloves *(optional)*
- Mask, goggles, or face shield
- Pulse oximeter and stethoscope

Implementation
STEPS

1 Complete preprocedure protocol and perform assessment.
2 Identify patient using two identifiers (e.g., name and birthday or name and account number) according to agency policy. Compare identifiers with information on patient's MAR or medical record.
3 Explain the procedure to patient and the importance of coughing during the suctioning procedure. Even if patients cannot speak, provide information regarding the procedure.
4 Help patient assume a position of comfort, usually semi- or high-Fowler's position. Place towel across patient's chest.
5 ⚡ Perform hand hygiene, apply clean gloves and face shield, and attach suction.
  a In many agencies a respiratory therapist attaches the catheter to the mechanical ventilator circuit. If catheter is not already in place, open suction catheter package using aseptic technique and attach closed-suction catheter to ventilator circuit by removing swivel adapter and placing closed-suction catheter apparatus on ET or TT. Connect Y on mechanical ventilator circuit to closed-suction catheter with flex tubing (Fig. 72-1).
  b Connect one end of connecting tubing to suction machine; connect other end to the end of a closed-system or in-line suction catheter. Turn suction device on, set vacuum regulator to appropriate negative pressure, and check pressure. Many closed-system suction catheters require slightly higher suction pressures (consult manufacturer's guidelines).
6 Hyperoxygenate the patient's lungs (usually 100% oxygen) by adjusting the FiO_2 setting on the ventilator or by using a temporary oxygen-enrichment program available on microprocessor ventilators (AARC, 2010). Manual ventilation is not recommended.

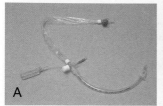 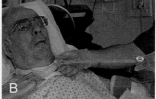

Fig. 72-1 **A,** Closed-system suction catheter attached to endotracheal tube. **B,** Suctioning tracheostomy with closed-system suction catheter.

STEPS

7 Pick up suction catheter enclosed in plastic sleeve with dominant hand.

8 Wait until patient inhales to insert catheter. Use a repeating maneuver of pushing catheter and sliding (or pulling) plastic sleeve back between thumb and forefinger until resistance is felt or patient coughs. Pull back 1 cm ($\frac{1}{2}$ inch) before applying suction to avoid tissue damage to carina.

9 Encourage patient to cough, and apply suction by squeezing on suction control mechanism while withdrawing catheter. Apply continuous suction for no longer than 10 seconds as you remove the suction catheter. Be sure to withdraw catheter completely into plastic sheath so it does not obstruct airflow.

10 Reassess cardiopulmonary status, including pulse oximetry and ventilator measures, to determine any complications or need for subsequent suctioning. Repeat Steps 5 to 9 one more time to clear secretions. Allow adequate time (at least 1 full minute) between suction passes for ventilation and reoxygenation.

11 When airway is clear, withdraw catheter completely into sheath. Be sure that colored indicator line on catheter is visible in the sheath. Squeeze vial or push syringe while applying suction to rinse inner lumen of catheter. Use at least 5 to 10 mL of saline to rinse the catheter until it is clear of retained secretions, which can cause bacterial growth and increase the risk for infection. Lock suction mechanism if applicable and turn off suction.

12 Hyperoxygenate the patient for at least 1 minute by following the same technique used to preoxygenate (AARC, 2010).

13 If patient requires oral or nasal suctioning, perform Skill 73 with separate standard suction catheter.

14 Reposition patient. Remove gloves and face shield, discard into appropriate receptacle, and perform hand hygiene.

STEPS

15 Compare patient's respiratory assessments before and after suctioning, observe airway secretions, and document findings.
16 Complete postprocedure protocol.

Recording and Reporting

- Record respiratory assessment findings before and after suctioning; size and route of catheter used; amount, consistency, and color of secretions obtained; frequency of suctioning.
- Report patient's intolerance to procedure or worsening of oxygenation.

UNEXPECTED OUTCOMES	RELATED INTERVENTIONS
1 Respiratory status worsens.	• Limit length of suctioning. • Determine need for more frequent suctioning, possibly of shorter duration. • Determine need for supplemental oxygen. Supply oxygen between suctioning passes. • Notify physician.
2 Bloody secretions return.	• Determine amount of suction pressure used. Suction pressure may need to be decreased. • Ensure suction is completed correctly using intermittent suction and catheter rotation. • Evaluate suctioning frequency. • Provide more frequent oral hygiene.
3 Paroxysms of coughing occur.	• Administer supplemental oxygen. • Allow patient to rest between passes of suction catheter. • Consult with physician regarding need for inhaled bronchodilators or topical anesthetics.

Suctioning:
Nasopharyngeal, Nasotracheal, and Artificial Airway

Oropharyngeal suctioning removes secretions only from the back of the throat. Tracheal airway suctioning extends into the lower airway to remove respiratory secretions and maintain optimum ventilation and oxygenation in patients who are unable to independently remove these secretions. When a patient's oxygen saturation measurement falls below 90%, it is a good indicator of the need for suctioning. Assess patients to determine frequency and depth of suctioning. Some patients require suctioning every 1 or 2 hours, whereas others need it only once or twice a day (AARC, 2004).

Delegation Considerations

The skills of nasotracheal suction and suctioning a new artificial airway tube cannot be delegated to nursing assistive personnel (NAP). When the patient has an established tracheostomy and is stable, you can delegate suctioning. The nurse directs the NAP about:

- Any unique modifications of the skill, such as the need for supplemental oxygen or the use of a clean-versus-sterile suction technique.
- Appropriate suction limits for suctioning tracheostomy tubes (TTs) and risks of applying excessive or inadequate suction pressure.
- Signs and symptoms of hypoxemia, such as a change in the patient's respiratory status, confusion, and restlessness, and to report these signs immediately to the nurse.
- Reporting any change in secretion quality, quantity, and color.

Equipment

- Appropriate-size suction catheter (smallest diameter that will remove secretions effectively)
- Nasal or oral airway (if indicated)
- Two sterile gloves or one sterile and one clean glove
- Clean towel or paper drape
- Suction machine/source
- Mask, goggles, or face shield
- Connecting tubing (6 feet)

- Small Y-adapter (if catheter does not have a suction control port)
- Water-soluble lubricant
- Sterile basin
- Sterile normal saline solution or water, about 100 mL
- Pulse oximeter and stethoscope

Implementation

STEP	RATIONALE
1 Complete preprocedure protocol.	
2 Assess signs and symptoms of upper and lower airway obstruction requiring airway suctioning, including wheezes, crackles, or gurgling on inspiration or expiration; restlessness; ineffective coughing; absent or diminished breath sounds; tachypnea; hypertension or hypotension; cyanosis; decreased level of consciousness, especially acute; or excess nasal secretions, drooling, or gastric secretions or vomitus in mouth (AARC, 2004).	Physical signs and symptoms result from decreased oxygen to tissues and pooling of secretions in upper and lower airways. Assessment is necessary before and after the suction procedure (AARC, 2004).
3 Determine the presence of apprehension, anxiety, decreased ability to concentrate, lethargy, decreased level of consciousness (especially acute), increased fatigue, dizziness, behavioral changes (especially irritability), pallor, cyanosis, dyspnea, or use of accessory muscles.	Signs and symptoms indicate hypoxia (low oxygen concentration at the cellular or tissue level), hypoxemia, or hypercapnia. Anxiety and pain consume oxygen and in turn worsen the signs of hypoxia. Patients with conditions such as acute respiratory distress syndrome, pulmonary edema, and heart failure are at particular risk for hypoxia.
4 Assess for risk factors for upper or lower airway	Presence of these risk factors can impair patient's ability to clear

STEP	RATIONALE
obstruction including obstructive lung disease, pulmonary infections, impaired mobility, sedation, decreased level of consciousness, seizures, presence of feeding tube, decreased gag or cough reflex, and decreased swallowing ability.	secretions from airway and necessitate nasopharyngeal or nasotracheal suctioning.
5 Assess factors that affect volume and consistency of secretions:	Thickened or copious secretions increase risk for airway obstruction.
a Fluid balance	Fluid overload increases amount of secretions. Dehydration promotes thicker secretions.
b Lack of humidity	The environment influences secretion formation and gas exchange.
c Infection (e.g., pneumonia)	Patients with respiratory tract infections are prone to increased secretions that are thicker and sometimes more difficult to expectorate.
d Allergies, sinus drainage	Increases volume of secretions in pharynx.

6 Weigh the patient's need for suction, and consider contraindications to nasotracheal suctioning (AARC, 2004):
  a Facial or neck trauma/ surgery
  b Bleeding disorders
  c Nasal bleeding
  d Epiglottitis or croup
  e Laryngospasm
  f Irritable airway
  h Gastric surgery
  g Acute head injuries
	Consider these conditions only if suctioning appears to be hazardous. Passage of catheter through nasal route causes additional trauma, increases nasal bleeding, or causes severe bleeding in presence of bleeding disorders. In the presence of epiglottitis, croup, laryngospasm, or irritable airway, entrance of suction catheter via the nasal route may cause intractable coughing, hypoxemia, and

STEP	RATIONALE
	severe bronchospasm; this may necessitate emergency intubation or tracheostomy.
7 Place pulse oximeter on patient's finger. Take reading, and leave oximeter in place.	Provides continuous SpO$_2$ value to determine patient's response to suctioning.
8 Perform hand hygiene, and apply mask, goggles, or face shield if splashing is likely.	Reduces transmission of microorganisms.
9 Attach one end of connecting tubing to suction machine, and place other end in convenient location near patient. Turn suction device on and set suction pressure to as low a level as possible that is yet able to effectively clear secretions (AARC, 2010). Occlude end of suction to check pressure.	Excessive negative pressure damages nasopharyngeal and tracheal mucosa and induces greater hypoxia. Lowest possible suction pressure is recommended; less than 150 mm Hg in adults (AARC, 2010; Pedersen et al., 2009).
10 Prepare suction catheter. a One-time-use catheter: (1) Using aseptic technique, open suction kit or catheter. If sterile drape is available, place it across patient's chest or on the over-bed table. Do not allow the suction catheter to touch any nonsterile surfaces.	Prepares catheter, maintains asepsis, and reduces transmission of microorganisms. Provides sterile surface on which to lay catheter between passes.
(2) Unwrap or open sterile basin, and place on bedside table. Be careful not to touch inside of basin. Fill with about 100 mL of sterile	Saline or water is used to clean tubing after each suction pass.

STEP	RATIONALE
normal saline solution or water (Fig. 73-1).	
(3) Open lubricant. Squeeze small amount onto open sterile catheter package without touching package. **NOTE:** *Lubricant is not necessary for artificial airway suctioning.*	Prepares lubricant while maintaining sterility. Using water-soluble lubricant helps avoid lipoid aspiration pneumonia. Excessive lubricant occludes catheter.
b Closed (in-line) suction catheter: See Skill 72.	
11 Apply sterile glove to each hand, or apply nonsterile glove to nondominant hand and sterile glove to dominant hand.	Reduces transmission of microorganisms and maintains sterility of suction catheter.
12 Pick up suction catheter with dominant hand without touching nonsterile surfaces. Pick up connecting tubing with nondominant hand. Secure catheter to tubing (Fig. 73-2).	Maintains catheter sterility. Connects catheter to suction.
13 Check that equipment is functioning properly by suctioning small amount of normal saline solution from basin.	Ensures equipment function. Lubricates internal catheter and tubing.
14 Suction airway:	
a Nasopharyngeal and nasotracheal suctioning:	
(1) Increase oxygen flow rate for face masks as ordered by health care provider (Lewis et al., 2011). Have patient deep breathe slowly, if possible.	Hyperoxygenation is recommended, especially in patients who are hypoxemic (AARC, 2010).

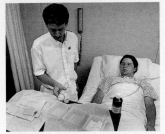

Fig. 73-1 Pouring sterile saline into tray.

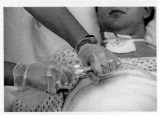

Fig. 73-2 Attaching catheter to suction.

STEP	RATIONALE
(2) Lightly coat distal 6 to 8 cm (2 to 3 inches) of catheter with water-soluble lubricant.	Lubricates catheter for easier insertion.
(3) Remove oxygen delivery device, if applicable, with nondominant hand. Without applying suction and using dominant thumb and forefinger, gently but quickly insert catheter into naris. Instruct patient to deep breathe and insert catheter following natural course of naris. Slightly slant the catheter downward or through mouth. Do not force through naris (Fig. 73-3).	Application of suction pressure while introducing catheter into trachea increases risk for damage to mucosa and increases risk for hypoxia. Passing catheter during inhalation improves likelihood of entering trachea.
(a) *Nasopharyngeal* (without applying suction): In adults, insert catheter about 16 cm (6.4	Ensures that catheter tip reaches pharynx for suctioning.

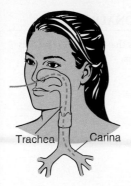

Fig. 73-3 Pathway for nasotracheal catheter progression.

Trachea Carina

STEP	RATIONALE
inches); in older children, 8 to 12 cm (3 to 5 inches); in infants and young children, 4 to 7.5 cm (1.6 to 3 inches). Rule of thumb is to insert catheter distance from tip of nose (or mouth) to angle of mandible. Apply intermittent suction for no more than 15 seconds by placing and releasing non-dominant thumb over catheter vent. Slowly withdraw catheter while rotating it back and forth between thumb and forefinger.	Intermittent suction removes pharyngeal secretions.

STEP	RATIONALE
(b) *Nasotracheal* (without applying suction): In adults, insert catheter about 20 cm (8 inches); in older children, about 16 to 20 cm (6 to 8 inches); and in young children and infants, 8 to 14 cm (3 to 5½ inches).	Ensures that catheter tip reaches trachea.

SAFETY ALERT When there is difficulty passing the catheter, ask patient to cough or say "ahh" or try to advance the catheter during inspiration. Both measures help to open the glottis to permit passage of the catheter into the trachea.

Apply intermittent or continuous suction for no more than 10 seconds by placing nondominant thumb over vent of catheter and slowly withdrawing catheter while rotating it back and forth between dominant thumb and forefinger. Encourage patient to cough. Replace oxygen device, if applicable, and have patient deep breathe.	Both intermittent and continuous suction can cause tracheal tissue damage (Lynn-McHale Wiegand, 2011; Pedersen et al., 2009). Suctioning longer than 10 seconds causes cardiopulmonary compromise, usually from hypoxemia or vagal overload (AARC, 2010).

STEP	RATIONALE
(4) Positioning: In some instances turning patient's head helps you suction more effectively. If you feel resistance after insertion of catheter, use caution; it has probably hit carina. Pull catheter back 1 to 2 cm (0.4 to 0.8 inch) before applying suction (AARC, 2004).	Turning the patient's head to side elevates bronchial passage on opposite side. Turning head to right helps with suctioning of left main-stem bronchus; turning head to left helps you suction right main-stem bronchus. Suctioning too deep may cause tracheal mucosa trauma.

SAFETY ALERT Monitor patient's vital signs and oxygen saturation throughout suction procedure. If the patient's pulse rate drops more than 20 beats/min or increases more than 40 beats/min, or if SpO_2 falls below 90% or 5% from baseline, stop suctioning.

STEP	RATIONALE
(5) Rinse catheter and connecting tubing with normal saline or water until cleared.	Secretions that remain in suction catheter or connecting tubing decrease suctioning efficiency.
(6) Assess for need to repeat suctioning procedure. Do not perform more than two passes with catheter. Observe for alterations in cardiopulmonary status. When possible, allow adequate time (at least 1 minute) between suction passes for ventilation and oxygenation. Encourage patient to deep breathe with oxygen mask in place (if ordered) and cough.	Suctioning can induce hypoxemia, dysrhythmias, laryngospasm, and bronchospasm. Deep breathing ventilates and reoxygenates alveoli. Repeated passes clear airway of excessive secretions but can also remove oxygen and may induce laryngospasm (Higgins, 2009a).

STEP	RATIONALE
b Artificial airway suctioning:	
(1) Hyperoxygenate patient with 100% oxygen for 30 to 60 seconds before suctioning by adjusting fractional inspired oxygen (FiO$_2$) setting on a mechanical ventilator or using an oxygen-enrichment program on microprocessor ventilators (AARC, 2010). Manual ventilation of a patient is not recommended; it is ineffective for providing FiO$_2$ of 1.0 (AARC, 2010).	Preoxygenation converts large proportion of resident lung gas to 100% oxygen to offset amount used in metabolic consumption while ventilation or oxygenation is interrupted and volume is lost during suctioning (Lewis et al., 2011; Pedersen et al., 2009).
(2) If patient is receiving mechanical ventilation, open swivel adapter, or, if necessary, remove oxygen or humidity delivery device with nondominant hand.	Exposes artificial airway.
(3) Without applying suction, gently but quickly insert catheter into artificial airway using dominant thumb and forefinger (it is best to try to time catheter insertion into the artificial airway with inspiration) until you meet resistance or patient coughs; then	Application of suction pressure while introducing catheter into trachea increases risk for damage to tracheal mucosa and increased hypoxia. Pulling back stimulates cough and removes catheter from mucosal wall so catheter is not resting against tracheal mucosa during suctioning. Shallow suctioning is recommended to prevent tracheal mucosa trauma (AARC, 2010).

STEP	RATIONALE
pull back 1 cm (0.4 inch) (Pedersen et al., 2009).	
(4) Apply continuous suction by placing nondominant thumb over vent of catheter; slowly withdraw catheter while rotating it back and forth between dominant thumb and forefinger (Fig. 73-4). Encourage patient to cough. Watch for respiratory distress.	Continuous suction and rotation of catheter are recommended because studies show that tracheal tissue damage from intermittent and continuous suctioning is similar (Pedersen et al., 2009). If catheter "grabs" mucosa, remove thumb to release suction.
(5) If patient is receiving mechanical ventilation, close swivel adapter, or replace oxygen delivery device.	Reestablishes artificial airway.
(6) Encourage patient to deep breathe, if able. Hyperoxygenate for at least 1 minute following same technique used to preoxygenate (AARC, 2010).	Reoxygenates and reexpands alveoli. Suctioning causes hypoxemia and atelectasis. Hyperventilation should not be used routinely (AARC, 2010).

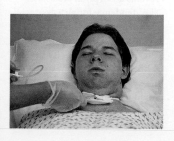

Fig. 73-4 Suctioning tracheostomy.

STEP	RATIONALE
(7) Rinse catheter and connecting tubing with normal saline until clear. Use continuous suction.	Removes catheter secretions. Secretions left in tubing decrease suctioning efficiency and provide environment for microorganism growth.
(8) Assess patient's vital signs, cardiopulmonary status, and ventilator measurements for secretion clearance. Repeat Steps (1) to (7) once or twice more to clear secretions. Allow adequate time (at least 1 full minute) between suction passes.	Suctioning can induce dysrhythmias, hypoxia, and bronchospasm and impair cerebral circulation or adversely affect hemodynamic stability (Higgins, 2009a).
(9) When pharynx and trachea are sufficiently cleared of secretions, perform oropharyngeal suctioning to clear mouth of secretions. Do not suction nose again after suctioning mouth.	Removes upper airway secretions. More microorganisms are generally present in mouth. Upper airway is considered "clean" and lower airway is considered "sterile." You can use the same catheter to suction from sterile to clean areas (e.g., tracheal suctioning to oropharyngeal suctioning) but not from clean to sterile areas.
15 Complete postprocedure protocol.	
16 If indicated, readjust oxygen to original level because patient's blood oxygen level should have returned to baseline.	Prevents absorption atelectasis (i.e., tendency for airways to collapse if proximally obstructed by secretions). Prevents oxygen toxicity while allowing patient time to reoxygenate blood.
17 Place unopened suction kit on suction machine table or at head of bed.	Provides immediate access to suction catheter for next procedure.

STEP	RATIONALE
18 Ask patient if breathing is easier and if congestion is decreased.	Provides subjective confirmation that suctioning procedure has relieved airway.

Recording and Reporting

- Record the amount, consistency, color, and odor of secretions; size of catheter and route of suctioning; and patient's response to suctioning.
- Document patient's presuctioning and postsuctioning vital signs, cardiopulmonary status, and ventilation measures.

UNEXPECTED OUTCOMES	RELATED INTERVENTIONS
1 Patient's respiratory status does not improve.	• Limit length of suctioning. • Determine need for more frequent suctioning, possibly of shorter duration. • Determine need for supplemental oxygen. Supply oxygen between suctioning passes. • Notify health care provider.
2 Bloody secretions are returned after suctioning.	• Determine amount of suction pressure used. May need to be decreased. • Ensure suction completed correctly using proper suction technique and catheter rotation. • Evaluate suctioning frequency. • Provide more frequent oral hygiene.
3 Unable to pass suction catheter through naris at first attempt.	• Try other naris or oral route. • Increase lubrication of catheter. • Insert nasal airway, especially if suctioning through patient's nares frequently.

Continued

UNEXPECTED OUTCOMES	RELATED INTERVENTIONS
	• If obstruction is mucus, apply suction to relieve obstruction but not to mucosa. If you think obstruction is a blood clot, consult with health care provider.
4 Patient has paroxysms of coughing.	• Administer supplemental oxygen.
	• Allow patient to rest between passes of suction catheter.
	• Consult with physician regarding need for inhaled bronchodilators or topical anesthetics.
5 No secretions obtained during suctioning.	• Evaluate patient's fluid status and adequacy of humidification on oxygen delivery device.
	• Assess for signs of infection. Determine need for chest physiotherapy.

Suprapubic Catheter Care

A suprapubic catheter is a urinary drainage tube inserted surgically into the bladder through the abdominal wall above the symphysis pubis. The catheter may be sutured to the skin, secured with an adhesive material, or retained in the bladder with a fluid-filled balloon similar to an indwelling catheter. Suprapubic catheters are placed when there is blockage of the urethra (e.g., enlarged prostate, urethral stricture, after urological surgery) and in situations when a long-term urethral catheter causes irritation or discomfort or interferes with sexual functioning.

Delegation and Collaboration

The skill of caring for a newly established suprapubic catheter cannot be delegated to nursing assistive personnel (NAP); however, care of an established suprapubic catheter may be delegated (refer to agency policy). The nurse directs the NAP to:

- Report patient's discomfort related to the suprapubic catheter.
- Empty drainage bag and document urinary output on intake and output (I&O) record.
- Report any change in the amount and character of the urine.
- Report any signs of redness, foul odor, or drainage around catheter insertion site.

Equipment

- Clean gloves (sterile may be needed in some cases, see agency policy)
- Cleaning agent (sterile normal saline solution)
- Sterile cotton-tipped applicators
- Sterile surgical drainage gauze (split gauze)
- Sterile gauze dressing
- Washcloth, towel, soap, and water
- Tape
- Velcro tube holder or tube stabilizer (optional)

Implementation

STEP	RATIONALE
1 Complete preprocedure protocol	

STEP	RATIONALE
2 Assess urine in drainage bag for amount, clarity, color, odor, and sediment.	Abnormal findings indicate potential complications such as urinary tract infection (UTI), decreased urinary output, and catheter occlusion.
3 Observe dressing for drainage and intactness.	Drainage indicates potential complication such as infection. Dressing may become nonocclusive because of tape choice or drainage.
4 Assess catheter insertion site (may be deferred until you clean site) for signs of inflammation (i.e., pain, erythema, edema, and drainage) and for the growth of over-granulation tissue. Ask patient if there is any pain at site; if so, have him or her rate on scale of 0 to 10.	If insertion is new, slight inflammation may be expected as part of normal wound healing but can also indicate infection. Over-granulation tissue can develop at insertion site as reaction to catheter. In some instances intervention may be needed (Rigby, 2009).
5 Explain procedure to patient.	Reduces anxiety and promotes cooperation.
6 ⬧ Perform hand hygiene. Apply clean gloves. Loosen tape and remove existing dressing. Note type and presence of drainage. Remove gloves and perform hand hygiene.	Provides baseline for condition of suprapubic wound. Reduces transmission of infection from dressing.
7 Clean insertion site using sterile aseptic technique for newly established catheter (option used less frequently; review agency policy or consider individual patient need).	Catheter site is made surgically and therefore is treated similarly to other incisions, using either aseptic or sterile technique as designated by agency policy.
a **Apply sterile gloves.**	
b Without creating tension, hold catheter up with nondominant hand while cleaning. Use	Moves from area of least contamination to area of most contamination. Tension on catheter may cause discomfort

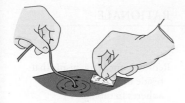

Fig. 74-1 Cleaning around suprapubic catheter in circular pattern.

STEP	RATIONALE
sterile gauze moistened in saline, and clean skin around insertion site in circular motion, starting near insertion site and continuing in outward widening circles for approximately 5 cm (2 inches) (Fig. 74-1).	or damage to wall of bladder or catheter to slip out of place.
c With fresh, moistened gauze, gently clean base of catheter, moving up and away from site of insertion (proximal to distal).	Removes microorganisms that reside on any drainage that adheres to tubing.
d Once insertion site is dry, use sterile gloved hand to apply drain dressing (split gauze) around catheter. Tape in place.	Collects drainage that develops around catheter insertion site.
8 Clean using medical aseptic technique for new or established catheter:	
a ✋ Apply clean gloves.	
b Without creating tension, hold catheter up with nondominant hand while cleaning. Clean with soap and water in circular motion, starting near catheter insertion site and continuing in outward widening circles	Cleansing and drying suprapubic insertion site requires general hygienic measures; dressing is an option if drainage is not present (Newman and Wein, 2009).

STEP	RATIONALE
for approximately 5 cm (2 inches).	
c With a fresh washcloth or gauze, gently clean base of catheter, moving up and away from site of insertion (proximal to distal).	Removes microorganisms that reside in any drainage that adheres to tubing.
d *Option:* Apply drain dressing (split gauze) around catheter and tape in place.	
9 Secure catheter to lateral abdomen with tape or Velcro multipurpose tube holder.	Secures catheter and reduces risk of excessive tension on suture and/or catheter.
10 Coil excess tubing on bed. Keep drainage bag below level of bladder at all times.	Maintains free flow of urine, thus decreasing risk for catheter-associated urinary tract infection (CAUTI) (Gould et al., 2009).
11 Complete postprocedure protocol.	

Recording and Reporting

- Record and report character of urine and type of dressing change, including assessments of insertion site and patient's comfort level with the catheter and dressing change, in nurses' notes and electronic health record (EHR).
- Record urine output on I&O flow sheet. When there is both a suprapubic and a urethral catheter, record outputs from each catheter separately.

UNEXPECTED OUTCOMES	RELATED INTERVENTIONS
1 Patient develops symptoms of UTI or catheter site infection.	• Increase fluid intake to at least 2200 mL in 24 hours (unless contraindicated). • Monitor vital signs, I&O; observe amount, color, consistency of urine; assess site. • Notify health care provider.

UNEXPECTED OUTCOMES	RELATED INTERVENTIONS
2 Urine leaks around catheter.	• Check catheter and drainage tubing for kinks or other causes of occlusion. • Monitor vital signs; assess urine for signs of infection. • Change dressing frequently; protect skin from moisture. • Notify health care provider.
3 Suprapubic catheter becomes dislodged.	• Cover site with sterile dressing. • Notify health care provider. If newly established catheter, it will need to be reinserted immediately.
4 Skin surrounding catheter exit site becomes red or irritated and/or develops open areas.	• Notify health care provider. • Change dressing (if used) more frequently to keep site dry. • Consult with wound care nurse.

Suture and Staple Removal

Sutures and staples are removed generally within 7 to 14 days after surgery if healing is adequate (Whitney, 2012). Retention sutures usually remain in place 14 to 21 days. Timing the removal of sutures and staples is important. They must remain in place long enough to ensure that the initial wound closure has enough strength to support internal tissues and organs. Sutures retained longer than 14 days generally leave suture marks (Whitney, 2012). The health care provider determines and orders removal of all sutures or staples at one time or removal of every other suture or staple as the first phase, with the remainder removed in the second phase.

Delegation Considerations

The skill of staple and/or suture removal cannot be delegated to nursing assistive personnel (NAP). The nurse directs NAP by:

- Instructing to report to the nurse drainage, bleeding, swelling at the site, or an elevation in patient's temperature.
- Instructing to report to the nurse patient's complaints of pain.
- Providing information about any special hygiene practices following suture removal.

Equipment

- Disposable waterproof bag
- Sterile suture removal set (forceps and scissors) or sterile staple extractor
- Sterile applicators or antiseptic swabs
- Steri-Strips or butterfly adhesive strips
- Clean gloves
- Sterile gloves

Implementation

STEP	RATIONALE
1 Complete preprocedure protocol.	
2 Identify patient with need for suture or staple removal:	
a Check health care provider's order.	Health care provider's order is required for removal of sutures.

STEP	RATIONALE
b Review specific directions related to suture or staple removal.	Indicates specifically which sutures are to be removed (e.g., every other suture).
c Determine history of conditions that may pose risk for impaired wound healing: advanced age, cardiovascular disease, diabetes, immunosuppression, radiation, obesity, smoking, poor cellular nutrition, very deep wounds, and infection.	Preexisting health disorders affect speed of healing and sometimes result in dehiscence.
3 Assess patient for history of allergies.	Determines if patient is sensitive to antiseptic or latex.
4 Assess patient's comfort level or pain on a scale of 0 to 10.	Provides baseline of patient's comfort level to determine response to therapy.
5 Assess healing ridge and skin integrity of suture line for uniform closure of wound edges, normal color, and absence of drainage and inflammation.	Indicates adequate wound healing for support of internal structures without continued need for sutures or staples.

SAFETY ALERT If wound edges are separated or signs of infection are present, the wound has not healed properly. Notify the health care provider because sutures or staples may need to remain in place and/or other wound care may need to be initiated.

STEP	RATIONALE
6 Place cuffed waterproof disposal bag within easy reach.	Provides for easy disposal of contaminated dressings and prevents passing items over sterile work area.
7 Prepare materials needed for suture/staple removal: a Open sterile suture removal kit or staple extractor kit.	

STEP	RATIONALE
b Open sterile antiseptic swabs and place on inside surface of kit.	
c Obtain gloves (sterile gloves if policy indicates).	
8 🖐 Perform hand hygiene. Apply clean or sterile gloves as required by agency policy.	Reduces transmission of infection.
9 Clean sutures or staples and healed incision with antiseptic swabs.	Removes surface bacteria from incision and sutures or staples.
10 Remove staples:	
a Place lower tips of staple extractor under first staple. As you close handles, upper tip of extractor depresses center of staple, causing both ends of staple to be bent upward and simultaneously exit their insertion sites in the dermal layer (Fig. 75-1).	Avoids excess pressure to suture line and secures smooth removal of each staple.
b Carefully control staple extractor.	Avoids suture-line pressure and pain.
c As soon as both ends of staple are visible, move it away from skin surface, and continue until staple is over refuse bag (Fig. 75-2).	Prevents scratching tender skin surface with sharp points of staple, promoting comfort and infection control.
d Release handles of staple extractor, allowing staple to drop into refuse bag.	Avoids contaminating sterile field with used staples.
e Repeat Steps a to d until all staples are removed.	
11 Remove intermittent sutures (Fig. 75-3):	
a Place gauze a few inches from suture line. Hold scissors in dominant hand and forceps (clamp) in nondominant hand.	Gauze serves as receptacle for removed sutures. Placement of scissors and forceps allows for efficient suture removal.

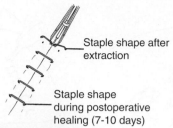

Staple shape after extraction

Staple shape during postoperative healing (7-10 days)

Fig. 75-1 Staple extractor placed under staple.

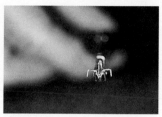

Fig. 75-2 Metal staple removed by extractor.

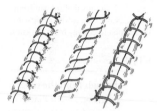

Fig. 75-3 Types of sutures. *Left*, Intermittent; *middle*, continuous; *right*, blanket.

STEP	RATIONALE

SAFETY ALERT Placement of scissors and forceps is very important. Avoid pinching the skin around the wound when lifting up the suture. Likewise, avoid cutting the skin around the wound by accident when snipping the suture.

b Grasp knot of suture with forceps, and gently pull up knot while slipping tip of scissors under suture near skin (Fig. 75-4).	Releases suture.
c Snip suture as close to the skin as possible at end distal to the knot.	

SAFETY ALERT Never snip both ends of suture; there will be no way to remove the part of the suture situated below the surface.

d Grasp knotted end with forceps, and in one continuous smooth action pull the suture	Smoothly removes suture without additional tension to suture line.

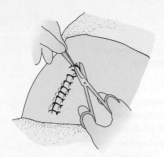

Fig. 75-4 Removal of intermittent suture. Nurse cuts suture as close to skin as possible, away from the knot.

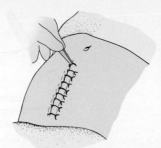

Fig. 75-5 Nurse removes suture and never pulls the contaminated stitch through tissues.

STEP	RATIONALE
through from the other side (Fig. 75-5). Place removed suture on gauze.	
e Repeat Steps a through d until you have removed every other suture.	
f Observe healing level. Based on observations of wound response to suture removal and health care provider's original order, determine whether remaining sutures will be removed at this time. If so, repeat Steps a to d until you have removed all sutures.	Determines status of wound healing and if suture line will remain closed after all sutures are removed.
g If any doubt, stop and notify health care provider.	
12 Remove continuous and blanket stitch sutures:	
a Place sterile gauze a few inches from suture line. Grasp scissors in dominant hand and forceps in nondominant hand.	Gauze serves as receptacle for removed sutures. Placement of scissors and forceps allows for efficient suture removal.

STEP	RATIONALE
b Snip first suture close to skin surface at end distal to knot.	Releases suture.
c Snip second suture on same side.	Releases interrupted sutures from knot.
d Grasp knotted end, and gently pull with continuous smooth action, removing suture from beneath the skin. Place suture on gauze compress.	Smoothly removes sutures without additional tension to suture line. Prevents pulling of contaminated portion of suture through the skin.
e Repeat Steps a through d in consecutive order until the entire line is removed.	
13 Inspect incision site to make sure that all sutures are removed, and identify any trouble areas. Gently wipe suture line with antiseptic swab to remove debris and cleanse wound.	Reduces risk for further incision line separation.
14 Apply Steri-Strips if *any* separation greater than two stitches or two staples in width is apparent to maintain contact between wound edges.	Supports wound by distributing tension across wound and eliminates closure technique scarring.
a Cut Steri-Strips to allow strips to extend 4 to 5 cm (1½ to 2 inches) on each side of the incision.	
b Remove from backing and apply across incision.	
c Instruct patient to take showers rather than soak in bathtub according to health care provider's preference.	Steri-Strips are not removed and are allowed to fall off gradually.
15 Apply light dressing or expose to air if no clothing	Healing by primary intention eliminates need for dressing.

STEP	RATIONALE
will come in contact with suture line. Instruct patient about applying own dressing if it will be needed at home.	
16 Complete postprocedure protocol.	

Recording and Reporting

- Record the time the sutures or staples were removed and the number of sutures or staples removed. Also document the cleansing of the suture line, appearance of the wound, level of healing of the wound, and type of dressing applied. Document patient's response to suture or staple removal.
- Immediately report to health care provider if suture line separation, dehiscence, evisceration, bleeding, or purulent drainage occurs.

UNEXPECTED OUTCOMES	RELATED INTERVENTIONS
1 Retained suture is present.	• Notify health care provider. • Instruct patient to notify health care provider if signs of suture line infection develop following discharge from agency.
2 Patient experiences wound separation or drainage secondary to healing problems.	• Leave remaining sutures or staples in place. • Place supportive butterfly closures across suture line. • Notify health care provider.

Topical Skin Applications

Topical administration of medication involves applying drugs locally to the skin, mucous membranes, or tissues. Topical drugs such as lotions, patches, pastes, and ointments primarily produce local effects; but they can create systemic effects if absorbed through the skin. To protect from accidental exposure, apply topical drugs using gloves and applicators. Always clean the skin or wound thoroughly before applying a new dose of a topical medication. Apply each type of medication, whether an ointment, lotion, powder, or patch, in a specific way to ensure proper penetration and absorption.

Delegation Considerations

The skill of administering topical medications cannot be delegated to nursing assistive personnel (NAP). However, some agencies (e.g., long-term care) may allow NAP to apply some forms of topical agents (e.g., skin barriers) to irritated skin or for the protection of the perineum during morning or perineal care. Check agency policies. The nurse directs NAP about:

- The expected therapeutic effects and potential side effects of medications and the importance of reporting their occurrence.

Equipment

- Clean gloves (for intact skin) or sterile gloves (for nonintact skin)
- *Option:* Cotton-tipped applicators or tongue blades.
- Ordered medication (powder, cream, lotion, ointment, spray, patch)
- Basin of warm water, washcloth, towel, nondrying soap
- *Option:* Sterile dressing, tape
- Felt-tip pen
- Medication administration record (MAR) or computer printout
- *Option:* Plastic wrap, transparent dressing

Implementation

STEP	RATIONALE
1 Complete preprocedure protocol.	
2 Check accuracy and completeness of each medication administration record (MAR) with health	The health care provider's order is the most reliable source and only legal record of drugs that the patient should receive.

STEP	RATIONALE
care provider's medication order. Check patient's name, drug name and dosage, route of administration, and time for administration. Clarify incomplete or unclear orders with health care provider before administration.	Ensures patient receives correct medication. Handwritten MARs are a source of medication errors (ISMP, 2010; Jones and Treiber, 2010).
3 Assess condition of skin or membrane where medication is to be applied. If there is an open wound, perform hand hygiene and apply clean gloves. First wash site thoroughly with mild, nondrying soap and warm water; then rinse and dry. Also remove any blood, body fluids, secretions, or excretions. Assess for symptoms of skin irritation such as pruritus or burning. Remove gloves when finished.	Cleaning site thoroughly promotes a proper assessment of skin surface. Assessment provides baseline to determine change in condition of skin after therapy. Application of certain topical agents can lessen or aggravate these symptoms.
4 Determine amount of topical agent required for application by assessing skin site, reviewing health care provider's order, and reading application directions carefully (a thin, even layer is usually adequate).	An excessive amount of topical agent can chemically irritate skin, negate effectiveness of drug, and/or cause adverse systemic effects such as decreased white blood cell (WBC) counts.
5 Perform hand hygiene. If skin is broken (e.g., wound), apply sterile gloves. Otherwise apply clean gloves.	Reduces transmission of microorganisms.
6 Apply topical creams, ointments, and oil-based lotions.	

STEP	RATIONALE
a Expose affected area while keeping unaffected areas covered.	Provides visualization for application and protects privacy.
b Wash, rinse, and dry affected area before applying medication.	Cleaning removes microorganisms from remaining debris.
c If skin is excessively dry and flaking, apply topical agent while skin is still damp.	Retains moisture within skin layers.
d ✋ Remove gloves, perform hand hygiene, and apply new clean or sterile gloves.	Sterile gloves are used when applying agents to open, noninfectious skin lesions. Changing gloves prevents cross-contamination of infected or contagious lesions and protects you from drug effects.
e Place required amount of medication in palm of gloved hand and soften by rubbing briskly between hands.	Softening of topical agent makes it easier to spread on skin.
f Tell patient that initial application of agent may feel cold. Once medication is softened, spread it evenly over skin surface, using long, even strokes that follow direction of hair growth. Do not vigorously rub skin. Apply to the thickness specified by manufacturer's instructions.	Ensures even distribution and sufficient dosage of medication. Technique prevents irritation of hair follicles.
g Explain to patient that skin may feel greasy after application.	Ointments often contain oils.
7 **Apply antianginal (nitroglycerin) ointment.**	
a Remove previous dose paper. Fold used paper	Prevents overdose that can occur with multiple dose papers

STEP	RATIONALE
containing any residual medication with used sides together and dispose of it in biohazard trash container. Wipe off residual medication with tissue.	left in place. Proper disposal protects others from accidental exposure to medication.
b Write date, time, and nurse's initials on new application paper.	Label provides reference to prevent missing doses.
c Antianginal (nitroglycerin) ointments are usually ordered in inches and can be measured on small sheets of paper marked off in 1.25 cm ($\frac{1}{2}$ inch) markings. Unit-dose packages are available. Apply desired number of inches of ointment to paper-measuring guide (Fig. 76-1).	Ensures correct dose of medication.
d Select application: Apply nitroglycerin to chest area, back, abdomen, or anterior thigh (Lehne, 2010). Do not apply on hairy surfaces or over scar tissue.	Application on hairy surfaces or scar tissue may interfere with absorption.
e Be sure to rotate application sites.	Minimizes skin irritation.
f Apply ointment to skin surface by holding edge or back of the paper measuring guide and placing ointment and wrapper directly on skin. Do not rub or massage ointment into skin (Fig. 76-2).	Minimizes chance of ointment covering gloves and later touching nurse's hands. Medication is designed to absorb slowly over several hours; massaging increases absorption rate.

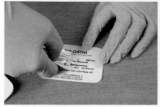

Fig. 76-1 Ointment spread in inches over measuring guide.

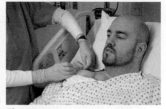

Fig. 76-2 Nurse applies wrapper with medication to patient's skin.

STEP	RATIONALE
g Secure ointment and paper with a transparent dressing or strip of tape. Plastic wrap may be used as an occlusive dressing.	Prevents staining of clothing or inadvertent removal of the medication.
8 **Apply transdermal patches (e.g., analgesic, nicotine, nitroglycerin, estrogen).**	
a If old patch is present, remove it and clean area. Be sure to check between skinfolds for patch.	Failure to remove the old patch can result in overdose. Many patches are small, clear, or flesh colored and can be easily hidden between skinfolds. Cleaning removes traces of previous patch.
b Dispose of old patch by folding in half with sticky sides together. Some agencies require patch to be cut before disposal (see agency policy). Dispose of it in biohazard trash bag.	Proper disposal prevents accidental exposure to medication.
c Date and initial outer side of new patch before applying it, and note time of administration. Use a soft-tip or felt-tip marker pen.	Visual reminder prevents missing or extra doses. Ballpoint pen damages patch and alters medication delivery.
d Choose a new site that is clean, dry, and free of hair.	Ensures complete medication absorption.

STEP	RATIONALE
Some patches have specific instructions for placement locations (e.g., Testoderm patches are placed on scrotum; a scopolamine patch is placed behind the ear; never apply an estrogen patch to breast tissue or waistline). Do not apply patch on skin that is oily, burned, cut, or irritated in any way.	

SAFETY ALERT Never apply heat, such as with a heating pad, over a transdermal patch because this results in an increased rate of absorption with potentially serious adverse effects.

e	Carefully remove the patch from its protective covering by pulling off liner. Hold the patch by the edge without touching adhesive edges.	Touching only edges ensures that the patch will adhere and that medication dose has not changed. Removing the protective covering allows the medication to be absorbed through skin.
f	Apply patch. Hold palm of one hand firmly over patch for 10 seconds. Make sure it sticks well, especially around the edges. Apply overlay if provided with patch.	Adequate adhesion prevents loss of patch, which results in decreased dose and effectiveness.
g	Do not apply to previously used sites for at least 1 week.	Rotation of sites reduces skin irritation from medication and adhesive.
h	Instruct patient that transdermal patches are never to be cut in half; a change in dose would require prescription for new strength of transdermal medication.	Cutting transdermal patch in half would alter intended medication delivery of transdermal system, resulting in inadequate or altered drug levels.

STEP	RATIONALE

SAFETY ALERT It is recommended to have a daily "patch free" interval of 10 to 12 hours because tolerance develops if patches are used 24 hours a day every day (Lehne, 2010). Apply a new patch each morning, leave in place for 12 to 14 hours, and remove in the evening.

STEP	RATIONALE
9 Administer aerosol sprays (e.g., local anesthetic sprays).	
a Shake container vigorously. Read container label for distance recommended to hold spray away from area (usually 15 to 30 cm [6 to 12 inches]).	Mixing ensures delivery of fine, even spray. Proper distance ensures that fine spray hits skin surface. Holding container too close results in thin, watery distribution.
b Ask patient to turn face away from spray or briefly cover face with towel while spraying neck or chest.	Prevents inhalation of spray.
c Spray medication evenly over affected site (in some cases, time the spray for a period of seconds).	Ensures that affected area of skin is medicated.
10 Apply suspension-based lotion.	
a Shake container vigorously.	Mixes powder throughout liquid to form well-mixed suspension.
b Apply small amount of lotion to small gauze dressing or pad, and apply to skin by stroking evenly in direction of hair growth.	Method of application leaves protective film of powder on skin after water base of suspension dries. Technique prevents irritation to hair follicles.
c Explain to patient that area will feel cool and dry.	Water evaporates to leave thin layer of powder.
11 Apply powder.	
a Be sure that skin surface is thoroughly dry. With your nondominant hand, fully spread apart any skinfolds such as between toes or under axilla and dry with towel.	Minimizes caking and crusting of powder. Fully exposes skin surface for application.

STEP	RATIONALE
b If area of application is near face, ask patient to turn face away from powder or briefly cover face with towel.	Prevents inhalation of powder.
c Dust skin site lightly with dispenser so area is covered with fine, thin layer of powder. *Option:* Cover skin area with dressing if ordered by health care provider.	Thin layer of powder has slight lubricating properties to reduce friction and promote drying (Lilley et al., 2011).
12 Complete postprocedure protocol.	

Recording and Reporting

- Record actual time each drug was administered, type and strength of agent applied, and site of application in nurses' notes and electronic health record (EHR) and on MAR immediately after administration, not before. Include initials or signature. Record patient teaching and validation of understanding in nurses' notes. If you withhold a drug, record reason in nurses' notes and follow agency policy for noting withheld doses.
- Describe condition of skin before each application in nurses' notes and EHR.
- Report adverse effects, patient response, and/or withheld drugs to nurse in charge or health care provider. Depending on medication, immediate notification of health care provider may be required.

UNEXPECTED OUTCOMES	RELATED INTERVENTIONS
1 Skin site appears inflamed and edematous with blistering and oozing of fluid from lesions.	• Hold medication. • Notify health care provider; alternative therapies may be needed.
2 Patient is unable to explain information about drug or does not administer as prescribed.	• Identify possible reasons for noncompliance and explore alternative approaches or options.

Tracheostomy Care

A tracheostomy is a 51- to 76-mm (2- to 3-inch) curved metal or plastic tube inserted into a stoma through the neck and into the trachea to maintain a patent airway. Some patients with a tracheostomy tube are able to cough secretions out of the tube completely, whereas others are only able to cough secretions up into it. Standards for care include properly securing the tube, inflating the cuff to an appropriate pressure, maintaining patency by suctioning, and providing oral hygiene. A tracheostomy tube can cause granulation tissue to form on the vocal cords, epiglottis, or trachea secondary to inappropriate cuff inflation.

Delegation Considerations

The skill of performing tracheostomy care is not routinely delegated to nursing assistive personnel (NAP). In some settings, patients who have well-established tracheostomy tubes may have the care delegated to an NAP. The nurse is responsible for assessing a patient and evaluating for proper artificial airway care. The nurse directs the NAP to:

- Immediately report any changes in patient's respiratory status, level of consciousness, confusion, restlessness, irritability, or level of comfort.
- Immediately report any dislodgment or excessive movement of the tracheostomy tube.
- Immediately report abnormal color of tracheal stoma and drainage.

Equipment

- Bedside table
- Towel
- Tracheostomy suction supplies
- Sterile tracheostomy care kit, if available (be sure to collect supplies listed that are not available in kit), or two sterile 4 × 4–inch gauze pads
- Sterile cotton-tipped applicators
- Sterile tracheostomy dressing (precut and sewn surgical dressing)
- Sterile basin
- Small sterile brush (pipe cleaner) (or disposable inner cannula)
- Roll of twill tape, tracheostomy ties, or tracheostomy holder
- Scissors
- Pulse oximeter
- Clean gloves (two pair)
- Mask, goggles, or face shield

Implementation

STEP	RATIONALE
1 Complete preprocedure protocol.	
2 Observe for excess peristomal secretions, excess intratracheal secretions, soiled or damp tracheostomy ties, soiled or damp tracheostomy dressing, diminished airflow through tracheostomy tube, or signs and symptoms of airway obstruction requiring suctioning.	Indicate need for tracheostomy care caused by presence of secretions at stoma site or within tracheostomy tube.
3 ✋ Perform hand hygiene, and apply clean gloves and face shield if applicable.	Reduces transmission of microorganisms.
4 Apply pulse oximeter sensor.	Provides monitoring for oxygen desaturation during procedure.
5 Suction tracheostomy (see Skill 73). Before removing gloves, remove soiled tracheostomy dressing, and discard in glove with coiled catheter.	Removes secretions to avoid occluding outer cannula while inner cannula is removed. Reduces need for patient to cough.
6 Perform hand hygiene. Prepare equipment on bedside table.	Allows for smooth, organized completion of tracheostomy care.
a Open sterile tracheostomy kit. Open two 4 × 4–inch gauze packages using aseptic technique, and pour normal saline on one package. Leave second package dry. Open two cotton-tipped swab packages, and pour normal saline on one package. Do not recap normal saline.	

STEP	RATIONALE
b Open sterile tracheostomy dressing package.	
c Unwrap sterile basin, and pour about 1 to 2 cm ($\frac{1}{2}$ to 1 inch) of normal saline into it.	
d Open small sterile brush package, and place aseptically into sterile basin.	
e Prepare length of twill tape long enough to encircle patient's neck 2 times, about 60 to 75 cm (24 to 30 inches) for an adult. Cut ends on diagonal. Lay aside in dry area.	Cutting ends of tie on diagonal aids in inserting tie through eyelet.
f If using commercially available tracheostomy tube holder, open package according to manufacturer's directions.	
7 Hyperoxygenate patient's lungs using ventilator setting or by applying oxygen source loosely over tracheostomy.	Required if patient has oxygen saturation levels less than 92% (Higgins, 2009b). Helps to reduce amount of oxygen desaturation.
8 **Apply sterile gloves.** Keep dominant hand sterile throughout procedure.	Reduces transmission of microorganisms.
9 Care of tracheostomy with inner cannula:	
a While touching only the outer aspect of tube, unlock and remove inner cannula with nondominant hand. Drop inner cannula into normal saline basin.	Removes inner cannula for cleaning. Normal saline loosens secretions from inner cannula.

STEP	RATIONALE
b Place tracheostomy collar, T tube, or ventilator oxygen source over outer cannula. (**NOTE:** May not be able to attach T tube and ventilator oxygen devices to all outer cannulas when the inner cannula is removed.)	Maintains supply of oxygen to patient as needed.
c To prevent oxygen desaturation in affected patients, quickly pick up inner cannula and use small brush to remove secretions inside and outside inner cannula.	Tracheostomy brush provides mechanical force to remove thick or dried secretions.
d Hold inner cannula over basin, and rinse with normal saline, using nondominant hand to pour normal saline.	Removes secretions and normal saline from inner cannula.
e Replace inner cannula, and secure "locking" mechanism (Fig. 77-1). Reapply ventilator after hyperventilating the patient's lungs if needed.	Secures inner cannula and reestablishes oxygen supply.
10 Tracheostomy with disposable inner cannula:	
a Remove new cannula from manufacturer's packaging.	

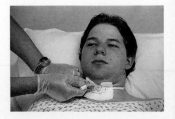

Fig. 77-1 Reinserting the inner cannula.

STEP	RATIONALE
b While touching only the outer aspect of the tube, withdraw inner cannula, and replace with new cannula. Lock into position.	
c Dispose of contaminated cannula in appropriate receptacle, and reconnect to ventilator or oxygen supply.	Prevents transmission of infection. Restores oxygen delivery.
11 Using normal saline–saturated cotton-tipped swabs and 4 × 4–inch gauze, clean exposed outer cannula surfaces and stoma under faceplate extending 5 to 10 cm (2 to 4 inches) in all directions from stoma. Clean in circular motion from stoma site outward using dominant hand to handle sterile supplies.	Aseptically removes secretions from stoma site. Moving in outward circle pulls mucus and other contaminants from stoma to periphery.
12 Using dry 4 × 4–inch gauze, pat lightly at skin and exposed outer cannula surfaces.	Dry surfaces prohibit formation of moist environment for microorganism growth and skin excoriation (Higgins, 2009b).
13 Secure tracheostomy.	
a Tracheostomy tie method:	
(1) Instruct assistant, if available, to apply gloves and securely hold tracheostomy tube in place. With assistant holding tracheostomy tube, cut old ties.	Promotes hygiene and reduces transmission of microorganisms. Secures tracheostomy tube. Reduces risk for incidental extubation.

SAFETY ALERT Assistant must not release hold on tracheostomy tube until new ties are firmly tied. If working without an assistant, do not cut old ties until new ties are in place and securely tied (Lewis et al., 2011).

STEP	RATIONALE
(2) Take prepared tie, insert one end of tie through faceplate eyelet, and pull ends even (Fig. 77-2).	
(3) Slide both ends of tie behind the head and around neck to other eyelet, and insert one tie through second eyelet.	
(4) Pull snugly.	Secures tracheostomy tube.
(5) Tie ends securely in double square knot, allowing space for only one loose or two snug finger widths in tie.	One finger width of slack prevents ties from being too tight when tracheostomy dressing is in place and also prevents movement of tracheostomy tube in lower airway (Frace, 2010).
(6) Insert fresh 4 × 4–inch tracheostomy dressing under clean ties and faceplate.	Absorbs drainage. Dressing prevents pressure on clavicle heads (Frace, 2010; Regan and Dallachiesa, 2009).
b **Tracheostomy tube holder method:**	
(1) While wearing gloves, maintain secure hold on the tracheostomy tube. This can be done with an assistant or, when an assistant is not available, by leaving the old tracheostomy tube holder in place until the new device is **secure.**	Prevents incidental dislodgment of tube.
(2) Align strap under patient's neck. Be sure that the Velcro attachments are on	

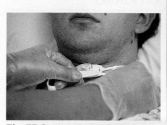

Fig. 77-2 Replacing tracheostomy tube ties. Do not remove old tracheostomy tube ties until new ones are secure.

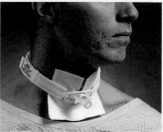

Fig. 77-3 Tracheostomy tube holder in place. (Courtesy Dale Medical Products, Plainesville, Mass.)

STEP	RATIONALE
either side of the tracheostomy tube.	
(3) Place narrow end of ties under and through the faceplate eyelets. Pull ends even, and secure with the Velcro closures.	
(4) Verify that there is space for only one loose or two snug finger widths under neck strap (Fig. 77-3).	
14 Position patient comfortably, and assess respiratory status.	Promotes comfort. Some patients require post–tracheostomy care suctioning.
15 Be sure that oxygen or humidification delivery sources are in place and set at correct levels.	Humidification provides moisture for airway, makes it easier to suction secretions, and decreases risk of mucus plugs (Frace, 2010; Regan and Dallachiesa, 2009).
16 Assess fit of new tracheostomy ties and ask patient if tube feels comfortable.	Tracheostomy ties are uncomfortable and place patient at risk for injury when they are too loose or too tight.

STEP	RATIONALE
17 Inspect inner and outer cannulas for secretions.	Presence of secretions on cannulas indicates need for more frequent tracheostomy care.
18 Assess stoma for signs of inflammation, edema, or discolored secretions.	Broken skin places patient at risk for infection. Stoma infection necessitates change in tracheostomy skin care plan.
19 Complete postprocedure protocol.	

Recording and Reporting

- Record respiratory assessments before and after care; type and size of tracheostomy tube; frequency and extent of care; type, color, and amount of secretions; patient tolerance and understanding of procedure; and special care in event of unexpected outcomes.
- Report accidental decannulation or respiratory distress to the health care provider.

UNEXPECTED OUTCOMES	RELATED INTERVENTIONS
1 Excessively loose or tight tracheostomy ties/ tracheostomy holder.	• Adjust ties, or apply new ties/tracheostomy holder.
2 Inflammation of the tracheostomy stoma.	• Increase frequency of tracheostomy care. • Apply topical antibacterial solution, and allow it to dry and provide bacterial barrier. • Apply hydrocolloid or transparent dressing just under stoma to protect skin from breakdown. Consult with skin care specialist.
3 Pressure area around tracheostomy tube.	• Increase frequency of tracheostomy care, and keep dressing under faceplate at all times. • Consider using double dressing or applying

UNEXPECTED OUTCOMES	RELATED INTERVENTIONS
	hydrocolloid or stoma adhesive dressing around stoma.
4 Accidental decannulation.	• Call for assistance.
	• Replace old tracheostomy tube with new tube. Some experienced nurses or respiratory therapists may be able to quickly reinsert tracheostomy tube.
	• Keep spare tracheostomy tube of same size and kind at bedside in event of emergency replacement (Weber-Jones, 2010).
	• Same-size endotracheal (ET) tube can be inserted in stoma in an emergency.
	• Insert suction catheter to confirm that the new tube is in the trachea.
	• Be prepared to manually ventilate lungs of patients in whom respiratory distress develops with Ambu bag until tracheostomy is replaced.
	• Notify health care provider.
5 Respiratory distress from mucous plug in cannula.	• Remove inner cannula, if applicable, for cleaning, or suction cannula.
	• Notify health care provider if tracheostomy tube requires replacement (Weber-Jones, 2010).

Urinary Catheter Insertion

Urinary catheterization is the placement of a tube through the urethra into the bladder to drain urine. This is an invasive procedure that requires a medical order and aseptic technique in institutional settings (Gould et al., 2009; Lo et al., 2008). Urinary catheterization may be short term (2 weeks or less) or long term (more than 1 month) (Parker et al., 2009). The steps for inserting an indwelling and a single-use straight/intermittent catheter are the same. The difference lies in the inflation of a balloon to keep the indwelling catheter in place and the presence of a closed drainage system.

For patients with urinary retention or critical illness and who require long-term catheterization, catheter changes should be individualized, not routine (Gould et al., 2009; Green et al., 2008; Willson et al., 2009). They should be changed for leaking, for blockage, and before obtaining a sterile specimen for urine culture (Smith et al., 2008). Long-term catheterization should be avoided because of its association with urinary tract infection (UTI) (Green et al., 2008). Make every attempt to remove catheters as soon as a patient can void.

An indwelling catheter is attached to a urinary drainage bag to collect the continuous flow of urine. Always hang the bag below the level of the bladder on the bed frame or a chair so that urine drains down, out of the bladder. The bag should never touch the floor.

Delegation Considerations

The skill of inserting a straight or indwelling urinary catheter cannot be delegated to nursing assistive personnel (NAP). The nurse directs the NAP to:

- Help with patient positioning, focus lighting for the procedure, maintain privacy, empty urine from collection bag, and help with perineal care.
- Report postprocedure patient discomfort or fever to the nurse.
- Report abnormal color, odor, or amount of urine in drainage bag and if the catheter is leaking or causes pain.

Equipment

- Catheter kit containing the following sterile items: (Catheter kits vary; thus it is important to check the list of contents on the package.)

- Catheter of correct size and type for procedure or patient condition (i.e., indwelling [double lumen 14 or 16 French (Fr)] or intermittent [usually 12 to 14 Fr]). Some kits contain a catheter with attached drainage bag; others contain only a catheter; others have no catheter.
- Drapes (one fenestrated—has an opening in the center)
- Sterile gloves
- Lubricant
- Antiseptic cleaning solution such as chlorhexidine or povidone-iodine incorporated in an applicator or to be added to cotton balls (forceps to pick up cotton balls)
- Specimen container
- Prefilled syringe with sterile water for balloon inflation of an indwelling catheter
- Sterile drainage tubing and collection bag (Some kits come preconnected; others do not, and a separate package is required.)
- Sterile drainage tubing and bag (if not included in the kit)
- Device to secure catheter (i.e., strap)
- Extra sterile gloves and catheter (*optional*)
- Bath blanket
- Waterproof absorbent pad
- Clean gloves; basin with warm water, soap or perineal cleaner, washcloth; and towel for perineal care
- Additional lighting as needed (such as a flashlight or procedure light)
- Measuring container for urine

Implementation

STEP	RATIONALE
1 Complete preprocedure protocol.	
2 Assess for pain and bladder fullness. Palpate bladder over symphysis pubis, or use bladder scanner (if available).	Palpation of full bladder causes pain and/or urge to void, indicating full or overfull bladder.
3 Perform hand hygiene.	Reduces transmission of microorganisms.
4 Raise bed to appropriate working height. If side rails	Promotes good body mechanics. Use of side rails in this

STEP	RATIONALE
in use, raise side rail on opposite side of bed and lower side rail on working side.	manner promotes patient safety.
5 Position patient: a **Female patient:**	
(1) Help to dorsal recumbent position (on back with knees flexed). Ask patient to relax thighs so you can rotate hips.	Exposes perineum and allows hip joints to be externally rotated.
(2) Alternate female position: Position patient in side-lying (Sims') position with upper leg flexed at knee and hip. Support patient with pillows if necessary to maintain position.	Alternate position is more comfortable if patient cannot abduct leg at hip joint (e.g., patient has arthritic joints or contractures).
b **Male patient:**	
(1) Position supine with legs extended and thighs slightly abducted.	Comfortable position for patient aids in visualization of penis.
6 Perform perineal care: a **Female patient:**	
(1) Drape with bath blanket. Place blanket diamond fashion over patient, with one corner at patient's midsection, side corners over each thigh and abdomen, and last corner over perineum.	Protects patient dignity by avoiding unnecessary exposure of body parts.

STEP	RATIONALE
b Male patient:	
(1) Drape patient by covering upper part of body with small sheet or towel; drape with separate sheet or bath blanket so that only perineum is exposed.	
7 ⚡ Apply clean gloves. Wash perineal area with soap and water, rinse, and dry. Use gloves to examine patient and identify urinary meatus. Remove and discard gloves.	Hygiene before initiating aseptic catheter insertion removes secretions, urine, and feces that could contaminate sterile field and increase risk for catheter-associated urinary tract infection (CAUTI).
8 Position light to illuminate genitals, or have assistant available to hold light source to visualize urinary meatus.	Adequate visualization of urinary meatus helps with speed and accuracy of catheter insertion.
9 Open outer wrapping of catheterization kit. Place inner wrapped catheter kit tray on clean, accessible surface such as bedside table or, if possible, between patient's open legs. Patient's size and positioning dictate exact placement.	Provides easy access to supplies during catheter insertion.
10 Open inner sterile wrap covering tray containing catheterization supplies, using sterile technique. Fold back each flap of sterile covering one at a time, with the last flap opened toward patient.	Sterile wrap serves as sterile field.

STEP	RATIONALE
a Indwelling catheterization open system: Open separate package containing drainage bag, check to make sure that clamp on drainage port is closed, and place drainage bag and tubing in an easily accessible location. Open outer package of sterile catheter, maintaining sterility of inner wrapper.	Open drainage bag systems have separate sterile packaging for sterile catheter, drainage bag and tubing, and insertion kit.
b Indwelling catheterization closed system: All supplies are in sterile tray and are arranged in sequence of use.	Closed drainage bag systems have catheter preattached to drainage tubing and bag.
c Straight catheterization: All needed supplies are in sterile tray that contains supplies and can be used for urine collection.	
11 **Put on sterile gloves.** (Or apply sterile drape with ungloved hands when drape is packed as first item. Touch only edges of drape. Then apply clean gloves.)	Maintains surgical asepsis.
12 Drape perineum, keeping gloves sterile.	Sterile drapes provide sterile field over which you will work during catheterization.
a Drape female: (1) Pick up square sterile drape touching only edges (2.5 cm [1 inch]).	

STEP	RATIONALE
(2) Allow drape to unfold without touching unsterile surfaces. Allow top edge of drape (2.5 to 5 cm [1 to 2 inches]) to form cuff over both hands.	When creating the cuff over sterile gloved hands, sterility of gloves and workspace is maintained.
(3) Place drape with shiny side down on bed between patient's thighs. Slip cuffed edge just under buttocks as you ask patient to lift hips. Take care not to touch contaminated surfaces with sterile gloves.	
(4) Pick up fenestrated sterile drape out of tray. Allow drape to unfold without touching unsterile surfaces. Allow top edge of drape to form cuff over both hands. Apply drape over perineum, exposing labia.	Opening in drape creates sterile field around labia.
b **Drape male:**	
(1) Use of square sterile drape is optional; you may apply a fenestrated drape instead.	
(2) Pick up edges of square drape and unfold without touching unsterile surfaces. Place over	Creates sterile field.

STEP	RATIONALE
thighs, with shiny side down, just below penis.	
(3) Place fenestrated drape with opening centered over penis.	
13 Move tray closer to patient. Arrange remaining supplies on sterile field, maintaining sterility of gloves. Place sterile tray with cleaning medium (premoistened swab sticks or cotton balls, forceps, and solution), lubricant, catheter, and prefilled syringe for inflating balloon (indwelling catheterization only) on sterile drape.	
a If kit contains sterile cotton balls, open package of sterile antiseptic solution and pour over cotton balls. Some kits contain a package of premoistened swab sticks. Open end of package for easy access.	Use of sterile supplies and antiseptic solution reduces risk of CAUTI (Gould et al., 2009; Lo et al., 2008).
b Open sterile specimen container if specimen will be obtained.	Makes container accessible to receive urine from catheter if specimen is needed.
c For indwelling catheterization, open sterile wrapper of catheter and leave catheter on sterile field. If part of a closed system kit, remove tray with catheter and preattached drainage bag and place on sterile drape. Make sure that clamp on drainage	Indwelling catheterization trays vary. Some have preattached catheters; others need to be attached but are part of the sterile tray; others do not have catheter or drainage system as part of tray.

STEP	RATIONALE
port of bag is closed. If needed and if part of sterile tray, attach catheter to drainage tubing.	
d Open packet of lubricant and squeeze out on sterile field. Lubricate catheter tip by dipping it into water-soluble gel 2.5 to 5 cm (1 to 2 inches) for women and 12.5 to 17.5 cm (5 to 7 inches) for men.	Lubrication minimizes trauma to urethra and discomfort during catheter insertion.
14 Cleanse urethral meatus:	
a Female patient:	
(1) Separate labia with fingers of nondominant hand (now contaminated) to fully expose urethral meatus.	Optimal visualization of urethral meatus is possible.
(2) Maintain position of nondominant hand throughout procedure.	Closure of labia during cleaning means that area is contaminated and requires cleaning procedure to be repeated.
(3) Holding forceps in dominant hand, pick up one moistened cotton ball or pick up one swab stick at a time. Clean labia and urinary meatus from clitoris toward anus. Use new cotton ball or swab for each area that you clean. Clean by wiping labial fold,	Front-to-back cleaning moves from area of least contaminated toward highly contaminated area. Follows principles of medical asepsis. Dominant gloved hand remains sterile.

STEP	RATIONALE
near labial fold, and directly over center of urethral meatus.	
b Male patient:	
(1) With nondominant hand (now contaminated) retract foreskin (if uncircumcised) and gently grasp penis at shaft just below glans. Hold shaft of penis at right angle to body. This hand remains in this position for remainder of procedure.	When grasping shaft of penis, avoid pressure on dorsal surface to prevent compression of urethra. Losing grasp during cleaning means that area is contaminated and requires cleaning procedure to be repeated.
(2) Using uncontaminated dominant hand, clean the meatus with cotton balls/swab sticks, using circular strokes, beginning at the meatus and working outward in a spiral motion.	Circular cleaning pattern follows principles of medical asepsis.
(3) Repeat cleansing three times using clean cotton ball/swab stick each time.	
15 Pick up and hold catheter 7.5 to 10 cm (3 to 4 inches) from catheter tip with catheter loosely coiled in palm of hand. If catheter is not attached to drainage bag, make sure to position urine tray so end of catheter can be placed there once insertion begins.	Holding catheter near tip allows for easier manipulation during its insertion. Coiling cather in palm prevents distal end from striking nonsterile surface.

STEP	RATIONALE
16 Insert catheter:	
a Female patient:	
(1) Ask patient to bear down gently and slowly; insert catheter through urethral meatus (Fig. 78-1).	Bearing down may help visualize urinary meatus and promotes relaxation of external urinary sphincter, aiding in catheter insertion.
(2) Advance catheter total of 5 to 7.5 cm (2 to 3 inches) or until urine flows out of catheter. When urine appears, advance catheter another 2.5 to 5 cm (1 to 2 inches). Do not use force to insert catheter.	Urine flow indicates that catheter tip is in bladder or lower urethra.
(3) Release labia and hold catheter securely with nondominant hand.	
b Male patient:	
(1) Lift penis to position perpendicular to patient's body, and apply light traction (Fig. 78-2).	Straightens urethra to ease catheter insertion.
(2) Ask patient to bear down as if to void and slowly insert catheter through urethral meatus.	Relaxation of external sphincter aids in insertion of catheter.
(3) Advance catheter 17 to 22.5 cm (7 to 9 inches) or until urine flows out end of catheter.	There are variations in length of male urethra. Flow of urine indicates that tip of catheter is in bladder or urethra but not necessarily that the balloon portion of an indwelling catheter is in bladder.

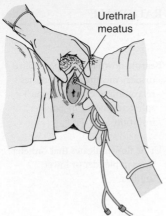

Fig. 78-1 Inserting the catheter.

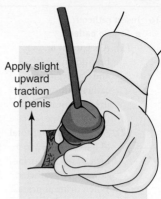

Fig. 78-2 Inserting catheter into male urinary meatus.

STEP	RATIONALE
(4) Stop advancing with a straight catheter. When urine appears in an indwelling catheter, advance it to bifurcation (inflation and deflation ports exposed) (Fig. 78-3).	Further advancement of catheter to bifurcation of drainage and balloon inflation port ensures that balloon portion of catheter is not still in prostatic urethra (D'Cruz et al., 2009; Méndez-Probst et al., 2012; Newman and Wein, 2009).
(5) Lower penis, and hold catheter securely in nondominant hand.	Prevents accidental dislodgment of catheter.
17 Inflate catheter balloon fully with amount of fluid designated by manufacturer.	Indwelling catheter balloons should not be underinflated. Underinflation causes balloon distortion and potential bladder damage (Newman and Wein, 2009).
a Continue to hold catheter with nondominant hand.	Holding on to catheter before inflating balloon prevents expulsion of catheter from urethra.

In image 1: Urethral meatus

In image 2: Apply slight upward traction of penis

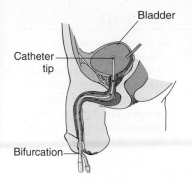

Fig. 78-3 Male anatomy with correct catheter insertion to the bifurcation of the drainage and balloon inflation port.

STEP	RATIONALE
b With free dominant hand, connect prefilled syringe to injection port at end of catheter.	
c Slowly inject total amount of solution.	
d After inflating balloon, release catheter from nondominant hand. Gently pull catheter until resistance is felt. Then advance catheter slightly.	By moving catheter slightly back into bladder, pressure on bladder neck is avoided.
e Connect drainage tubing to catheter if it is not already preconnected.	

SAFETY ALERT If patient complains of sudden pain during inflation of a catheter balloon or resistance is felt when inflating the balloon, stop inflation, allow the fluid from the balloon to flow back into the syringe, advance catheter further, and reinflate balloon. The balloon may have been inflating in the urethra. If pain continues, remove catheter and notify health care provider.

STEP	RATIONALE
18 Secure indwelling catheter with catheter strap or other securement device. Leave enough slack to allow leg movement. Attach securement device at tubing just above catheter bifurcation.	Securing catheter reduces risk of urethral erosion, CAUTI, or accidental catheter removal (Gould et al., 2009). Attachment of securement device at catheter bifurcation prevents occlusion of catheter (Gray, 2008).
a Female patient: (1) Secure catheter tubing to inner thigh, allowing enough slack to prevent tension.	
b Male patient: (1) Secure catheter tubing to upper thigh or lower abdomen (with penis directed toward chest). Allow slack in catheter so that movement does not create tension on catheter.	Anchoring catheter reduces traction on urethra and minimizes urethral injury (Stoller, 2008).
(2) If retracted, replace foreskin over glans penis.	Leaving foreskin retracted can cause discomfort and dangerous edema.
19 Clip drainage tubing to edge of mattress. Position drainage bag lower than bladder by attaching to bed frame. Do not attach to side rails of bed.	Drainage bags that are below level of bladder ensure free flow of urine, thus decreasing risk for CAUTI (Gould et al., 2009; Lo et al., 2008). Bags attached to movable objects such as a side rail increase risk for urethral trauma because of pulling or accidental dislodgment.
20 Check to make sure that there is no obstruction to urine flow. Coil excess tubing on bed, and fasten to bottom sheet with clip or other securement device.	

STEP	RATIONALE
21 Provide hygiene as needed. Help patient to comfortable position.	
22 Observe character and amount of urine in drainage system.	Determines if urine is flowing adequately.
23 Complete postprocedure protocol.	

Recording and Reporting

- Record and report the reason for catheterization, type and size of catheter inserted, amount of fluid used to inflate balloon, specimen collection (if applicable), characteristics and amount of urine, patient's response to procedure, and any education in nurses' notes and electronic health record (EHR).
- Record amount of urine on intake and output (I&O) flow sheet record.
- Report persistent catheter-related pain, inadequate urine output, and discomfort to health care provider.

UNEXPECTED OUTCOMES	RELATED INTERVENTIONS
1 Catheter goes into vagina	• Leave catheter in vagina. • Clean urinary meatus again. Using another catheter kit, reinsert sterile catheter into meatus (check agency policy). **NOTE:** If gloves become contaminated, start procedure over. • Remove catheter in vagina once functional catheter is inserted.
2 Sterility is broken during catheterization by nurse or patient.	• Replace gloves if contaminated and start over. • If patient touches sterile field but equipment and supplies remain sterile, avoid touching that part of sterile field.

Continued

UNEXPECTED OUTCOMES	RELATED INTERVENTIONS
	• If equipment and/or supplies become contaminated, replace with sterile items or start over with new sterile kit.
3 Patient complains of bladder discomfort, and catheter is patent as evidenced by adequate urine flow.	• Check catheter to ensure that there is no traction on it.
	• Notify health care provider. Patient may be experiencing bladder spasms or symptoms of UTI.
	• Monitor catheter output for color, clarity, odor, and amount.

Urinary Catheter Care and Removal

Bacterial growth is common where the catheter enters the urethral meatus in both men and women. Perform catheter care each shift as part of routine perineal care, after bowel incontinence, or if secretions accumulate around the urinary meatus. Removal of a retention catheter requires the use of clean technique. You deflate the retention balloon before removal. If the retention catheter balloon remains even partially inflated, its removal will result in trauma and subsequent swelling of the urethral meatus. Always remove an indwelling catheter as soon as possible after insertion because of risk for catheter-associated urinary tract infection (CAUTI).

Delegation Considerations

The skill of performing routine catheter care and removing a catheter can be delegated to nursing assistive personnel (NAP). The nurse instructs NAP to:

- Report characteristics of the urine output from the catheter, including color, odor, and amount.
- Report the condition of the patient's perineum (color, discharge, contamination from fecal incontinence).
- Check the size of the balloon and the size of the syringe needed to deflate the balloon, and to report if balloon does not deflate and/ or if there is bleeding or excessive burning.
- Measure first voiding and report time and amount voided.

Equipment

- Clean gloves (needed for care and removal)
- Waterproof pad
- Bath blanket

For Catheter Care

- Soap, washcloth, towel, and basin filled with warm water

For Removing a Catheter

- 10-mL or larger syringe without needle—information on balloon size (mL) is printed directly on balloon inflation valve (Fig. 79-1)
- Correctly labeled sterile specimen container
- Alcohol or other disinfectant swab

Fig. 79-1 Size of balloon printed on catheter inflation valve.

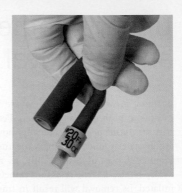

- 25-gauge ½-inch needle (if not a needleless system) or Luer-Lok syringe for a needleless catheter port (if culture and sensitivity are to be obtained before catheter removal)
- Washcloth and warm water to perform perineal care after removal
- Graduated cylinder
- Available urinal for male patients, bedside commode or urine output commode pan for female patients for urine collection after catheter is removed

Implementation

STEP	RATIONALE
1 Complete preprocedure protocol.	
2 Preparation for catheter care:	
a Observe urinary output and urine characteristics.	Encrustation, the formation of hard deposits around the tip and inside of the drainage lumen of the catheter, leads to blockage of the drainage lumen and causes urinary retention.
b Assess patient's knowledge of catheter care.	Patients who perform own catheter care may be unsure of touching the catheter. Assess patient's ability and knowledge in order to provide instruction as needed (Leaver, 2007).

STEP	RATIONALE
c Observe any discharge or redness around urethral meatus.	Indicates inflammatory process and possible infection.
3 Preparation for catheter removal:	
a Assess need for Foley catheter removal. Determine how long catheter has been in place. Check agency policy to determine time frame for Foley catheter change. Check medical record for order to remove, or obtain order as needed.	The duration of catheterization is an important risk factor for development of nosocomial urinary tract infection (UTI) and gram-negative urosepsis.
b Determine size of catheter inflation balloon by looking at balloon inflation valve. (See Figure 79-1.)	Determines amount of water to remove from balloon.
c Observe any discharge or redness around urethral meatus.	Indicates inflammatory process and possible infection. Provides information for perineal care after catheter removal.
4 ![] Perform hand hygiene, and apply clean gloves.	Reduces transmission of microorganisms.
5 Position patient, and cover with bath blanket, exposing only perineal area.	Reduces patient's embarrassment. Ensures easy access to perineal tissues.
a Female in dorsal recumbent position.	
b Male in supine position.	
6 Catheter care:	
a Place waterproof pad under patient. Provide routine perineal care with soap and water. Application of topical antimicrobial agents is not recommended.	Perineal care with soap and water is sufficient to keep the area clean (Leaver, 2007). The application of topical antimicrobial products is not effective in reducing meatal bacterial flora and reducing risk

STEP	RATIONALE
	for UTI. Do not include them as a part of routine catheter care (Leaver, 2007; Gould et al., 2009).
b Assess urethral meatus and surrounding tissues for inflammation, swelling, and discharge, and ask patient if burning or discomfort is present.	Determines condition of perineum and the frequency and type of ongoing care required.
c Using a clean washcloth, soap, and water, cleanse the catheter in a circular motion along its length for about 10 cm (4 inches) (Fig. 79-2). Start cleansing where the catheter enters the meatus and down toward the drainage tubing. Make sure to remove all traces of soap.	Reduces presence of secretions or drainage on outside catheter surface.
d Replace, as necessary, the adhesive tape (remove any adhesive residue from skin) or multipurpose tube holder that anchors catheter to patient's leg or abdomen.	
e Avoid placing tension on the catheter.	Tension causes urethral trauma.
f Check drainage tubing and bag for the following:	Ensuring unobstructed flow of urine is one of the most effective measures to prevent CAUTI (Gould et al., 2009).
(1) Tubing does not have dependent loops, and it is not positioned above level of bladder.	Prevents pooling of urine and reflux of urine into the bladder.

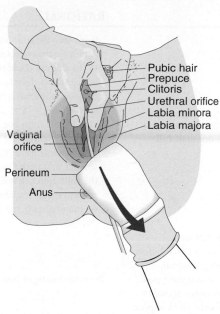

- Pubic hair
- Prepuce
- Clitoris
- Urethral orifice
- Labia minora
- Labia majora

Vaginal orifice

Perineum

Anus

Fig. 79-2 The catheter is cleansed starting at the meatus. About 4 inches of the catheter is cleansed.

STEP	RATIONALE
(2) Tubing is coiled and secured onto bed linen.	Promotes free drainage of urine; prevents dependent loops of tubing and subsequent urine stasis.
(3) Tube is without kinks, tube is not clamped, and patient is not lying on tubing.	Promotes free flow of urine and prevents stasis of urine in bladder, which increases risk for infection.
(4) The collection bag is lower than the bladder level at all times. Hook the catheter on the bed frame, not on the side rail.	Reflux of urine from the contaminated drainage bag has been associated with infection (Cipa-Tatum, 2011). When the catheter is lower than the bladder, urine can drain

STEP	RATIONALE
	freely into the collection bag. Attaching the collection bag to the side rail could result in inadvertently dislodging the catheter as the rail is raised or lowered.
g Empty collection bag when one-half full.	Urine in collection bag is excellent medium for growth of microorganisms. Having smaller volumes of urine in the collection bag will help to prevent excess trauma/traction on the urethra (Cipa-Tatum, 2011).
7 Catheter removal: Follow Steps 1 to 6 before catheter removal.	
a Place waterproof pad: (1) Between female's thighs (if in supine position). (2) Over male's thighs.	Prevents soiling of bed linen.
b Obtain sterile urine specimen if required.	Determines if bacteria are present in urine.
c Remove adhesive tape or Velcro tube holder used to secure and anchor catheter.	Allows for positioning of catheter for removal.
d Insert hub of syringe into inflation valve (balloon port). Allow sterile water to return into syringe by gravity until the plunger stops moving and the amount instilled is removed.	Many manufacturers recommend that fluid return to syringe by gravity. Manual aspiration leads to increased discomfort when removing catheter, resulting in the development of creases or ridges in balloon. A balloon that is not completely deflated will cause discomfort and trauma to urethral wall, which will result in bleeding as the catheter is removed.

STEP	RATIONALE
e Pull catheter out slowly and gently while wrapping contaminated catheter in waterproof pad. Unhook collection bag and drainage tubing from bed.	Slow and gentle removal prevents possible trauma caused by deflated balloon deformation and accumulated encrustation.

SAFETY ALERT Catheter should slide out very easily. Do not use force. If you note any resistance, repeat Step 7d to remove any remaining fluid in inflation port. Notify prescriber.

---

f Reposition patient as necessary. Cleanse perineum. Lower level of bed, and position side rails accordingly.	Promotes patient comfort and safety.
g Empty, measure, and record urine present in drainage bag.	Records urinary output.
8 Complete postprocedure protocol.	
9 Observe time the patient urinates, and measure the urine; assess urine characteristics.	Urinary retention is a common occurrence after removal of an indwelling Foley catheter.
10 Evaluate the patient for dysuria; small, frequent voidings; or bleeding during urination.	UTI can develop after catheter removal.

Recording and Reporting

- Record times for catheter care in the nursing care plan.
- Record in nurses' notes times of catheter care and removal of catheter, condition of urethral meatus, and character and amount of urine.
- Record urine emptied from drainage bag on intake and output form.

UNEXPECTED OUTCOMES	RELATED INTERVENTIONS
1 Urethral or perineal irritation is present.	• Observe for leaking from around catheter; catheter may need replacement. • Make sure catheter (if not removed) is anchored and secured appropriately.
2 Patient has fever and/or urine is malodorous; patient has small, frequent voidings; or bleeding or burning occurs with urination after catheter is removed.	• Monitor vital signs and urine. • Report findings to prescriber, because any of these symptoms/signs indicates a UTI.
3 Patient is unable to void after catheter removal or voids in small, frequent amounts.	• Assess for bladder distention. • Assist to a normal position for voiding. • Provide privacy. • Perform bladder ultrasonography to assess for residual urine. Notify prescriber if residual volume is greater than 150 mL. Catheterization may be indicated. • If patient is unable to void within 6 to 8 hours of catheter removal, notify prescriber.

Urinary Catheter Irrigation

There are two types of irrigation: closed catheter irrigation and open irrigation. Closed catheter irrigation provides intermittent or continuous irrigation of a urinary catheter without disrupting the sterile connection between the catheter and the drainage system (Fig. 80-1). Intermittent irrigation involves insertion of a sterile catheter into a catheter port to irrigate a bolus of fluid.

Open catheter irrigation is used only when intermittent irrigation of the catheter and bladder is required. The skill involves breaking or opening the closed drainage system at the connection between the catheter and the drainage system. **This procedure should be avoided unless irrigation is needed to relieve or prevent obstruction** (Senese et al., 2005). Strict asepsis is required throughout the procedure to minimize contamination and subsequent development of a urinary tract infection (UTI).

Delegation Considerations

The skill of catheter irrigation cannot be delegated to nursing assistive personnel (NAP). The nurse directs the NAP to:

- Report if the patient complains of pain, discomfort, or leakage of fluid around the catheter.
- Monitor and record intake and output (I&O); report immediately any decrease in urine output.
- Report any change in the color of the urine, especially the presence of blood clots.

Equipment

- Sterile irrigation solution at room temperature (as prescribed)
- Antiseptic swabs
- Clean gloves

Closed Intermittent Irrigation

- Sterile container
- Sterile 30- to 60-mL irrigation syringe (piston type)
- Syringe to access system (Luer-Lok syringe without needle for needleless access port per manufacturer's directions)
- Screw clamp or rubber band (used to temporarily occlude catheter while irrigant is instilled)

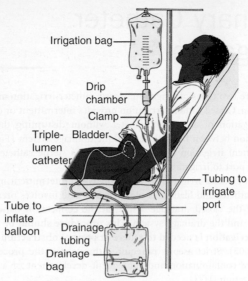

Fig. 80-1 Closed continuous bladder irrigation.

Closed Continuous Irrigation

- Irrigation tubing with clamp to regulate irrigation flow rate
- Y connector *(optional)* to connect irrigation tubing to double-lumen catheter
- Intravenous (IV) pole (closed continuous or intermittent)

Open Intermittent Irrigation

- Disposable sterile irrigation kit that contains solution container, collection basin, drape, sterile gloves, 30- to 60-mL irrigation syringe (piston type)
- Sterile catheter plug
- Sterile gloves *(optional)*

Implementation

STEP	RATIONALE
1 Complete preprocedure protocol.	

STEP	RATIONALE
2 Verify in medical record: a Order for irrigation method (continuous or intermittent), type (sterile saline or medicated solution), and amount of irrigant.	Health care provider's order is required to initiate therapy. Frequency and volume of solution used for irrigation may be in the order or standardized as part of agency policy.
b Type of catheter in place.	Single- and double-lumen catheters are used with open irrigation. Triple-lumen catheters are used for both intermittent and continuous closed irrigation.
3 Observe urine for color, amount, clarity, and presence of mucus, clots, or sediment.	Indicates if patient is bleeding or sloughing tissue, which would require increased irrigation rate or frequency of catheter irrigation.
4 Monitor I&O. If continuous bladder irrigation (CBI) is being used, amount of fluid draining from bladder should exceed amount of fluid infused into bladder.	If output does not exceed irrigant infused, catheter obstruction (i.e., blood clots, kinked tubing) should be suspected, irrigation stopped, and prescriber notified (Lewis et al., 2011).
5 🕊 Organize supplies according to type of irrigation prescribed. Apply clean gloves.	Ensures efficient procedure.
6 **Closed continuous irrigation:** a Close clamp on new irrigation tubing, and hang bag of irrigating solution on IV pole. Insert (spike) tip of sterile irrigation tubing into designated port of irrigation solution bag using aseptic technique.	Prevents air from entering tubing. Air can cause bladder spasms. Technique prevents transmission of microorganisms.

STEP	RATIONALE
b Fill drip chamber half full by squeezing chamber; then open clamp and allow solution to flow (prime) through tubing, keeping end of tubing sterile. Once fluid has completely filled tubing, close clamp and recap end of tubing.	Priming tubing with fluid prevents introduction of air into bladder.
c Using aseptic technique, connect tubing securely to drainage port of Y connector on double/triple-lumen catheter.	Reduces transmission of microorganisms.
d Adjust clamp on irrigation tubing to begin flow of solution into bladder. If set volume rate is ordered, calculate drip rate and adjust rate at roller clamp. If urine is bright red or has clots, increase irrigation rate until drainage appears pink (according to ordered rate or agency protocol).	Continuous drainage is expected. It helps to prevent clotting in presence of active bleeding in bladder and flushes clots out of bladder.
e Observe for outflow of fluid into drainage bag. Empty catheter drainage bag as needed.	Discomfort, bladder distention, and possible injury can occur from overdistention of bladder when bladder irrigant cannot adequately flow from bladder. Bag will fill rapidly and may need to be emptied every 1 to 2 hours.
7 Closed intermittent irrigation:	Fluid is instilled through catheter in a bolus, flushing system. Fluid drains out after irrigation is complete.
a Pour prescribed sterile irrigating solution in sterile container.	

STEP	RATIONALE
b Draw prescribed volume of irrigant (usually 30 to 50 mL) into syringe using aseptic technique. Place sterile cap on tip of needleless syringe.	Ensures sterility of irrigating fluid.
c Clamp catheter tubing below soft injection port with screw clamp (or fold catheter tubing onto itself and secure with rubber band).	Occluding catheter tubing below the point of injection allows irrigating solution to enter catheter and flow upward toward bladder.
d Using circular motion, clean catheter port (specimen port) with antiseptic swab.	Reduces transmission of infection.
e Insert tip of needleless syringe using twisting motion into port.	Ensures that catheter tip enters lumen of catheter.
f Inject solution using slow, even pressure.	Gentle instillation of solution minimizes trauma to the bladder mucosa.
g Remove syringe and remove clamp (or rubber band), allowing solution to drain into urinary drainage bag. (**Note:** Some medicated irrigants may need to dwell in bladder for prescribed period, requiring catheter to be clamped temporarily before being allowed to drain.)	Allows drainage to flow via gravity. Medications must be instilled long enough to be absorbed by lining of bladder. Clamped drainage tubing and bag should not be left unattended.
8 Open intermittent irrigation:	
a ✈ Apply clean or sterile gloves (see agency policy).	Prevents introduction of microorganisms into urinary catheter and drainage system.
b Open sterile irrigation tray. Establish sterile field, and pour required amount	Maintains sterile field.

STEP	RATIONALE
of sterile solution into sterile solution container. Replace cap on large container of solution. Add sterile irrigation syringe (piston type) to sterile field. Have antiseptic wipe open and ready for use.	
c Position sterile waterproof drape under catheter.	Creates sterile field on which to work and prevents soiling of bed linen.
d Aspirate prescribed volume of irrigation solution into irrigating syringe (usually 30 mL). Place syringe in sterile solution container until ready to use.	Prepares solution for instillation into catheter. Maintains sterility of irrigating syringe.
e Move sterile collection basin close to patient's thigh.	Prevents soiling of bed linen and reaching over sterile field.
f Wipe connection point between catheter and drainage tubing with antiseptic wipe before disconnecting.	Reduces transmission of microorganisms.
g Disconnect catheter from drainage tubing, allowing any urine to flow into sterile collection basin. Cover open end of drainage tubing with sterile protective cap, and position tubing so it stays coiled on top of bed with end resting on sterile drape.	Maintains sterility of inner aspect of catheter lumen and drainage tubing. Reduces potential of infection by way of microorganism contamination.
h Insert tip of syringe into lumen of catheter, and gently push plunger to instill solution.	Gentle instillation of irrigating solution minimizes trauma to the bladder.

STEP	RATIONALE
i Remove syringe, lower catheter, and allow solution to drain into basin. Amount of drainage solution should be equal to or greater than amount instilled. If ordered, repeat sequence of instilling solution and draining until drainage is clear of clots and sediment.	If clot has been removed, solution will drain freely into basin.
j After irrigation is complete, remove protector cap from urinary drainage tubing end, clean end of tubing with antiseptic wipe, and reinsert into lumen of catheter.	Restores sterile system.
9 Anchor catheter with catheter securement device (see Skill 79).	Prevents trauma to urethral tissue.
10 Help patient to safe and comfortable position. Lower bed and place side rails accordingly.	Promotes patient comfort and safety.
11 Inspect urine for blood clots and sediment, and ensure that tubing is not kinked or occluded.	Decrease in blood clots means that therapy is successful in maintaining catheter patency.
12 Complete postprocedure protocol.	

Recording and Reporting

- Record irrigation method, amount and type of irrigation solution, amount returned as drainage, characteristics of output, urine output, and patient tolerance to procedure in nurses' notes.
- Report catheter occlusion, sudden bleeding, infection, or increased pain to health care provider.
- Record I&O on appropriate flow sheet.

UNEXPECTED OUTCOMES	RELATED INTERVENTIONS
1 Irrigating solution does not return (intermittent irrigation) or is not flowing at prescribed rate (CBI).	• Examine tubing for clots, sediment, and kinks. • Notify health care provider if irrigant does not flow freely from the bladder, patient complains of pain, or bladder distention occurs.
2 Drainage output is less than amount of irrigation solution infused.	• Examine drainage tubing for clots, sediment, or kinks. • Inspect urine for presence of or increase in blood clots and sediment. • Evaluate patient for pain and distended bladder. • Notify health care provider.
3 Bright-red bleeding with the irrigation (CBI) infusion wide open.	• Assess for hypovolemic shock (vital signs, skin color and moisture, anxiety level). • Leave irrigation infusion wide open and notify health care provider.
4 Patient experiences pain with irrigation.	• Examine drainage tubing for clots, sediment, or kinks. • Evaluate urine for presence of or increase in blood clots and sediment. • Evaluate for distended bladder. • Notify health care provider.
5 Signs of possible infection: fever; cloudy, foul-smelling urine; abdominal pain; change in mental status.	• Notify health care provider. • Monitor vital signs and character of urine.

Urinary Diversion:
Pouching an Incontinent Urinary Diversion

Because urine flows continuously from an incontinent urinary diversion, placement of the pouch is more challenging than with the fecal diversion. In the immediate postoperative period urinary stents extend out from the stoma (Fig. 81-1). A surgeon places the stents to prevent stenosis of the ureters at the site where the ureters are attached to the conduit. The stents will be removed during the hospital stay or at the first postoperative visit with the surgeon. The stoma is normally red and moist. It is made from a portion of the intestinal tract, usually the ileum. It should protrude above the skin. An ileal conduit is usually located in the right lower quadrant. While the patient is in bed, the pouch may be connected to a bedside drainage bag to decrease the need for frequent emptying. When the patient goes home, the bedside drainage bag may be used at night to avoid having to get up to empty the pouch. Each type of urostomy pouch comes with a connector for the bedside drainage bag.

Delegation Considerations

The skill of pouching a new incontinent urinary diversion cannot be delegated to nursing assistive personnel (NAP). In some agencies, care of an established urostomy (4 to 6 weeks or more after surgery) can be delegated to NAP. The nurse directs the NAP about:

- Expected appearance of the stoma.
- Expected amount and character of the output and when to report changes.
- Changes in patient's stoma and surrounding skin integrity that should be reported.
- Special equipment needed to complete the procedure.

Equipment

- Urinary pouch (with antireflux flap and skin barrier; clear, drainable one- or two-piece, cut-to-fit or precut size) (Fig. 81-2)
- Appropriate adapter for connection to bedside drainage bag
- Measuring guide
- Bedside urinary drainage bag
- Clean gloves

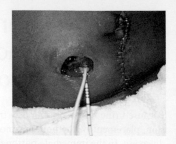

Fig. 81-1 Urostomy with stents in place. (Courtesy Jane Fellows.)

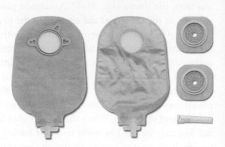

Fig. 81-2 Urostomy pouching system with adapter to connect pouch to bedside drainage bag. (Courtesy Hollister Incorporated, Libertyville, Ill.)

- Washcloth
- Towel or disposable waterproof barrier
- Basin with warm tap water
- Scissors
- Adhesive remover
- Absorbent wick made from gauze rolled tightly in the shape of a tampon
- Waterproof bag for disposal of pouch
- Gown and goggles (used if there is risk of splashing when emptying pouch)

Implementation

STEP	RATIONALE
1 Complete preprocedure protocol and apply clean gloves.	
2 Observe existing skin barrier and pouch for leakage and length of time in place. Pouch should be changed	Assesses effectiveness of pouching system and allows for early detection of potential problems. To minimize skin

STEP	RATIONALE
every 3 to 7 days, not daily (Colwell et al., 2004). If urine is leaking under wafer, change pouch.	irritation, avoid changing entire pouching system unnecessarily. Repeated leakage may indicate need for different type of pouch to provide a reliable seal.
3 Observe urine in pouch or bedside drainage bag. Empty pouch if it is more than one-third to one-half full by opening the valve and draining it into a container for measurement.	Urine output provides information about renal status and whether volume is within acceptable limits (≥30 mL/hr). Weight of pouch can disrupt seal. Urine for ileal conduit will contain mucus because of flow through intestinal segment.
4 Observe stoma for color, swelling, presence of sutures, trauma, and healing of the peristomal skin. Assess type of stoma. Remove and dispose of gloves.	Consider stoma characteristics in selecting appropriate pouching system. Convexity in the skin barrier is often necessary with a flush or retracted stoma.
5 Position patient in a semireclining or supine position. If possible, provide patient a mirror for observation.	When patient is semireclining, there are fewer skin wrinkles, which allows for ease of pouch application.
6 ✋ Perform hand hygiene, and apply clean gloves.	Reduces transmission of microorganisms.
7 Place towel or disposable waterproof barrier under patient and across patient's lower abdomen.	Protects bed linen; maintains patient's dignity.
8 Remove used pouch and skin barrier gently by pushing skin away from barrier. If stents are present, pull pouch gently around them, and lay towel underneath. Empty each pouch and measure output. Dispose of pouch in appropriate receptacle.	Reduces risk for trauma to skin and for dislodging stents. Keeps urine from leaking onto skin.

STEP	RATIONALE
9 Place rolled gauze wick at stomal opening. Maintain gauze at the stoma opening continuously during pouch measurement and change.	Using a wick at stoma opening prevents peristomal skin from becoming wet with urine during pouch change.
10 While keeping rolled gauze in contact with the stoma, cleanse peristomal skin gently with warm tap water using washcloth; do not scrub skin. If you touch stoma, minor bleeding is normal. Pat the skin dry.	Avoid soap. It leaves residue on skin, which can irritate it. Pouch does not adhere to wet skin.
11 Measure stoma. Be sure that opening is at least $\frac{1}{8}$ inch larger than stoma to avoid pressure on stoma. Expect size of stoma to change for first 4 to 6 weeks after surgery.	Allows for proper fit of pouch that will protect peristomal skin.
12 Trace pattern on pouch backing or skin barrier.	Prepares for cutting opening in the pouch.
13 Cut opening in pouch.	Customizes pouch to provide appropriate fit over stoma.
14 Remove protective backing from adhesive surface. Remove rolled gauze from stoma.	Prepares pouch for application to skin.
15 Apply pouch. Press firmly into place around stoma and outside edges. Have patient hold hand over pouch 1 to 2 minutes to apply heat to secure seal.	Pouch adhesives are heat activated and will hold more securely at body temperature.
16 Use adapter provided with pouches to connect pouch to bedside urinary bag. Keep tubing below level of bag.	Provides for collection and measurement of urine. Allows patient to rest without frequent emptying of the pouch.
17 Complete postprocedure protocol.	

STEP	RATIONALE
18 Observe appearance of stoma, peristomal skin, and suture line during pouch change.	Determines condition of stoma and peristomal skin and progress of wound healing.
19 Evaluate character and volume of urinary drainage.	Determines if stoma and/or stents are patent. Character of urine reveals degree of concentration and alterations in renal function.
20 Observe patient's and family caregiver's willingness to view stoma and ask questions about procedure.	Determines level of adjustment and understanding of stoma care and pouch application.

Recording and Reporting

- Record type of pouch, time of change, condition and appearance of stoma and peristomal skin, and character of urine.
- Record urinary output on intake and output form.
- Record patient's and family caregiver's reaction to stoma and level of participation.
- Report abnormalities in stoma or peristomal skin and absence of urinary output to nurse in charge or health care provider.

UNEXPECTED OUTCOMES	RELATED INTERVENTIONS
1 Skin around stoma is irritated, blistered, or bleeding, or a rash is noted, as a result of chronic exposure to urine.	• Check stoma size and opening in skin barrier. Resize skin barrier opening if necessary. • Remove pouch more carefully. • Consult ostomy care nurse.
2 There is no urine output for several hours, or output is less than 30 mL/hr. Urine has foul odor.	• Increase fluid intake. • Notify health care provider. • Obtain urine specimen for culture and sensitivity as ordered.
3 Patient and family caregiver are unable to observe stoma, ask questions, or participate in care.	• Consult ostomy care nurse. • Allow patient to express feelings. • Encourage family support.

Vaginal Instillations

Vaginal medications are available in foam, jelly, cream, or suppository form. Medicated irrigations or douches can also be given. However, their excessive use can lead to vaginal irritation. Vaginal suppositories are oval shaped and individually packaged in foil wrappers. They are larger and more oval than rectal suppositories. Storage in a refrigerator prevents the solid suppositories from melting.

Delegation Considerations

The skill of administering vaginal medications cannot be delegated to nursing assistive personnel (NAP). The nurse directs the NAP about:

- Potential side effects of medications and to report their occurrence.
- Reporting any change in comfort level or any new or increased vaginal discharge or bleeding to the nurse for further assessment.

Equipment

- Vaginal cream, foam, jelly, tablet, or suppository, or irrigating solution
- Applicators (if needed)
- Clean gloves
- Tissues
- Towels and/or washcloths
- Perineal pad; drape or sheet
- Water-soluble lubricants
- Bedpan
- Irrigation or douche container (if needed)
- Medication administration record (MAR) or computer printout

Implementation

STEP	RATIONALE
1 Complete preprocedure protocol.	
2 Check accuracy and completeness of each medication administration record (MAR) with health care provider's medication order. Check patient's	The health care provider's order is the most reliable source and only legal record of drugs that patient is to receive. Ensures that patient receives correct medication. Handwritten

STEP	RATIONALE
name, drug name and dosage, route, and time for administration. Clarify incomplete or unclear orders with health care provider before administration.	MARs are a source of medication errors (ISMP, 2010; Jones and Treiber, 2010).
3 ⬛ Perform hand hygiene and apply clean gloves. During perineal care inspect condition of vaginal tissues; note if drainage is present. Remove gloves and perform hand hygiene.	Prevents transmission of microorganisms. Identifies symptoms of vaginal irritation or infection.
4 Assess patient's ability to manipulate applicator, suppository, or irrigation equipment and to properly position self to insert medication (may be done just before insertion).	Presence of mobility restrictions indicates need for assistance from nurse.
5 Prepare suppository for administration. Check label of medication against MAR 2 times. Preparation usually involves taking suppository out of refrigerator and taking to patient room. Check expiration date on container.	*These are the first and second checks for accuracy.* Process ensures that right patient receives right medication.
6 Identify patient using at least two patient identifiers (e.g., name and birthday or name and account number) according to agency policy. Compare identifiers with information on patient's MAR or medical record.	Ensures correct patient. Complies with The Joint Commission requirements for patient safety (TJC, 2014).

STEP	RATIONALE
7 At patient's bedside again compare MAR or computer printout with names of medications on medication labels and patient name. Ask patient if he or she has allergies.	*This is the third check for accuracy* and ensures that patient receives correct medication. Confirms patient's allergy history.
8 Discuss purpose of each medication, action, and possible adverse effects. Allow patient to ask any questions about the drugs. Explain procedure if patient plans to self-administer medication.	Patient has right to be informed, and patient's understanding of each medication improves adherence to drug therapy.
9 ![hand icon] Close door or pull curtain. Perform hand hygiene, arrange supplies at bedside, and apply clean gloves.	Reduces transfer of microorganisms; helps nurse perform procedure smoothly.
10 Have patient void. Help her lie in dorsal recumbent position. Patients with restricted mobility in knees or hips may lie supine with legs abducted.	Voiding prevents passing of urine during insertion of suppository. Position provides easy access to and good exposure of vaginal canal. Dependent position also allows suppository to completely dissolve in vagina
11 Keep abdomen and lower extremities draped.	Minimizes patient's embarrassment by limiting exposure.
12 Be sure vaginal orifice is well illuminated by room light. Otherwise, position portable gooseneck lamp.	Proper insertion requires visualization of external genitalia if not self-administered.
13 **Insert suppository:**	
a Remove suppository from wrapper, and apply liberal amount of water-soluble lubricant to smooth or rounded end. Be sure that	Lubrication reduces friction against mucosal surfaces during insertion. Use of petroleum jelly may leave a residue that harbors bacteria and yeast fungi.

STEP	RATIONALE
suppository is at room temperature. Lubricate gloved index finger of dominant hand.	
b With nondominant gloved hand, gently separate labial folds in the front-to-back direction.	Exposes vaginal orifice.
c With dominant gloved hand, insert rounded end of suppository along posterior wall of vaginal canal the entire length of finger (7.5 to 10 cm [3 to 4 inches]) (Fig. 82-1).	Proper placement of suppository ensures equal distribution of medication along walls of vaginal cavity.
d Withdraw finger and discard remaining lubricant from around orifice and labia with tissue or cloth.	Maintains comfort.
14 Apply cream or foam:	
a Fill cream or foam applicator following package directions.	Dose is based on volume in applicator.
b With nondominant gloved hand, gently separate labial folds.	Exposes vaginal orifice.
c With dominant gloved hand, insert applicator approximately 5 to 7.5 cm (2 to 3 inches). Push applicator plunger to deposit medication into vagina (Fig. 82-2).	Allows equal distribution of medication along vaginal walls.
d Withdraw applicator, and place on paper towel. Remove residual cream from labia or vaginal or-ifice with a tissue or cloth.	Maintains patient comfort.

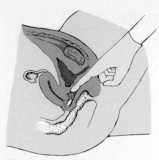

Fig. 82-1 Angle of vaginal suppository insertion.

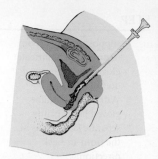

Fig. 82-2 Applicator inserted into vaginal canal. Plunger pushed to instill medication.

STEP	RATIONALE
15 Administer irrigation and douche:	
a Place patient on bedpan with absorbent pad underneath.	Allows hips to be higher than shoulders, and solution reaches posterior wall of vagina. Bedpan collects solution.
b Be sure that irrigation or douche fluid is at body temperature. Run fluid through container nozzle (priming the tubing).	Body temperature promotes patient comfort. Priming tubing removes air and moistens the nozzle tip.
c Gently separate labial folds, and direct nozzle toward sacrum, following the floor of the vagina.	Correct angle allows nozzle access into the vagina.
d Raise container approximately 30 to 50 cm (12 to 20 inches) above level of vagina. Insert nozzle 7 to 10 cm (3 to 4 inches). Allow solution to flow while rotating nozzle. Administer all irrigating solution.	Rotating nozzle allows irrigation of all areas in vagina.

STEP	RATIONALE
e Withdraw nozzle, and assist patient to a comfortable sitting position.	Remaining solution drains by gravity.
f Allow patient to remain on bedpan for a few minutes. Cleanse perineum with soap and water.	Ensures all solution drains from vagina. Provides comfort for the patient.
g Help patient off bedpan. Dry perineal area.	Provides comfort.
16 Instruct patient who received suppository, cream, or tablet to remain on her back for at least 10 minutes.	Allows melting and spreading of the medication throughout vaginal cavity and prevents loss through the vaginal orifice.
17 If using an applicator, wash with soap and warm water, rinse, and store for future use.	Vaginal cavity is not sterile. Soap and water assist in removal of bacteria and residual cream from applicator.
18 Offer perineal pad when patient resumes ambulation.	Provides patient comfort.
19 Complete postprocedure protocol.	
20 Observe patient demonstrate administration of next dose.	Reflects learning of technique.

Recording and Reporting

- Record drug (or solution if vaginal instillation), dose, type of instillation, and time administered on MAR immediately after administration, not before. Include initials or signature. Record patient teaching and validation of understanding and ability to self-administer medication in nurses' notes and electronic health record (EHR).
- Report to health care provider if patient states that symptoms do not disappear or if symptoms worsen.
- Report adverse effects, patient response, and/or withheld drugs to nurse in charge or health care provider.

UNEXPECTED OUTCOMES	RELATED INTERVENTIONS
1 Patient reports localized pruritus and burning.	• Are symptoms of infection or inflammation, but may also be a possible side effect of some medications (such as miconazole).
	• Monitor symptoms; report to health care provider.
2 Patient is unable to discuss drug therapy correctly.	• Repeat instructions, or assess whether patient is able to learn.
	• Include family caregiver when appropriate.
3 Patient is unable to self-administer medications.	• Reinstruction is necessary.

Venipuncture: Collecting Blood Specimens and Cultures by Syringe and Vacutainer Method

You are often responsible for collecting blood specimens; however, many agencies have specially trained phlebotomists who are responsible for drawing venous blood. Be familiar with your agency policies and procedures and your state Nurse Practice Act regarding guidelines for drawing blood samples.

The three methods of obtaining blood specimens are (1) skin puncture, (2) venipuncture, and (3) arterial puncture. Venipuncture is the most common method of obtaining blood specimens. This involves inserting a hollow-bore needle into the lumen of a large vein to obtain a specimen using either a needle and syringe or a Vacutainer device that allows the drawing of multiple samples. Because veins are major sources of blood for laboratory testing and routes for intravenous (IV) fluid or blood replacement, maintaining their integrity is essential. You need to be skilled in venipuncture to avoid unnecessary injury to veins.

Blood cultures aid in detection of bacteria in the blood. It is important that at least two culture specimens be drawn from two different sites. Because bacteremia may be accompanied by fever and chills, blood cultures should be drawn when the patient is experiencing these clinical signs (Pagana and Pagana, 2011). Bacteremia exists when both cultures grow the infectious agent. If only one culture grows bacteria, the bacteria are considered contaminated.

Draw cultures before antibiotic therapy begins since the antibiotic may interrupt the organism's growth in the laboratory. If the patient is receiving antibiotics, notify the laboratory of the specific antibiotics the patient is receiving (Pagana and Pagana, 2011).

Delegation Considerations

The skill of collecting blood specimens by venipuncture can be delegated to specially trained nursing assistive personnel (NAP). In some agencies, phlebotomists obtain the venipuncture samples. Agency and governmental regulations and policies differ regarding personnel who may draw blood specimens. The nurse informs the NAP to:

- Report any patient discomfort or signs of excessive bleeding from the puncture site to the nurse.

Equipment

All Procedures

- Chlorhexidine or antiseptic swab (check agency policy for use of 70% alcohol)
- Clean gloves
- Small pillow or folded towel
- Sterile 2 × 2–inch gauze pads
- Tourniquet
- Adhesive bandage or adhesive tape
- Completed identification labels with proper patient identifiers
- Completed laboratory requisition (appropriate patient identification, date, time, name of test, and source of culture)
- Small plastic biohazard bag for delivery of specimen to laboratory (or container specified by agency)
- Sharps container

Venipuncture with Syringe

- Sterile safety needles (20 to 21 gauge for adults; 23 to 25 gauge for children)
- Sterile 10- to 20-mL Luer-Lok safety syringes
- Needle-free blood transfer device
- Appropriate blood specimen tubes

Venipuncture with Vacutainer

- Vacutainer and safety access device with Luer-Lok adapter
- Sterile double-ended needles (20 to 21 gauge for adults; 23 to 25 gauge for children)
- Appropriate blood specimen tubes

Blood Cultures

- Sterile double needles (20 to 21 gauge for adults; 23 to 25 gauge for children)
- Two 20-mL sterile syringes
- Anaerobic and aerobic culture bottles (check agency policy)

Central Venous Catheter Collection

- Two empty 10-mL sterile syringes
- Sterile 10-mL normal saline flushes
- Vacutainer and safety access device with Luer-Lok adapter
- Appropriate blood specimen tubes

Implementation

STEP	RATIONALE
1 Complete preprocedure protocol.	
2 Determine if special conditions need to be met before specimen collection (e.g., patient allowed nothing by mouth [NPO], specific time for collection in relation to medication given, need to ice specimen).	Some tests require meeting specific conditions to obtain accurate measurement of blood elements (e.g., fasting blood glucose, drug peak and trough levels, and timed endocrine hormone levels).
3 Assess patient for possible risks associated with venipuncture: anticoagulant therapy, low platelet count, bleeding disorders (history of hemophilia). Review medication history.	Patient history may include abnormal clotting abilities caused by low platelet count, hemophilia, or medications that increase risk for bleeding and hematoma formation.
4 Assess patient for contraindicated sites for venipuncture: presence of IV fluids, hematoma at potential site, arm on side of mastectomy, or hemodialysis shunt.	Drawing specimens from such sites can result in false test results or may injure patient. Samples taken from vein near IV infusion may be diluted or may contain concentrations of IV fluids. Postmastectomy patient may have reduced lymphatic drainage in arm on operative side, increasing risk for infection from needlesticks. Never use arteriovenous shunt to obtain specimens because of risks of clotting and bleeding. Hematoma indicates existing injury to vessel wall.
5 Apply tourniquet so it can be removed by pulling an end with a single motion.	Tourniquet blocks venous return to heart from extremity, causing veins to dilate for easier visibility.

STEP	RATIONALE
a Position tourniquet 5 to 10 cm (2 to 4 inches) above venipuncture site selected (antecubital fossa site is most often used).	
b Cross tourniquet over patient's arm. May place tourniquet over gown sleeve to protect skin.	Older adult's skin is very fragile.
c Hold tourniquet between your fingers close to arm. Tuck loop between patient's arm and tourniquet so you can grasp free end easily.	Pull free end to release tourniquet after venipuncture.

SAFETY ALERT Palpate distal pulse (e.g., brachial) below tourniquet. If pulse is not palpable, remove tourniquet, wait 60 seconds, and reapply tourniquet more loosely. If tourniquet is too tight, pressure will impede arterial flow.

6 **Do not** keep tourniquet on patient longer than 1 minute.	Prolonged tourniquet application causes stasis, localized acidemia, and hemoconcentration (Pagana and Pagana, 2011).
7 Ask patient to open and close fist several times, finally leaving fist clenched.	Facilitates distention of veins by forcing blood up from distal veins. Vigorous opening and closing may cause erroneous laboratory results of hemoconcentration (Pagana and Pagana, 2011).
8 Quickly inspect extremity for best venipuncture site, looking for straight, prominent vein without swelling or hematoma.	Straight and intact veins are easiest to puncture.

STEP	RATIONALE
9 Apply clean gloves. Palpate selected vein with finger (Fig. 83-1). Note if vein is firm and rebounds when palpated or if it feels rigid or cordlike and rolls when palpated. Avoid vigorously slapping vein, which can cause vasospasm.	Patent, healthy vein is elastic and rebounds on palpation. Thrombosed vein is rigid, rolls easily, and is difficult to puncture.
10 Obtain blood specimen:	
a Syringe method	
(1) Have syringe with appropriate needle securely attached.	Needle must not dislodge from syringe during venipuncture.
(2) Cleanse venipuncture site with antiseptic swabs, with first swab moving back and forth on horizontal plane, another swab on vertical plane, and last in circular motion from site outward for about 5 cm (2 inches) for 30 seconds. Allow to dry.	Antimicrobial agent cleans skin surface of resident bacteria so organisms do not enter puncture site. Allowing antiseptic to dry completes its antimicrobial task and reduces "sting" of venipuncture. Alcohol left on skin can cause hemolysis of sample and retraction of tissue away from puncture site.
(a) If drawing sample for blood alcohol level or blood cultures, use only antiseptic swab, not alcohol swab.	Ensures accurate test results.

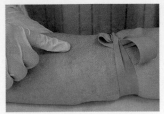

Fig. 83-1 Palpation of vein.

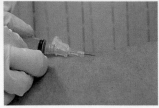

Fig. 83-2 Inserting needle into vein.

STEP	RATIONALE
(3) Remove needle cover, and inform patient that "stick" lasts only a few seconds.	Patient has better control over anxiety when prepared about what to expect.

SAFETY ALERT Observe needle for defects, such as burrs, which can cause increased discomfort and damage to the patient's vein (McCall and Tankersley, 2012).

(4) Place thumb or forefinger of nondominant hand 2.5 cm (1 inch) below site, and gently pull skin taut. Stretch skin steadily until vein is stabilized.	Stabilizes vein and prevents rolling during needle insertion.
(5) Hold syringe and needle at 15- to 30-degree angle from patient's arm with bevel up.	Reduces chance of penetrating both sides of vein during insertion. Bevel up decreases chance of contamination by not dragging bevel opening over the skin and allows point of needle to first puncture skin, reducing trauma.
(6) Slowly insert needle into vein (Fig. 83-2), stopping when "pop" is felt as needle enters vein.	Prevents puncture through vein to opposite side.

STEP	RATIONALE
(7) Hold syringe securely and pull back gently on plunger.	Syringe held securely prevents needle from advancing. Pulling on plunger creates vacuum needed to draw blood into syringe. If plunger is pulled back too quickly, pressure may collapse vein.
(8) Observe for blood return.	If blood flow fails to appear, needle may not be in vein.
(9) Obtain desired amount of blood, keeping needle stabilized.	Test results are more accurate when required amount of blood is obtained. You cannot perform some tests without minimal blood requirement. Movement of needle increases discomfort.
(10) After obtaining specimen, release tourniquet.	Reduces bleeding at site when needle is withdrawn.
(11) Apply 2 × 2–inch gauze pad without applying pressure. Quickly but carefully withdraw needle from vein, and apply pressure following removal of needle. Check for hematoma.	Pressure over needle can cause discomfort. Careful removal of needle minimizes discomfort and vein trauma. Hematoma may cause compression injury (McCall and Tankersley, 2012).
(12) Activate safety cover and immediately discard needle in appropriate container.	Prevents needlestick injury.
(13) Attach blood-filled syringe to needle-free blood transfer device. Attach tube and allow vacuum to	Additives prevent clotting. Shaking can cause hemolysis of red blood cells (RBCs).

STEP	RATIONALE
fill tube to specified level. Remove and fill other tubes as appropriate. Gently rotate each tube back and forth 8 to 10 times.	
b Vacutainer method (vacuum tube system method)	
(1) Attach double-ended needle to Vacutainer tube.	Long end of needle is used to puncture vein. Short end fits into blood tubes.
(2) Have proper blood specimen tube resting inside Vacutainer, but do not puncture rubber stopper.	Puncturing causes loss of tube's vacuum.
(3) Clean venipuncture site by following Step 10(2). Allow to dry.	Cleans skin surface of resident bacteria so that organisms do not enter puncture site. Drying maximizes effect of antiseptic.
(4) Remove needle cover and inform patient that "stick" will occur, lasting only a few seconds.	Patient has better control over anxiety when prepared about what to expect.
(5) Place thumb or forefinger of nondominant hand 2.5 cm (1 inch) below site, and gently pull skin taut. Stretch skin down until vein stabilizes.	Helps to stabilize vein and prevent rolling during needle insertion.
(6) Hold Vacutainer needle at 15- to 30-degree angle from arm with bevel up.	Smallest and sharpest point of needle will puncture skin first. Reduces chance of penetrating sides of vein during insertion. Keeping bevel up causes less trauma to vein.

STEP	RATIONALE
(7) Slowly insert needle into vein.	Prevents puncture on opposite side.
(8) Grasp Vacutainer securely, and advance specimen tube into needle of holder (do not advance needle in vein).	Pushing needle through stopper breaks the vacuum and causes flow of blood into tube. If needle in vein advances, vein may become punctured on other side.
(9) Note flow of blood into tube (should be fairly rapid) (Fig. 83-3).	Failure of blood to appear indicates that vacuum in tube is lost or needle is not in vein.
(10) After filling specimen tube, grasp Vacutainer firmly, and remove tube. Insert additional specimen tubes as needed. Gently rotate each tube back and forth 8 to 10 times.	Vacuum in tube stops flow at amount to be collected. Grasping prevents needle from advancing or dislodging. Tube should fill completely because additives in certain tubes are measured in proportion to filled tube. Ensures proper mixing with additive to prevent clotting.
(11) After last tube is filled and removed from Vacutainer, release tourniquet.	Reduces bleeding at site when needle is withdrawn.
(12) Apply 2 × 2–inch gauze pad over puncture site without applying	Pressure over needle can cause discomfort. Careful removal of needle minimizes discomfort and vein trauma.

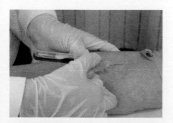

Fig. 83-3 Blood flowing into tube.

STEP	RATIONALE
pressure, and quickly but carefully withdraw needle with Vacutainer from vein.	
(13) Immediately apply pressure over venipuncture site with gauze or antiseptic pad for 2 to 3 minutes or until bleeding stops. Observe for hematoma. Tape gauze dressing securely.	Direct pressure minimizes bleeding and prevents hematoma formation. A hematoma may cause compression on nerve injury. Pressure dressing controls bleeding.
c Blood cultures	
(1) Clean venipuncture site as in Step 10(2) with antiseptic swab to follow agency policy. Allow to dry.	Antimicrobial agent cleans skin surface so that organisms do not enter puncture site or contaminate culture. Drying ensures complete antimicrobial action and decreases stinging.
(2) Clean bottle tops of culture bottles for 15 seconds with agency-approved cleaning solution. Allow to dry.	Ensures that bottle top is sterile.
(3) Collect 10 to 15 mL of venous blood using syringe method in 20-mL syringe from two different venipuncture sites.	Two blood cultures must be collected from two different sites to confirm culture growth (Pagana and Pagana, 2011).
(4) With each specimen, activate safety guard and discard needle. Replace with new sterile needle before injecting blood sample into culture bottle.	Maintains sterile technique and prevents contamination of specimen.

STEP	RATIONALE
(5) If both aerobic and anaerobic cultures are needed, fill anaerobic bottle first.	Anaerobic organisms may take longer to grow (Pagana and Pagana, 2011).
(6) Gently mix blood in each culture bottle.	Mixes medium and blood.
11 Check tubes for any sign of external contamination with blood. Decontaminate with 70% alcohol if necessary.	Prevents cross-contamination. Reduces risk for exposure to pathogens present in blood.
12 Remove gloves and perform hand hygiene after specimen is obtained and any spillage is cleaned.	Reduces risk for exposure to bloodborne pathogens.
13 Perform postprocedure protocol.	

Recording and Reporting

- Record method used to obtain blood specimen, date and time collected, type of test ordered, disposition of specimen, and description of venipuncture site.
- Report any STAT or abnormal test results to health care provider.

UNEXPECTED OUTCOMES	RELATED INTERVENTIONS
1 Hematoma forms at venipuncture site.	• Apply pressure using 2 × 2–inch gauze dressing. • Continue to monitor patient for pain and discomfort.
2 Bleeding at site continues.	• Apply pressure to site; patient may also apply pressure. • Monitor patient. • Notify health care provider.
3 Signs and symptoms of infection at venipuncture site occur.	• Notify health care provider. • Apply moist heat to site.
4 Laboratory tests reveal abnormal blood results.	• Notify health care provider.

Wound Drainage Devices:
Jackson-Pratt, Hemovac

If drainage accumulates in the wound bed, wound healing is delayed. Drainage is removed by using either a closed or an open drain system even if the amount of drainage is small. An open drain system (e.g., a Penrose drain [Fig. 84-1]) removes drainage from the wound and deposits it onto the skin surface. Insert a sterile safety pin through the drain, outside the skin, to prevent the tubing from moving into the wound. To remove the Penrose drain, the health care provider advances the tubing in stages as the wound heals from the bottom up.

A closed drain system, such as the Hemovac drain (Fig. 84-2) or Jackson-Pratt (JP) drain (Fig. 84-3), relies on the presence of a vacuum to withdraw accumulated drainage from around the wound bed into the collection device. The collection device is connected to a clear plastic drain with multiple perforations. Drainage collects in a closed reservoir, or a suction bladder.

Delegation Considerations

The assessment of wound drainage and maintenance of drains and the drainage system cannot be delegated to NAP. However, you may delegate emptying a closed drainage container or pouch, measuring the amount of drainage, and reporting the amount on the patient's intake and output (I&O) record to NAP. The nurse directs the NAP by:

- Discussing any increase in frequency of emptying the drain other than once a shift.
- Instructing to report to the nurse any change in amount, color, or odor of drainage.
- Reviewing the I&O procedure.

Equipment

- Graduated measuring cylinder
- Alcohol sponge
- Gauze sponges
- Goggles if needed
- Sterile specimen container, if culture is needed
- Sterile dressings or pouch, if drain is needed
- Clean gloves
- Safety pin(s)

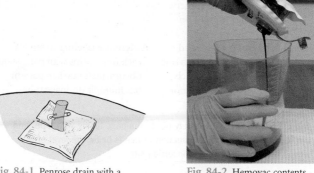

Fig. 84-1 Penrose drain with a drain-split gauze.

Fig. 84-2 Hemovac contents drained into sterile measuring container.

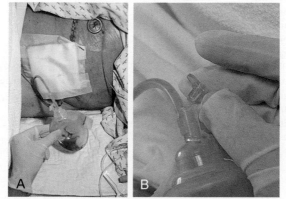

Fig. 84-3 **A,** Jackson-Pratt wound drainage system. **B,** Emptying Jackson-Pratt device.

Implementation

STEP	RATIONALE
1 Complete preprocedure protocol.	
2 Identify presence, location, and purpose of closed wound drain and drainage system as	Drainage tubing is usually placed near wound through small surgical incision.

STEP	RATIONALE
patient returns from surgery. Assess drainage present on patient's dressing.	
3 Identify number of wound drain tubes and what each one will be draining. Label each drain tube with a number or label.	Assigning a labeling system to each drain helps with consistent documentation when patient has multiple drainage tubes.

SAFETY ALERT Attach a safety pin to drainage tubing with tape, and pin to patient's gown so the suction device is below the level of the wound and does not pull on insertion site.

4 Be sure Penrose drain has a sterile safety pin in place. Penrose drains are sometimes covered with a gauze dressing or wound pouch. Use caution, and do not accidentally pull on drain while positioning gauze.	Pin prevents drain from being pulled below the skin's surface.
5 Place open specimen container or measuring graduate on bed between you and patient.	Permits measuring and discarding of wound drainage.
6 Empty Hemovac or ConstaVac:	Avoids entry of pathogens.
a Maintain asepsis while opening plug on port indicated for emptying drainage reservoir.	Vacuum will be broken, and reservoir will pull air in until chamber is fully expanded.
(1) Tilt suction container in direction of plug.	Drains fluid toward plug.
(2) Slowly squeeze two flat surfaces together, tilting toward measuring container.	Prevents splashing of contaminated drainage.
b Drain contents into measuring container.	Contents are counted as fluid output.
c Hold uncovered alcohol swab in dominant hand. Place suction device on flat surface with open outlet	Compression of surface of Hemovac creates vacuum.

STEP	RATIONALE
facing upward; continue pressing downward until bottom and top are in contact.	
d Holding surfaces together with one hand, and using an alcohol swab, quickly clean opening and plug with other hand and immediately replace plug; secure evacuator on patient's bed.	Cleansing of plug reduces transmission of microorganisms into drainage evacuation.
e Check suction device for reestablishment of vacuum, patency of drainage tubing, and absence of stress on tubing.	Facilitates wound drainage and prevents tension on drainage tubing.
7 Empty JP suction drain:	
a Open port on top of bulb-shaped reservoir (see Fig. 84-2, *B*).	Breaks vacuum for drain.
b Tilt bulb in direction of port, and drain toward opening. Empty drainage from suction device into measuring container. Clean end of emptying port and plug with alcohol wipe.	Reduces transmission of microorganisms.
c Compress bulb over drainage container. While compressing bulb, replace plug immediately.	Reestablishes vacuum.
8 Place and secure drainage system below site with safety pin on patient's gown. Be sure there is slack in tubing from reservoir to wound.	Pinning drainage tubing to patient's gown prevents tension or pulling on tubing and insertion site.
9 Complete postprocedure protocol.	

Recording and Reporting

- Record emptying the drainage suction device; reestablishing vacuum in suction device; amount, color, odor of drainage; dressing change to drain site; and appearance of drain insertion site.
- Record amount of drainage on I&O record.
- Immediately report a sudden change in amount of drainage, either output or absence of drainage flow, to the health care provider. Also report pungent odor of drainage or new evidence of purulence, severe pain, or dislodgment of the drainage tube to the health care provider.

UNEXPECTED OUTCOMES	RELATED INTERVENTIONS
1 Site where tube exits becomes infected.	• Notify health care provider about the presence of signs of infection: purulent drainage, odor, reddened site, increased white blood cell count, and temperature elevation. • Use aseptic technique when changing dressings.
2 Bleeding appears in or around drainage collector.	• Determine amount of bleeding, and notify health care provider if excessive. • Assess for tension on patient's drainage tubing. • Secure tubing to prevent pulling and pain.
3 Patient experiences pain.	• Assess patient's level of pain. • Medicate patient. • Stabilize drainage tubing to reduce tension and pulling against incision. • Notify health care provider if signs of wound infection are present.
4 Drainage suction device is not accumulating drainage.	• Assess drainage tubing for clots. • Assess drainage system for air leaks or kinks. • Notify health care provider.

Wound Irrigation

Wound irrigation cleanses and irrigates surgical or chronic wounds such as pressure ulcers (Table 85-1). Introduce the cleansing solution directly into the wound with a syringe, syringe and catheter, or pulsed lavage device. When using a syringe, the tip remains 2.5 cm (1 inch) above the wound. If a patient has a deep wound with a narrow opening, attach a soft catheter to the syringe to permit the fluid to enter the wound. Irrigation should not cause tissue injury or discomfort. Avoid fluid retention in the wound by positioning patient on his or her side to encourage the flow of the irrigant away from the wound.

Delegation Considerations

The skill of sterile wound irrigation cannot be delegated to nursing assistive personnel (NAP). However, you can delegate the cleansing of chronic wounds using clean technique. It is the nurse's responsibility to assess and document wound characteristics. The nurse directs the NAP to:

- Notify the nurse when the wound is exposed so an assessment can be completed.
- Report patient pain.

Equipment

- Irrigant/cleansing solution (volume 1.5 to 2 times the estimated wound volume)
- Irrigation delivery system (per order), depending on amount of pressure desired: sterile irrigation 35-mL syringe with sterile soft angiocatheter or 19-gauge needle (WOCN, 2010) or handheld shower.
- Protective equipment: sterile gloves, gown, and goggles (used when splash or spray from wound is a risk)
- Waterproof underpad, if needed
- Dressing supplies (see Skills 18, 19, and 20)
- Disposable waterproof biohazard bag
- Extra towels and padding (used to protect bed)
- Wound assessment supplies

TABLE 85-1 Wound Cleansing Considerations

| | Mechanical Force | |
	High Pressure	Low Pressure
Wound base characteristics	Presence of necrotic tissue (eschar, fibrin slough), debris, or other particulate matter Significant bacterial burden Moderate/large amount of exudates	Presence of granulation tissue or new epithelial cells Nonserous or minimally serous or serosanguineous exudate
Clinical outcomes	Loosen, soften, and remove devitalized tissue from wound Separate eschar from fibrotic tissue/fibrotic tissue from granulating base	Prevent trauma to viable wound tissue Remove wound care product residue
Solutions	Normal saline Volume of solution depends on size of wound	Normal saline Volume of solution depends on size of wound
Delivery systems	35-mL syringe/19-gauge angiocatheter	Pouring saline directly from a bottle Bulb syringe Piston syringe

Adapted from Spear M: Wound cleansing: solutions and techniques, *Plast Surg Nurs* 31(1):29, 2011.

Implementation

STEP	RATIONALE
1 Complete preprocedure protocol.	
2 If needed, administer analgesic 30 to 45 minutes before starting wound irrigation procedure.	Promotes pain control and permits patient to move more easily and be positioned to facilitate wound irrigation (Krasner, 2012).

STEP	RATIONALE
3 Close room door or bed curtains, perform hand hygiene, and position patient.	Maintains privacy. Frequent hand hygiene reduces microorganisms.
a Position comfortably to permit gravitational flow of irrigating solution over wound and into collection receptacle (Fig. 85-1).	Directing solution from top to bottom of wound and from clean to contaminated area prevents further infection. Position patient during planning stage, keeping in mind the bed surfaces needed for later preparation of equipment.
b Position patient so that wound is vertical to collection basin. Place container of irrigant/cleansing solution in basin of hot water to warm solution to body temperature.	Warmed solution increases comfort and reduces vascular constriction response in tissues.
4 Place padding or extra towel on bed under area where irrigation will take place.	Protects bedding from becoming wet.
5 Expose wound only.	Provides privacy and prevents chilling of patient.
6 ⚡ Apply gown and goggles. Apply sterile gloves for Steps 7 and 8, and use sterile precautions.	Protects nurse from splashes or sprays of blood and body fluids.
7 Irrigate wound with wide opening:	
a Fill 35-mL syringe with irrigation solution.	Flushing wound helps remove debris and facilitates healing by secondary intention.

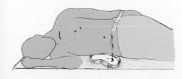

Fig. 85-1 Patient position for wound irrigation.

STEP	RATIONALE
b Attach a 19-gauge angiocatheter or 19-gauge needle.	Catheter lumen delivers ideal pressure for cleansing and removal of debris (Ramundo, 2012).
c Hold syringe tip 2.5 cm (1 inch) above upper end of wound and over area being cleansed.	Prevents syringe contamination. Careful placement of the syringe prevents unsafe pressure of the flowing solution.
d Using continuous pressure, flush wound; repeat Steps 7a to 7d until solution draining into basin is clear.	Clear solution indicates removal of all debris.
8 Irrigate deep wound with very small opening:	
a Attach soft catheter to filled irrigating syringe.	Catheter permits direct flow of irrigant into wound. Expect wound to take longer to empty when opening is small.
b Gently insert tip of catheter into opening about 1.3 cm (0.5 inch).	Prevents tip from touching fragile inner wall of wound.

SAFETY ALERT Do not force catheter into wound because this will cause tissue damage.

c Using slow, continuous pressure, flush wound.	Use of slow mechanical force of stream of solution loosens particulate matter on wound surface and promotes healing (Ramundo, 2012).
d While keeping catheter in place, pinch it off just below syringe.	
e Remove and refill syringe. Reconnect to catheter and repeat until solution draining into basin is clear.	

STEP	RATIONALE
9 **Cleanse wound with handheld shower:**	
a Perform hand hygiene and apply clean gloves. With patient seated comfortably in shower chair, adjust spray to gentle flow; make sure water is warm.	Useful for patients able to shower with assistance or independently. May be accomplished at home.
b Shower for 5 to 10 minutes with showerhead 30 cm (12 inches) from wound.	Ensures wound is thoroughly cleansed.
10 When indicated, obtain cultures after cleansing with nonbacteriostatic saline.	WOCN (2010) recommends using quantitative bacterial cultures (tissue biopsy or swab cultures).
11 Dry wound edges with gauze; dry patient after shower.	Prevents maceration of surrounding tissue from excess moisture.
12 Apply appropriate dressing (see Skills 18, 19, and 20) and label with time, date, and nurse's initials.	Maintains protective barrier and healing environment for wound.
13 Complete postprocedure protocol.	

Recording and Reporting

- Record wound assessment before and after irrigation; amount, color, and odor of drainage on dressing removed; amount and type of solution used; irrigation device used; patient's tolerance of the procedure; type of dressing applied after irrigation.
- Immediately report to attending health care provider any evidence of fresh bleeding, sharp increase in pain, retention of irrigant, or signs of shock.

UNEXPECTED OUTCOMES	RELATED INTERVENTIONS
1 Bleeding or serosanguineous drainage appears.	• Flush wound during next irrigation using less pressure. • Notify health care provider of bleeding.
2 Increased pain or discomfort occurs.	• Decrease force of pressure during wound irrigation. • Assess patient for need for additional analgesia before wound care.
3 Suture line opening extends.	• Notify health care provider. • Reevaluate amount of pressure to use for next wound irrigation.

Overview of CDC Hand Hygiene Guidelines

In 2002 the Centers for Disease Control and Prevention (CDC) released recommendations for hand hygiene in health care settings. *Hand hygiene* is a general term that applies to handwashing, antiseptic hand wash, antiseptic hand rub, or surgical hand antisepsis. *Handwashing* refers to washing hands thoroughly with plain soap and water. *Antiseptic hand wash* is defined as washing hands with water and soap containing an antiseptic agent. Antimicrobials effectively reduce bacterial counts on hands and often have residual antimicrobial effects for several hours. An *antiseptic hand rub* is an application of an antiseptic, alcohol-based waterless product to all surfaces of the hands to reduce the number of microorganisms present. *Surgical hand antisepsis* is an antiseptic hand wash or antiseptic hand rub performed preoperatively by surgical personnel.

Evidence suggests that hand antisepsis, the cleansing of hands with an antiseptic hand rub, is more effective in reducing health care–acquired infections (HAIs) than plain handwashing.

Guidelines in the Care of All Patients

Wash hands—preferably with an antimicrobial soap and water—when hands are visibly dirty, contaminated with proteinaceous material, or visibly soiled with blood or other body fluids. The recommended duration for lathering is *at least 15 seconds.*

- Wash hands with soap and water before eating.
- Wash hands with soap and water after using the restroom.
- Wash hands if exposed to spore-forming organisms such as *Clostridium difficile* or *Bacillus anthracis.* The physical action of washing and rinsing the hands is recommended because alcohols, chlorhexidine, iodophors, and other antiseptic agents have poor activity against spores.

If hands are not visibly soiled, use an alcohol-based hand rub for routinely decontaminating the hands in all of the following clinical situations:

- Before having direct contact with patients
- Before donning sterile gloves
- Before inserting indwelling urinary catheters, peripheral vascular catheters, or other invasive devices that do not require a surgical procedure
- After contact with a patient's intact skin (e.g., after taking a pulse or blood pressure, after lifting a patient)
- After contact with body fluids or excretions, mucous membranes, nonintact skin, and wound dressings *if hands are not visibly soiled*

- When moving from a contaminated body site to a clean body site during patient care
- After contact with inanimate objects (e.g., medical equipment) in the immediate vicinity of the patient
- After removing gloves

Note that antiseptic hand wash may be performed in all situations in which an alcohol-based hand rub is indicated. Antimicrobial-impregnated wipes (i.e., towelettes) are not a substitute for using an alcohol-based hand rub or antimicrobial soap.

Methods for Decontaminating Hands

When using an alcohol-based hand rub, apply product to the palm of one hand and rub hands together, covering all surfaces of hands and fingers, until hands are dry. Follow the manufacturer's recommendations regarding the volume of product to use.

Guidelines for Surgical Hand Antisepsis

Surgical hand antisepsis reduces the resident microbial count on the hands to a minimum.

- The CDC recommends using an antimicrobial soap and scrubbing hands and forearms for the length of time recommended by the manufacturer, usually 2 to 6 minutes. Long scrub times (e.g., 10 minutes) are not necessary. Refer to agency policy for time required.
- When using an alcohol-based surgical hand-scrub product with persistent activity, follow the manufacturer's instructions. Before applying the alcohol solution, prewash hands and forearms with a nonantimicrobial soap, and dry hands and forearms completely. After application of the alcohol-based product as recommended, allow hands and forearms to dry thoroughly before donning sterile gloves.

General Recommendations for Hand Hygiene

- Use hand lotions or creams to minimize the occurrence of irritant contact dermatitis associated with hand antisepsis or hand washing.
- Do not wear artificial fingernails or extenders when having direct contact with patients at high risk (e.g., those in intensive care units or operating rooms).
- Keep natural nail tips less than $\frac{1}{4}$ inch long.
- Wear gloves when contact with blood or other potentially infectious materials, mucous membranes, and nonintact skin could occur.

- Remove gloves after caring for a patient. Do not wear the same pair of gloves for the care of more than one patient.
- Change gloves during patient care if moving from a contaminated body site to a clean body site, even when working under isolation precautions.

Data from Centers for Disease Control and Prevention guideline for hand hygiene in healthcare settings: recommendations of the Healthcare Infection Control Practices Advisory Committee and the HICPAC/SHEA/APIC/ISDA Hand Hygiene Task Force. MMWR Recomm Rep 51 (RR16):1, 202, www.cdc.gov/handhygiene.

BIBLIOGRAPHY

Agency for Health Care Policy and Research: *Panel for the Treatment of Pressure Ulcers: Treatment of pressure ulcers, Clinical Practice Guideline No. 15, AHCPR Pub No. 95–0652*, Rockville, MD, 1994, US Department of Health and Human Services.

Agency for Healthcare Research and Quality (AHRQ): *Negative-pressure wound therapy devices*, Rockville, MD, 2009, AHRQ. Available at: http://www.ahrq.gov/clinic/ta/negpresswtd/negpresswtd.pdf. Accessed January 8, 2012.

Alexander M, et al: *Infusion Nursing: An Evidence-Based Approach*, ed 3, St Louis, 2009, Elsevier.

Al-shaikh G, et al: Accuracy of bladder scanning in the assessment of postvoid residual volume, *J Obstet Gynecol Can* 31(6):526, 2009.

American Academy of Orthopaedic Surgeons: *How to use crutches, canes, and walkers*, http://orthoinfo.aaos.org/topic/cfm/topic=A00181. Accessed December 2011.

American Association of Blood Banks: *Standards for blood banks and transfusion services*, ed 27, Bethesda, MD, 2011, The Association.

American Association of Critical Care Nurses (AACN): *Verification of feeding tube placement (blindly inserted)*, 2010, http://www.aacn.org/WD/Practice/Docs/PracticeAlerts/Verification_of_Feeding_Tube_Placement_05-2005.pdf. Accessed August 1, 2012.

American Association of Respiratory Care (AARC): *AARC clinical practice guideline: nasotracheal suctioning—2004 revision and update*, 2004, http://www.rcjournal.com/cpgs/pdf/09.04.1080.pdf. Accessed August 13, 2011.

American Association of Respiratory Care (AARC): AARC clinical practice guidelines: endotracheal suctioning of mechanically ventilated patients with artificial airways, *Respir Care* 55(6):758, 2010.

American Diabetes Association: *Foot complications*, 2011, http://www.diabetes.org/living-with-diabetes/complications/foot-complications/. Accessed February 21, 2012.

American Lung Association: *Supplemental oxygen*, 2012, http://www.lung.org/lung-disease/copd/living-with-copd/supplemental-oxygen.html. Accessed July 19, 2012.

American Pain Society (APS) and American Association of Pain Medicine (AAPM): Opioids guideline panel-Part 1, *J Pain* 10(2):113, 2009.

American Thoracic Society: *Home oxygen therapy*, 2012, http://www.thoracic.org/clinical/copd-guidelines/for-health-professionals/management-of-stable-copd/long-term-oxygen-therapy/home-oxygen-therapy.php. Accessed September 1, 2012.

Anthony K, et al: No interruption please: impact of a no-interruption zone on medication safety in intensive care units, *Crit Care Nurs* 30(3):21, 2010.

Aschenbrenner D, Venable S: *Drug therapy in nursing*, ed 3, Philadelphia, 2009, Lippincott, Williams & Wilkins.

Association of periOperative Registered Nurses (AORN): *Standards, recommended practices, and guidelines*, Denver, 2011, The Association.

Ayello EA, Braden B: How and why to do pressure ulcer risk assessment, *Adv Wound Care* 15(3):125, 2002.

Bankhead R, et al: Enteral nutrition administration: ASPEN enteral nutrition practice recommendations, *J Parenter Enteral Nutr* 33(2):158, 2009.

Barrons R, et al: Inhaler device selection: special considerations in elderly patients with chronic obstructive pulmonary disease, *Am J Health-System Pharmacy* 68(13):1221, 2011.

Bauman A, Handley C: Chest-tube care: the more you know the easier it gets, *Am Nurse Today* 6(9):27, 2011.

Beer C, et al: Quality use of medicines and health outcomes among a cohort of community dwelling older men: an observational study, *Br J Clin Pharmacol* 71(4):592, 2011.

Berg MD, et al: 2010 American Heart Association Guidelines for Cardiopulmonary Resuscitation and Emergency Cardiovascular Care. Part 13: Pediatric basic life support, *Circulation* 122(Suppl 3):S862, 2010.

Berry AM, et al: Effects of three approaches to standardized oral hygiene to reduce bacterial colonization and ventilator pneumonia in mechanically ventilated patients: a randomized control trial, *Int J Nurs Stud* 48(6):681, 2011.

Boullata J: Drug administration through an enteral feeding tube, *Am J Nurs* 109(10):34, 2009.

Bourgault AM, Halm MA: Feeding tube placement in adults: safe verification method for blindly inserted tubes, *Am J Crit Care* 18:73, 2009.

Boyd R, Stevens JA: Falls and fear of falling: burden, beliefs and behaviours, *Age Ageing* 38(4):423, 2009.

Braden BJ, Bergstrom N: Clinical utility of the Braden scale for predicting pressure sore risk, *Decubitus* 2(3):44, 1989.

Braden BJ, Bergstrom N: Predictive utility of the Braden scale for predicting pressure sore risk, *Res Nurs Health* 17:459, 1994.

Brady A: Managing the patient with dysphagia, *Home Healthc Nurse* 26(1):41, 2008.

Briggs D: Nursing care and management of patients with interpleural drains, *Nurs Stand* 24(21):47, 2010.

Brisko V: Isolation precautions. In Carrico R, et al, editors: *APIC text of infection control and epidemiology*, ed 3, Washington, DC, 2011, Association for Professionals in Infection Control and Epidemiology (APIC).

Btaiche IF, et al: Critical illness, gastrointestinal complications, and medication therapy during enteral feeding in critically ill adult patients, *Nutr Clin Pract* 25:32, 2010.

Campbell P, Smith G, Smith J: Retrospective clinical evaluation of gauze-based negative-pressure wound therapy, *Int Wound J* 5(2):280, 2008.

Centers for Disease Control and Prevention (CDC): *Guideline for isolation precautions: preventing transmission of infectious agents in healthcare settings*, 2007a, http://www.cdc.gov/ncidod/dhqp/gl_isolation.html. Accessed January 8, 2008.

Centers for Disease Control and Prevention (CDC): Hospital Infection Control Practices Advisory Committee: Guidelines for isolation precautions in hospitals, *MMWR Morb Mortal Wkly Rep* 57:RR–16, 2007b.

Centers for Disease Control and Prevention (CDC): *Epidemiology and prevention of vaccine-preventable diseases*, ed 12, Washington, DC, 2011a, Public Health Foundation.

Centers for Disease Control and Prevention (CDC): *Tuberculin skin test fact sheet*, 2011b, http://www.cdc.gov/tb/publications/factsheets/testing/skintesting.htm. Accessed July 11, 2011.

Centers for Medicare & Medicaid Services (CMS): *Revisions to Medicare conditions of participation, 37,* Bethesda, MD, 2008, US Department of Health and Human Services.

Centers for Medicare & Medicaid Services (CMS): *Updated guidance on medication administration, Hospital Appendix A of the State Operations Manual,* Baltimore, MD, 2011, US Department of Health and Human Services.

Cerfolio RJ: Recent advances in the treatment of air leaks, *Curr Opin Pulm Med* 11:319, 2005.

Chang C, Roberts B: Strategies for feeding patients with dementia, *Am J Nurs* 111(4):36, 2011.

Chang CM, et al: Medical conditions and medications as risk factors of falls in inpatient older people: a case-control study, *Int J Geriatr Psychiatry* 26(6):602, 2011.

Church N, Bjerke N: Surgical services. In Carrico R, editor: *APIC text of infection control and epidemiology,* revised, Washington, DC, 2009, Association for Professionals in Infection Control and Epidemiology (APIC).

Cicek HS, et al: Effect of nail polish and henna on oxygen saturation determined by pulse oximetry in healthy young adult females, *Emerg Med J* 28(9):783, 2011.

Cipa-Tatum J, et al: Urethral erosion: a case for prevention, *J Wound Ostomy Continence Nurs* 38(5):581, 2011.

Clore E: Seizure precautions for pediatric bedside nurses, *Pediatr Nurs* 36(4):191, 2010.

Colwell J, et al: *Fecal and urinary diversions: management principles,* St Louis, 2004, Mosby.

Costello E, Edelstein JE: Update on falls prevention for community-dwelling older adults: review of single and multifactorial intervention programs, *J Rehabil Res Dev* 45(8):1135, 2008.

Cullum N, et al: Beds, mattresses and cushions for pressure sore preventions and treatment, *Cochrane Database Syst Rev* 1(1), 2003.

Dandeles LM, Lodolce AE: Efficacy of agents to prevent and treat enteral feeding tube clogs, *Ann Pharmacother* 45:676, 2011.

D'Arcy Y: Keep your patient safe during PCA, *Nursing 2008* 38(1):50, 2008.

D'Arcy Y: Avoid the dangers of opioid therapy, *Am Nurse Today* 4(5):18, 2009.

D'Arcy Y: New thinking about postoperative pain management, *OR Nurse* 5(6):29, 2011.

D'Cruz R, et al: Catheter balloon-related urethral trauma in children, *J Paediatr Child Health* 45:564, 2009.

Delegge DH: Managing gastric residual volumes in the critically ill patient: an update, *Curr Opin Nutr Metab Care* 14:193, 2011.

Department of Health and Human Services, Centers for Medicare & Medicaid Services: *Updated guidance on medication administration, Hospital Appendix A of the State Operations Manual,* Baltimore, MD, 2011, Department of Health and Human Services.

Dietz D, Gates J: Basic ostomy management, part 1, *Nursing* 40(2):61, 2010a.

Dietz D, Gates J: Basic ostomy management, part 2, *Nursing* 40(5):62, 2010b.

Doughty DB, Sparks-Defriese B: Wound-healing physiology. In Bryant RA, Nix DP, editors: *Acute and chronic wounds: current management concepts,* ed 4, St Louis, 2012, Mosby.

Durai R, et al: Managing a chest tube and drainage system, *Nurs Stand* 91(2):275, 2010.

Durai R, Venkatraman R, Ng P: Nasogastric tubes 1: insertion technique and confirming the correct position, *Nurs Times* 105(16):12, 2009.

Eanarroch E: Orthostatic and postprandial hypotension. In Biller J, editor: *The interface of neurology and internal medicine*, Hagerstown, MD, 2007, Lippincott Williams and Wilkins.

Edmiaston J, et al: Validation of a dysphagia screening tool in acute stroke patients, *Am J Crit Care* 19(4):357, 2010.

Eliahu SF, et al: I. Status epilepticus, *South Med J* 101(4):400, 2008.

Evans LK, Cotter VT: Avoiding restraints in patients with dementia: understanding, prevention, and management are keys, *Am J Nurs* 108(3):40, 2008.

Ewy G, Kern K: Recent advances in cardiopulmonary resuscitation, *J Am Coll Cardiol* 53:149, 2009.

Farrington M, et al: Nasogastric tube placement verification in pediatric and neonatal patients, *Pediatr Nurs* 35(1):17, 2009.

Fox J, et al: Prophylactic hypothermia for traumatic brain injury: a quantitative systematic review, *CJEM* 12(4):355, 2010.

Frace M: Tracheostomy care on the medical-surgical unit, *Medsurg Nurs* 19(1):58, 2010.

Frey K, Ramsberger G: Comparison of outcomes before and after implementation of a water protocol for patients with cerebrovascular accident and dysphagia, *J Neurosci Nurs* 43(3):165, 2011.

Gabriel J: Infusion therapy part two: prevention and management of complications, *Nurs Standards* 22(32):41, 2008.

Garcia J, Chambers E: Managing dysphagia through diet modifications, *Am J Nurs* 110(11):26, 2010.

Gibney M, et al: Skin and subcutaneous adipose layer thickness in adults with diabetes at sites used for insulin injections: implications for needle length recommendation, *Curr Med Res Opin* 26(6):1520, 2010.

Giuliano K, Liu LM: Knowledge of pulse oximetry among critical care nurses, *Dimens Crit Care Nurs* 25(1):44, 2006.

Goldberg M, et al: *Management of the patient with a fecal ostomy: best practice guidelines for clinicians*, Mt Laurel, NJ, 2010, WOCN.

Gottschalk AW: Ice and cold application for musculoskeletal soft-tissue trauma, *Evid Based Pract* 14(5):13, 2011.

Gould CV, et al: *Guideline for prevention of catheter-associated urinary tract infections, Healthcare Infection Control Practices Advisory Committee*, 2009, http://www.cdc.gov/hicpac/cauti/001_cauti.html, 2009. Accessed August 2012.

Gray M: Securing the indwelling catheter, *Am J Nurs* 108(12):44, 2008.

Green L, Marx J, Oriola S: *Guide to the elimination of catheter-associated urinary tract infections, APIC*, 2008, www.apic.org/Resource_/Elimination GuideForm/c0790db8-2aca-4179-a7ae-676c27592de2/File/APIC-CAUTI-Guide.pdf. Accessed October 1, 2013.

Gribbin J, et al: Risk of falls associated with antihypertensive medication: population-based case-control study, *Age Ageing* 39(5):592, 2010.

Grodner, et al: *Foundations and clinical applications of nutrition: a nursing approach*, ed 4, St Louis, 2012, Mosby.

Hall LM, et al: Going blank: factors contributing to interruptions to nurses' work and related outcomes, *J Nurs Manage* 18(8):1040, 2010.

Halm MA: Hourly rounds: what does the evidence indicate? *Am J Crit Care* 18:581, 2009.

Harvard Health Publications: On the alert for deep-vein blood clots, *Harvard Heart Lett* 19(9):4, 2009.

Higgins D: Tracheostomy care: Part one—using suction, *Nurs Times* 105(4):16, 2009a.

Higgins D: Tracheostomy care: Part three—dressing, *Nurs Times* 105(6):12, 2009b.

Hockenberry M, Wilson D: *Wong's nursing care of infants and children*, ed 9, St Louis, 2011, Mosby.

Hoeman S: *Rehabilitation prevention, intervention, and outcomes*, ed 4, St Louis, 2007, Mosby.

Hopf H, et al: Managing wound pain. In Bryant RA, Nix DP, editors: *Acute and chronic wounds: current management concepts*, ed 4, St Louis, 2012, St Louis.

Howes D, et al: Stock your emergency departments with ice packs: a practical guide to therapeutic hypothermia for survivors of cardiac arrest, *Can Med Assoc J* 176(6):759, 2007.

Hunt C: Which site is best for an IM injection? *Nursing* 38(11):62, 2008.

Hunter K: Intramuscular injection technique, *Nurs Stand* 22(24):35, 2008a.

Hunter K: Subcutaneous injection technique, *Nurs Stand* 22(21):41, 2008b.

Institute for Clinical Systems Improvement (ICSI): *Prevention of falls (acute care)*, revised 2010, http://www.guideline.gov/summary/summary.aspx?ss=15&doc_id=13697&nbr=007031&string=patient+AND+falls#s23. Accessed May 2011.

Institute for Healthcare Improvement: *Implement the IHI Central Line Bundle*, Cambridge, Mass, 2011, http://www.ihi.org/knowledge/Pages/Changes/ImplementtheCentralLineBundle.aspx. Accessed August 20, 2012.

Infusion Nurses Society: Infusion nursing standards of practice, *J Infus Nurs* 34(Suppl 1):S93, 2011a.

Infusion Nurses Society: *Policy and procedures for infusion nursing*, ed 4, Norwood, Mass, 2011b, Author.

Institute for Safe Medication Practices (ISMP): *Splitting tablets challenges you and your patients*, 2008, http://www.ismp.org/newsletters/nursing/Issues/NurseAdviseERR200806.pdf. Accessed February 3, 2012.

Institute for Safe Medication Practices (ISMP): *Never use parenteral syringes for oral medications*, 2010, http://www.accessdata.fda.gov/psn/transcript.cfm?show=94#9. Accessed January 18, 2012.

Institute for Safe Medication Practices (ISMP): *Guidelines for standard order sets*, 2010, http://www.ismp.org/Tools/guidelines/StandardOrderSets.pdf, Accessed July 2011.

Institute for Safe Medication Practices (ISMP): *Acute care guidelines for timely administration of scheduled medications*, 2011, http://www.ismp.org/Tools/guidelines/acutecare/tasm.pdf. Accessed July 11, 2012.

Jones J, Treiber L: When 5 rights go wrong: medication errors from the nursing perspective, *J Nurs Care Qual* 25(3):240, 2010.

Jongerden I, et al: Effect of open and closed endotracheal suctioning on cross-contamination with gram-negative bacteria: a prospective crossover study, *Crit Care Med* 39(6):1313, 2011.

Justad M: Continuous subcutaneous infusion: an efficacious, cost-effective analgesia alternative at the end of life, *Home Healthc Nurse* 27(3):140, 2009.

LeFever Kee J, et al: *Fluids and electrolytes with clinical applications: a programmed approach*, ed 8, Clifton Park, NY, 2010, Delmar Cengage Learning.

Kelly J, et al: An analysis of two incidents of medicine administration to a patient with dysphagia, *J Clin Nurs* 20(1–2):146, 2011.

Kenny DJ, Goodman P: Care of the patient with enteral feeding: an evidence-based protocol, *Nurs Res* 59(Suppl):S22, 2010.

Khazzani H, et al: The relationship between physical performance measures, bone mineral density, falls, and the risk of peripheral fracture: a cross-sectional analysis, *BMC Public Health* 9:297, 2009.

Kiekkas P, et al: Physical antipyresis in critically ill adults, *Am J Nurs* 108(7):40, 2008.

Kiekkas P, et al: Postoperative hypothermia and mortality in critically ill adults: review and meta-analysis, *Aust J Adv Nurs* 28(4):60, 2011.

Kinetic Concepts: *The V.A.C. vacuum-assisted closure: V.A.C. therapy clinical guidelines: a reference source for clinicians, product information*, San Antonio, TX, 2012, Kinetic Concepts.

Kojima T, et al: Association of polypharmacy with fall risk among geriatric outpatients, *Geriatr Gerontol Int* 11(4):438, 2011.

Krasner DL: Wound pain: impact and assessment. In Bryant RA, Nix DP, editors: *Acute and chronic wounds: current management concepts*, ed 4, St Louis, 2012, Mosby.

Krenitsky J: Blind bedside placement of feeding tubes: treatment or threat? *Pract Gastroenterol* XXXV(3), 32, 2011.

Labeau SO, et al: Prevention of ventilator-associated pneumonia with oral antiseptics: a systematic review and meta-analysis, *Lancet Infect Dis* 11(11):845, 2011.

Leaver R: The evidence for urethral meatal cleansing, *Nurs Stand* 21(41):29, 2007.

Lehne R: *Pharmacology for nursing care*, ed 7, St Louis, 2010, Saunders.

LePorte L, et al: Effect of distraction-free environment on medication errors, *Am J Health-System Pharmacy* 66(9):795, 2009.

Lewis ML, et al: *Medical-surgical nursing: assessment and management of clinical problems*, ed 8, St Louis, 2011, Mosby.

Lilley LL, et al: *Pharmacology and the nursing process*, ed 6, St Louis, 2011, Mosby.

Linares G, Mayer SA: Hypothermia for the treatment of ischemic and hemorrhagic stroke, *Crit Care Med* 37(7 Suppl):S243, 2009.

Link MS, et al: American Heart Association Guidelines for Cardiopulmonary Resuscitation and Emergency Cardiovascular Care. Part 6: Electrical therapies: automated external defibrillators, defibrillation, cardioversion, and pacing, *Circulation* 122(Suppl 3):S706, 2010.

Lo E, et al: Strategies to prevent catheter-associated urinary tract infections in acute care hospitals, *Infect Control Hospital Epidemiol* 19(Suppl 1):S41, 2008.

Lynn-McHale, Wiegand D: *AACN procedure manual for critical care*, ed 6, St Louis, 2011, St Louis.

Malkin B, Berridge P: Guidance on maintaining personal hygiene in nail care, *Nurs Stand* (41):35, 23, 2009.

Markert S: The use of cryotherapy after a total knee replacement: a literature review, *Orthop Nurs* 30(10):29, 2011.

Martindell D: The safe use of negative-pressure wound therapy, *AJN* 112(6):61, 2012.

McCall R, Tankersley C: *Phlebotomy essentials*, ed 5, Philadelphia, 2012, Lippincott Williams & Wilkins.

Meiner SE: *Gerontologic nursing*, ed 4, St Louis, 2011, Mosby.

Méndez-Probst CE, et al: Fundamentals of instrumentation and urinary tract drainage. In Wein A, editor: *Campbell-Walsh Urology*, ed 10, Philadelphia, 2012, Saunders.

Mermel L, et al: Clinical practice guidelines for the diagnosis and management of intravascular catheter-related infection: 2009 update by the Infectious Diseases Society of America, *Clin Infect Dis* 49:1, 2009.

Metheny NA, et al: Gastric residual volume and aspiration in critically ill patients receiving gastric feeding, *Am J Crit Care* 17:512, 2008.

Metheny NA: Inconclusive evidence regarding the volume of gastric aspirate that can be safely reintroduced following residual volume measurements, *Evid Based Nurs* 13:71, 2010.

Metheny NA, et al: Relationship between feeding tube site and respiratory outcomes, *JPEN J Parenter Enteral Nutr* 35:346, 2011.

Middleman A, et al: Effect of needle length when immunizing obese adolescents with hepatitis B vaccine, *Pediatrics* 125(3):508, 2010.

Mininni NC, et al: Pulse oximetry: an essential tool for the busy med-surg nurse, *Am Nurs Today* 4(9):31, 2009.

Molinari J, Harte J: Dental services. In *APIC text of infection control and epidemiology*, revised, Washington, DC, 2009, Association for Professionals in Infection Control and Epidemiology (APIC).

NANDA International: *NANDA International: nursing diagnoses, definitions and classification, 2012-2014*, Philadelphia, 2012, NANDA International.

National High Blood Pressure Education Program (NHBPEP): National Heart, Lung, and Blood Institute; National Institutes of Health: The seventh report of the Joint National Committee on Detection, Evaluation, and Treatment of High Blood Pressure, *JAMA* 289(19):2560, 2003.

National Library of Medicine: *Medline Plus: Eye Emergencies*, 2011, http://www.nlm.nih.gov/medlineplus/ency/article/000054.htm, updated December 14 2011. Accessed December 2011.

National Pressure Ulcer Advisory Panel (NPUAP) and European Pressure Ulcer Advisory Panel (EPUAP): *Prevention and treatment of pressure ulcers*, Washington, DC, 2009, National Pressure Ulcer Advisory Board.

National Quality Forum (NQF): *National voluntary consensus standards for public reporting of patient safety event information*, 2011, http://www.qualityforum.org/Publications/2011/02/National_Voluntary_Consensus_Standards_for_Public_Reporting_of_Patient_Safety_Event_Information.aspx. Accessed June 24 2011.

Netsch DSL: Negative-pressure wound therapy. In Bryant RA, Nix DP, editors: *Acute and chronic wounds: nursing management*, ed 4, St Louis, 2011, Mosby.

Newman DK, Wein AJ: *Managing and treating urinary incontinence*, ed 2, Baltimore, 2009, Health Professions Press.

Ney D, et al: Senescent swallowing: impact, strategies, and interventions, *Nutr Clin Practice* 24:395, 2009.

Nguyen E, et al: Medication safety initiative in reducing medication errors, *J Nurs Care Qual* 25(3):224, 2010.

Nicholl L, Hesby A: Intramuscular injection: an integrative research review and guideline for evidence-based practice, *Appl Nurs Res* 16(2):159, 2002.

Nix DP: Skin and wound inspection and assessment. In Bryant RA, Nix DP, editors: *Acute and chronic wounds: current management concepts*, ed 4, St Louis, 2012, Mosby.

Occupational Safety and Health Administration (OSHA): *Bloodborne pathogens and needlestick injuries*, 77 FR 19934, 2012, http://www.osha.gov/pls/oshaweb/owadisp.show_document?p_table=STANDARDS&p_id=10051. Accessed July 2012.

O'Driscoll BR, Howard LS, Davison AG: British Thoracic Society guidelines for emergency oxygen use in adult patients, *Thorax* 63(Suppl VI):2008.

Oliver D, Healey F, Haines TP: Preventing falls and fall-related injuries in hospitals, *Clin Geriatr Med* 26(4):645, 2010.

Orgill D, et al: The mechanisms of action of vacuum-assisted closure: more to learn, *J Surg* 146(1):40, 2009.

Pagana K, Pagana T: *Mosby's diagnostic and laboratory test reference*, ed 10, St Louis, 2011, Mosby.

Parker D, et al: Evidence-based report card: nursing interventions to reduce the risk of catheter-associated urinary tract infection. Part 1: Catheter selection, *J Wound Ostomy Continence Nurs* 36(1):23, 2009.

Pasero C, McCaffery M: *Pain assessment and pharmacologic management*, St Louis, 2011, Mosby.

Pedersen C, et al: Endotracheal suctioning of the adult intubated patient— what is the evidence? *Intensive Crit Care Nurs* 25:21, 2009.

Petkar KS, et al: A prospective randomized controlled trial comparing negative-pressure dressing and conventional dressing methods on split-thickness skin grafts in burned patients, *Burns* 37(6):925, 2011.

Phillips NM, Endacott R: Medication administration via enteral tubes: a survey of nurses' practices, *J Adv Nurs* 67(12):2586, 2011.

Physiotherapy Canada: 6. Superficial Heat, *Physiother Can* 62(5):47, 2010.

Pieper B: Pressure ulcers: impact, etiology, and classification. In Bryant RA, Nix DP, editors: *Acute and chronic wounds: current management concepts*, ed 4, St Louis, 2012, Mosby.

Pierson F, Fairchild S: *Principles & techniques of patient care*, ed 4, St Louis, 2008, Saunders.

Polderman KH: Induced hypothermia and fever control for prevention and treatment of neurological injuries, *Lancet* 371:1955, 2008.

Polderman KH, Herold I: Therapeutic hypothermia and controlled normothermia in the intensive care unit: practical considerations, side effects and cooling methods, *Crit Care Med* 37(3):1101, 2009.

Pomfret I: The use of sheaths in male urinary incontinence, *Continence Essentials* (1):70, 2008.

Poon EG, et al: Effect of bar-code technology on the safety of medication administration, *New Engl J Med* 362(18):1698, 2010.

Popescu A, et al: Multifactorial influences on and deviations from medication administration safety and quality in the acute medical/surgical context, *Worldviews Evidence-Based Nurs* 8(1):15, 2011.

Ramundo J: Wound debridement. In Bryant RA, Nix DP, editors: *Acute and chronic wounds: current management concepts*, ed 4, St Louis, 2012, Mosby.

Regan E, Dallachiesa L: How to care for a patient with a tracheostomy, *Nursing 09* 39(8):34, 2009.

Rigby D: An overview of suprapubic catheter care in community practice, *Br J Commun Nurs* 14(7):278, 2009.

Rodden A, et al: Does fingernail polish affect pulse oximeter readings? *Intensive Crit Care Nurs* 23(1):51, 2007.

Rolstad BS, Bryant RA, Nix DP: Topical management. In Bryant RA, Nix DP, editors: *Acute and chronic wounds: nursing management*, ed 4, St Louis, 2011, Mosby.

Sanofi-Aventis: *Lovenox injections at home*, http://www.lovenox.com/consumer/prescribed-lovenox/lovenox-at-home.aspx, 2010. Accessed July 5, 2012.

Scheffer AC, et al: Fear of falling: measurement strategy, prevalence, risk factors, and consequences among older persons, *Age Aging* 37:19, 2008.

Schick L, Windle P, editors: *PeriAnesthesia nursing core curriculum: preoperative, phase I and phase II PACU nursing*, ed 2, St Louis, 2010, Saunders.

Senese V, et al: *SUNA clinical practice guidelines: care of the patient with an indwelling catheter*, 2005, http://www.suna.org/resources/indwelling Catheter.pdf. Accessed February 27, 2012.

Sheeja VS, et al: Insulin therapy in diabetes management, *Int J Pharm Sci Rev Res* 2(2):98, 2010.

Simmons D, et al: Tubing misconnections: normalization of deviance, *Nutr Clin Pract* 26:28, 2011.

Skirton H, et al: A systematic review of variability and reliability of manual and automated blood pressure readings, *J Clin Nurs* 20:614, 2011.

Smeltzer SC, et al: *Brunner & Suddharth's textbook of medical-surgical nursing*, ed 12, Philadelphia, 2009, Lippincott, Williams & Wilkins.

Smith PW, et al: SHEA/APIC guideline: infection prevention and control in the long-term care facility, *Am J Infect Control* 36:504, 2008.

Snyder E, et al: *Rossi's principles of transfusion medicine*, ed 4, St Louis, 2008, Mosby.

Stoller ML: Retrograde instrumentation of the urinary tract. In Tanagho EA, McAnanch JW, editors: *Smith's general urology*, ed 17, New York, 2008, Lange McGraw Hill.

Stotts N: Nutritional assessment and support. In Bryant RA, Nix DP, editors: *Acute and chronic wounds: current management concepts*, ed 4, St Louis, 2012, Mosby.

The Joint Commission: *Provision of care, treatment, and services: restraint/seclusion for hospitals that use TJC for deemed status purposes*, Chicago, 2009, The Commission.

The Joint Commission (TJC): *2012 Comprehensive accreditation manual for hospitals*, Oakbrook Terrace, IL, 2012, The Commission.

The Joint Commission (TJC): *National Patient Safety Goals*, Oakbrook Terrace, IL, 2014, The Commission. Available at: http://www.jointcommission.org/standards_information/npsgs.aspx.

VA National Center for Patient Safety (VA NCPS): *VHA NCPS escape and elopement management,* 2010, http://www4.va.gov/ncps/CogAids/ EscapeElope/index.html#page=page-13. Accessed May 2011.

Valdez-Lowe C, et al: Pulse oximetry in adults, *Am J Nurs* 109(6):52, 2009.

Viera ER, Freund-Heritage R, da Costa BR: Risk factors for geriatric patient falls in rehabilitation hospital settings: a systematic review, *Clin Rehabil* 25(9):788, 2011.

Weber-Jones J: Obstructed tracheostomy tubes: clearing the air, *Nursing 2010* 40(1):49, 2010.

Wells N, et al: Improving the quality of care through pain assessment and management. In Hughes RG, editor: *Patient safety and quality: an evidence-based handbook for nurses,* Rockville, MD, 2008, Agency for Healthcare Research and Quality (AHRQ).

Whitney JD: Surgical wounds and incisional care. In Bryant RA, Nix DP, editors: *Acute and chronic wounds: current management concepts,* ed 4, St Louis, 2012, Mosby.

Willson M, et al: Evidence-based report card: nursing interventions to reduce the risk of catheter-associated urinary tract infection. Part 2: Staff education, monitoring, and care techniques, *J Wound Ostomy Continence Nurs* 36(2):137, 2009.

Wooten MK, Hawkins K: *WOCN position statement: Clean versus sterile: management of chronic wounds,* Glenview, IL, 2005, Wound, Ostomy, and Continence Nurses Society.

Wound Ostomy and Continence Nurses (WOCN) Society: *Guideline for prevention and management of pressure ulcers,* WOCN clinical practice guidelines series, Mount Laurel, NJ, 2010, WOCN Society.

Zimmermann PG: Revisiting IM injections, *Am J Nurs* 110(2):60, 2010.

This logo identifies when the use of clean gloves is recommended. Clean gloves can protect both caregivers and patients from microbial transmission. However, gloves are not 100% effective. Personnel should wear clean, disposable gloves when touching blood, body fluids, mucous membranes, nonintact skin, secretions, excretions, and contaminated items. Gloves should be changed between skills on a patient involving contact with material that might contain a high concentration of microorganisms.

Preprocedure Protocol

1. Verify health care provider orders and need for consent form.
2. Introduce yourself to patient by both name and title or role, and explain what you plan to do.
3. **Patient identification**: Identify patient using two identifiers (e.g., name and birthday or name and account number) according to agency policy. Compare identifiers with information on patient's MAR or medical record.
4. Explain procedure and reason it is to be done in terms the patient can understand.
5. Assess patient to determine that the intervention is still appropriate and whether adaptations to skill steps are needed.
6. Gather equipment.
7. Perform hand hygiene before each new patient contact.
8. Adjust bed or chair to appropriate working height as needed.
9. Make sure that patient is comfortable and that you have sufficient room to perform procedure.
10. Make sure that you have sufficient lighting to perform procedure.
11. If patient is in bed and a side rail is raised, lower rail on side nearest you to access patient.
12. Provide privacy. Close door, use privacy curtain, and position and drape patient as needed.

During Skill Protocol

1. Promote patient involvement and comfort.
2. Communicate during skill to allay patient's anxiety, and explain source of any discomfort.
3. Assess patient's tolerance throughout procedure.